BANISH YOUR BELLY

The Ultimate Guide for Achieving a Lean, Strong Body—Now

BY KENTON ROBINSON AND THE EDITORS OF **Men'sHealth** BOOKS
WITH DRAGOMIR CIOROSLAN, HEAD COACH OF THE U.S. WEIGHTLIFTING
FEDERATION AND THE 1996 U.S. OLYMPIC WEIGHTLIFTING TEAM

Rodale Press, Inc.
Emmaus, Pennsylvania

Notice

The information here is designed to help you make decisions regarding your fitness and exercise program. It is not intended as a substitute for professional fitness and medical advice. As with all exercise programs, you should seek your doctor's approval before you begin.

Library of Congress Cataloging-in-Publication Data

Robinson, Kenton.
    Banish your belly : the ultimate guide for achieving a lean,
strong body—now / by Kenton Robinson and the editors of Men's
Health Books ; with Dragomir Cioroslan.
         p.   cm.
    Includes index.
    ISBN 0–87596–398–6 hardcover
    ISBN 0–87596–501–6 paperback
    1. Weight loss.   2. Men—Health and hygiene.   I. Cioroslan,
Dragomir. II. Men's Health Books.
    RM222.2.R62   1997
    613.7—dc21   97–2482

Distributed in the book trade by St. Martin's Press

      8 10 9 7   hardcover
4 6 8 10 9 7 5 3   paperback

──── OUR PURPOSE ────

*"We inspire and enable people to improve
their lives and the world around them."*

BANISH YOUR BELLY EDITORIAL STAFF

Editor: **Matthew Hoffman**

Managing Editor: **Jack Croft**

Writers: **Kenton Robinson, Ken McAlpine, Richard Laliberte, Doug Hill, Elizabeth A. Brown, R.D., Deborah Pedron**

Fitness Consultants: **Dragomir Cioroslan, head coach of the U.S. Weightlifting Federation and the 1996 U.S. Olympic weightlifting team, and Frank Eksten, strength coordinator in the Department of Athletics and visiting lecturer in kinesiology at Indiana University in Bloomington**

Assistant Research Manager: **Jane Unger Hahn**

Book Project Researcher: **Deborah Pedron**

Editorial Researchers: **Elizabeth A. Brown, R.D., Raymond M. DiCecco, Alice Drake, Jan Eickmeier, Sarah Wolfgang Heffner, Terry Sutton Kravitz, Sally A. Reith, Staci Ann Sander, Shea Zukowski**

Senior Copy Editor: **Amy K. Kovalski**

Copy Editor: **Karen Neely**

Associate Art Director: **Darlene Schneck**

Cover and Interior Designer: **Christopher R. Neyen**

Cover and Interior Photographer: **Mitch Mandel**

Technical Artists: **Thomas P. Aczel, J. Andrew Brubaker**

Manufacturing Coordinator: **Patrick T. Smith**

Office Manager: **Roberta Mulliner**

Office Staff: **Julie Kehs, Bernadette Sauerwine, Mary Lou Stephen**

RODALE HEALTH AND FITNESS BOOKS

Vice-President and Editorial Director: **Debora T. Yost**

Executive Editor: **Neil Wertheimer**

Design and Production Director: **Michael Ward**

Research Manager: **Ann Gossy Yermish**

Copy Manager: **Lisa D. Andruscavage**

Studio Manager: **Stefano Carbini**

Book Manufacturing Director: **Helen Clogston**

C O N T E N T S

PART I

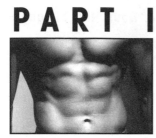

THE ART AND SCIENCE OF BELLY BANISHING

PART II

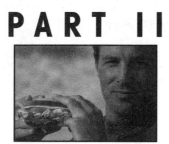

EATING FOR LEAN

PART III

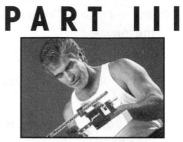

THE LEAN LIFESTYLE

PART IV

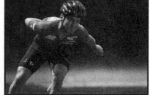

THE WORLD OF AEROBICS

PART V

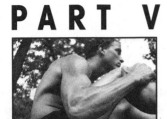

BUILDING A PROGRAM

PART VI

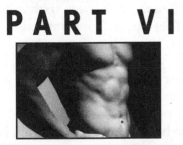

MIDBODY WORKOUTS

PART VII

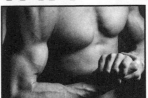

UPPER-BODY WORKOUTS

PART VIII

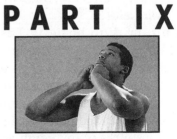

LOWER-BODY WORKOUTS

PART IX

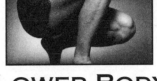

FLEXING AND STRETCHING

INTRODUCTION

Something happened to me in my late thirties. At 35, I quit smoking. At 36, I became the proud and sleep-deprived father of a baby girl. And at 38, the proud and even more sleep-starved father of a baby boy.

The upshot of all these blessed events is that I ate. I ate to make up for missing cigarettes, and I ate to make up for missing sleep. I sleepwalked and sleep-ate like this for a number of years until a snapshot of me at the beach got my attention: There was I, the former high-school beanpole, wading in the surf, lobster-red and eminently harpoonable. I couldn't fool myself any longer: I was 50 pounds heavier and my waist was 6 inches wider than ever before.

When I hit my 39th birthday, I acted out my midriff crisis by running—if you can call it that. It was a rude experience. The old high school cross-country star warn't what he used to be. I bounced my belly around the block on screaming knees.

In spite of the pain and that awful jiggling (not to mention the smirks of my neighbors), I kept at it. I dragged myself out on the street every other day of the week, often ending my runs by sitting in a tub of ice water to stop the swelling in my legs. On my days "off" I staggered my jogs with free-weight workouts and speed-bag boxing bouts.

I also stopped eating all the crap that I had eaten for so many years: the apple pies heaped with ice cream, the bags of corn chips, the double burgers with cheese. Instead, I ate as much as I wanted of good, low-fat, healthful foods: fruits, vegetables, lean meats, and whole grains.

The result?

By the time I hit 40, my belly was a mere shadow of its former self. I was 35 pounds lighter. I could run 12 miles without stopping. I had muscles in places where I had never had them before.

And I kept at it.

And then one hot spring day, as I was finishing up my fifth mile on the local high school track, three kids from the track team hopped on behind me. They started out half a lap behind, but within a lap I could hear their feet pounding the cinders.

"They're going to pass me," I thought. And then I thought again. "No they're not."

And I stepped on the gas.

As I pulled away, I heard one and then another utter an unprintable exclamation of disbelief.

They caught up in a couple laps and tried to pass me again. And once again I accelerated and left them behind. At the end of my sixth mile, they had given it up. They ran without conviction. And I was passing them.

Let me tell you how this felt: It was better than sex. (And sex, by the way, was better than ever minus the flab.)

Which brings me to the point of this story. The point isn't to boast about how I, an old fart, outran some teenagers. (I left out the part about how much my legs hurt the next day.) The point is this: If I can do it, you can do it, too.

Banish Your Belly will show you how.

If you're experiencing a midlife—or at least a midbody—crisis, we'll show you how to dump that gut once and for all.

If you're 50-plus and 50 pounds overweight, we'll help you roll back those pounds and, with them, the years.

Even if you're a lean, tough 20-something and simply want to stay that way, we'll show you how to do that, too.

How? First, we'll teach you how to eat better—without compromising taste or pleasure. We'll also explain how to make subtle shifts in your lifestyle that give surprisingly big payoffs in terms of health, weight, appearance, and attitude. Most of all, we'll show you how to exercise: smartly, safely, quickly, and effectively.

You don't have to lose weight and get in shape the way I did—in fact, you shouldn't. My path was physically painful and risky. Pick any of the eating or exercise programs we provide in this book; you'll be guaranteed that it is as safe as it is effective. Moreover, *Banish Your Belly* will give you all the information you need to put together a plan that works specifically for you. The bottom line is this: You, too, can banish your belly.

Kenton Robinson

PART I

THE ART AND SCIENCE OF BELLY BANISHING

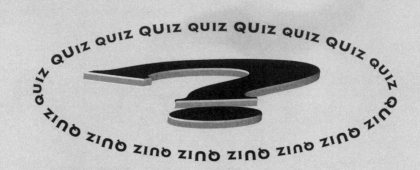

Is My Belly Too Big?

Lately, you've begun to wonder whether your stomach isn't getting the best of you.

Perhaps it's because the last time you bought a pair of pants, you didn't fit into your old size anymore. Or perhaps it's just the way your stomach hung out over your swimsuit the last time you hung out at the beach. Or maybe you have noticed that it has suddenly become harder to bend over and tie your shoes.

If any of these things have happened to you, chances are your belly is too big. In fact, the simplest answer to the question "Is my belly too big?" is "If you think it is, it probably is."

If you're still in doubt, take this quiz, answering yes or no to the following statements, to see how your middle measures up.

1. My dog is fat.

Yes   No

2. I always cruise the parking lot looking for the space closest to the door. And I always take the elevator because I really start to blow when I have to take the stairs.

Yes   No

3. I want to get in shape, but I can't find the time to exercise.

Yes   No

4. Television? Oh, I'd guess I watch a couple hours a day.

Yes   No

5. Sure, I nosh while watching the tube, but I stick to low-fat snacks.

Yes   No

6. And, uh, while you're up, I could use another beer.

Yes   No

7. I've had to let my belt out a couple of notches since college, but then, hey, hasn't everybody?

Yes   No

8. I used to be able to see all the way down to the ground, but lately my belt—and my feet—seem to have disappeared.

Yes   No

9. All of my friends make more money than I do.

Yes   No

10. I'm married.

Yes   No

11. And speaking of my wife, nowadays she always wants to be on top.

Yes   No

ANSWERS

1–2. Owners of fat dogs often tend to be fat themselves, says Karen J. Wolfsheimer, D.V.M., Ph.D., associate professor in the Department of Veterinary Physiology, Pharmacology, and Toxicology in the School of Veterinary Medicine at Louisiana State University in Baton Rouge. Which is not surprising, really, because if Bowser isn't taking any walks, neither are you, and both of you may be putting on the pounds. (For more on the diet/dog connection, see "Are You Too Fat? Do a 'Spot' Check" on page 23.)

3–4. "I just don't have time to exercise" is the most popular excuse for not doing it. And yet, Nielsen Media Research has found that the typical American man manages to find enough time to watch 3½ hours of television a day.

In addition, research has shown that the more TV you watch, the fatter you're likely to be. One study of more than 6,000 men found that those who viewed the tube more than 3 hours a day were twice as likely to be fat as those who viewed less than 1 hour.

5. Researchers have noted that even though we Americans are eating less fat than ever, we're still getting fatter. The reason, at least in part, may be that we're stuffing so much other stuff into our faces. Even if you're conscientious about eating nonfat or low-fat foods, they still have calories, and extra calories lead to pounds.

6. Research reveals a sad truth: They don't call a belly a beer gut for nothing. Of all the alcoholic beverages, beer is the highest in calories. Given the choice between a shot, a glass of wine, or a brew, you who choose the brew will put more rubber on your spare.

7. According to the U.S. Departments of Agriculture and Health and Human Services, if you have gained more than 10 pounds since you reached your adult height (since high school or college, say), you probably have the makings of a weight problem.

Of course, it's possible that you were a string bean in high school and have since worked out, adding about 10 pounds of muscle mass to your frame. But in most men those extra pounds don't come from muscle. Further, being 10 pounds too heavy today has an unfortunate way of turning into 15 pounds (or 20 or 30) next year.

8. One way to gauge the state of your stomach is to look at it when you're sitting down. If your stomach engulfs your belt, then you have more stomach than one man needs.

A more scientific way is to measure your waist-to-hip ratio: Take a tape measure to your waist and then to your hips. Divide your waist measurement by your hip measurement. If the number you get is .85 or greater, your belly's too big.

9. It may be an unfortunate commentary on the role physical appearance plays in our society, but research has shown that fatter people tend to make less money. A study of business school graduates found that men who were 20 percent or more overweight made $4,000 less a year than their thinner alums.

10. Beware: Wedded bliss can turn you into a wedded blimp. A Cornell University study found that married men were twice as likely to be obese as those who were single or divorced.

There are two speculations as to why this is so. It may be that married men eat more regularly because there is a woman feeding them. Or perhaps it's simply that having "caught" a wife and stepped out of the dating pool, they're more willing than their single peers to let appearances slip a bit.

11. What does having a belly have to do with sex? Studies have shown that when people lose weight, they feel better about themselves, and their sex lives often improve. In fact, one study found that when men started an aerobic exercise program, they started having sex about 30 percent more often than they had before.

WHY BELLIES GET FAT
BLAME IT ON BIOLOGY

"Why am I so soft in the middle, the rest of my life is so hard?" —Paul Simon

First of all, you're a mammal. Second, you're a human. Third, you're a man. And fourth, unlike your ancestors, who lived in the world God gave them, you live in a world of your own design.

It is a world for which you—as a mammal and a human and a man—were *not* designed.

In other words, the big-picture answer to the question of why bellies get fat really comes down to, but not only to, biology.

Man as Mammal

You are a mammal, and that makes you a homeotherm. What that means is that you come equipped with your own internal thermostat. Your thermostat warms you up or cools you down as needed, and fat is both your insulation and the fuel for your fire.

Burn a gram of protein or carbohydrate, and you'll get about 4 calories of heat; burn a gram of fat, and you get more than 9. No wonder people in cold climes look on blubber as a welcome snack.

Of course, there's a lot more to being a mammal than simply keeping warm. About 70 percent of the calories you burn in a day are burned to keep

your heart pumping, digest your food, and carry on the basic maintenance of keeping a body alive. Fat is an essential part of a very complex assortment of equipment that keeps your body running at a comfortable 98.6 degrees Fahrenheit (or thereabouts) regardless of the weather.

Animals that don't come with such equipment are known as poikilotherms. They don't have mechanisms for storing fat or burning it to keep warm, which means they have no choice but to be whatever the temperature around them happens to be. Your typical lizard, for example, can find out what temperature his body is going to be on any given day simply by tuning in to The Weather Channel.

Your Third Eye

But humans, as we have said, have their own personal thermostat, a tiny nodule of tissue called the hypothalamus buried at the base of the brain. You might call it your primitive brain, as the hypothalamus is the part of your brain that regulates what scientists call the vegetative functions of the body, such things as body temperature, arterial pressure, sleeping, eating, and more.

This primitive brain may be tiny—the hypothalamus represents less than 1 percent of your brain mass—but it plays a powerful role in regulating

Stone Age versus Phone Age

When it comes right down to it, you aren't built any differently than your great-great-great-grandfather some 100,000 grandfathers back. But the world you live in bears small resemblance to Grandpa's. He had to kill his lunch with a stone; you can get it delivered just by lifting a phone. Needless to say, he burned up a few more calories a day than you do.

Here's a sample of how many calories he might have burned in a typical Stone Age day compared to how many you, modern man, may burn in a typical day on the cusp of the twenty-first century.

	Grandpa's Day	Calories		Your Day	Calories
7–8 A.M.	Hunt for breakfast.	500	7–8 A.M.	Grab Egg McMuffin at drive-up window on way to work	166
8–9	Still hunting for breakfast	500	8–9	Eat Egg McMuffin at your desk and check e-mail	100
9–9:20	Run away from breakfast	901	9–10	Eat pineapple Danish. Read report on possible acquisition.	100
9:20–11	Hunt for smaller, more docile breakfast	832	10–12	Attend 2-hr. meeting to discuss need for more meetings	210
11–12	Kill breakfast and carry it back home	435	12–1:30 P.M.	Hop in car for lunch at Fat Boys Bar-B-Q	149
12–1 P.M.	Skin breakfast and chop wood for fire to cook it	650	1:30–2	Conference call with Los Angeles	50
1–2	Cook breakfast and eat it	124	2–2:30	Flirt with secretary at accounts receivable	55
2–2:30	Regale your fellows with tale about killing your breakfast	67	2:30–4	Type up the Gorsky proposal	172
2:30–3	Beat up fellow who calls you a liar	437	4–4:10	Grab candy bar from vending machine, eat it	17
3–5	Sit around in dazed torpor	49	4:10–5	Talk to old college friend on 800 line	83
5–6	Eat more breakfast	100	5–5:15	Drive to health club	27
6–7	Do dance in honor of the spirit of breakfast	305	5:15–5:45	Jog on treadmill	378
7–11	Sleep	299	5:45–6	Shower and get dressed	56
			6–7	Drive home, open brewdog, order and eat small pizza	112
Grandpa's Total Calories Burned: 5,199			7–11	Watch TV. Drink 2 more brewdogs. Eat tortilla chips and salsa	338
			Your Total Calories Burned: 2,013		

2025: Fat to the Future

If you think Americans are fat now, chances are we are going to be even fatter come the twenty-first century.

At least that's one possible future anticipated by Edward Cornish, president of the World Future Society and editor of The Futurist magazine.

It's well-established that Americans are getting fatter every year, and researchers lay a lot of the blame on our increasing idleness. Cornish foresees a cyber-future in which these trends will continue. As computer technology makes our lives easier and easier, we will contentedly grow heavier and heavier.

Here are some possible developments.

- **Where we now spend about 3½ hours a day watching television, we may spend even more time enjoying our new virtual-reality systems. In fact, Cornish says, we may come to prefer virtual reality to the real kind. "We will turn on our virtual-reality systems and lie back, experiencing heavenly pleasures of sight and sound in a snug electronic nest." Of course, we will still be eating real junk food.**
- **Controlled by infrared cameras and computers, our cars may drive themselves while we sit back and watch TV. No more having to jack up your blood pressure with flipping the bird at the jerk who dawdles in the passing lane. And no more burning calories by turning that pesky old steering wheel, let alone by shifting gears.**
- **In addition to TV sets, our cars may be equipped with computers, videoscreens, couches, wet bars, refrigerators, and hey, maybe even some exercise equipment.**
- **Not that we'll make much use of it. In fact, we will be more likely to be getting fatter at increasingly younger ages. Currently, the percentage of kids between ages 6 and 17 who are severely overweight has more than doubled since the 1960s. We shouldn't be surprised if we start seeing college kids lining up for bypass operations and heart transplants.**

The outlook may be grim, but, as Cornish stresses, none of this has to happen.

"There's always a possibility of a revolution that will counter the trend," he says. "People are a lot more health-conscious now than they were in the 1950s, say. In the 1950s people really didn't pay any attention to what they ate."

Of course, he also points out that although we have started paying attention to this stuff, we've still gotten a whole lot fatter.

---

how much you eat. It does this in conjunction with another, pea-size object in your brain called the pineal gland. It is thought that the pineal gland is a vestigial relic from the days when your most ancient ancestors were still crawling around on their bellies and had a third eye in the back of their heads.

It was, and still is, your third eye. Granted, it doesn't stick out of your head anymore, but scientists theorize it still "sees" by getting information piped to it from your optic nerves. And what the pineal gland is interested in "seeing" is how much daylight and darkness there is each day.

The less light there is, the less serotonin there is in your brain, and the less serotonin there is in your brain, the more your hypothalamus tells you to eat. Meanwhile, your pineal gland is pumping more and more melatonin into your body, making you more and more torpid.

This is why, if you look at a year in most any mammal's life—or at least in the life of any mammal living in a climate that gets cold in the winter—you'll see that as summer pivots around the solstice, a young mammal's thoughts turn to just one thing: food.

And he eats for just one reason: to get fat.

And as the days get colder and shorter and darker, he gets fatter and sleepier.

At its most extreme, this chemical reaction causes many humans to experience something called seasonal affective disorder, where in the fall and winter they sink into depression, desiring only to sleep and eat massive amounts of carbohydrates such as pasta and chocolate.

To put it another way, as the days narrow into fall, your most primitive brain, in conspiracy with your pineal gland, tells your body, "The days are getting shorter! Eat! Eat! Sleep! Sleep! Winter is coming!"

Meanwhile, your "higher" brain is saying, "You need to lose weight, man. You need to exercise. You don't want to have to strut that gut on the beach come summer, do you?"

Guess which brain wins?

Man as Human

Now you're saying, "Well, that may explain why I want to eat like a pig when the nights get long, but it doesn't explain why I want to eat so much in the spring and summer, too."

To understand that, you need to trace your family tree back through about 100,000 grandfathers.

Back when your greatest grandpa first climbed down from his family's tree, food was an elusive thing. It would hide in the thicket or a hole in the ground or run across the tundra at 20 miles an hour. Lunch was something that you had to chase down and stab with a sharp stick. And sometimes lunch picked up and moved to parts unknown and couldn't be found at all.

In short, for most of the past two million years, food played hard to get, and we got it by hunting and gathering it wherever we could find it.

Given that humans often lived hand to mammoth, there were obvious evolutionary advantages in eating fat when you could get it and being able to store it up for the times you couldn't. It was survival of the fattest.

Not that your ancestors were fat, mind you. They were more likely to be lean, for the simple reason that they burned calories like crazy, all the way from great-grandfather number 1, who chased (and was chased by) woolly rhinoceroses, to great-grandfather number 99,999, who busted sod with an ox in Kansas.

Those guys could eat just about anything that they wanted and do just fine, thank you very much, because they lived in a world that, whether they hunted and gathered their food or grew it, required considerable amounts of physical labor on a daily basis.

We, on the other hand, don't even have to lift our butts out of our bucket seats to gather our food from a drive-up window.

Man in Paradise

If our prehistoric forebears had a vision of heaven, it might have looked a lot like that drive-up window.

Think about it. If you lived in a world where your major preoccupation was getting enough to eat, a place where you could just roll up and be handed sacks of steaming meat would be a dream of inconceivable bliss.

Indeed, we are living in the heaven of our ancestors. We don't have to pursue our food; our food pursues us. Like a streetwalker, it hangs out on every corner and calls to us, "Hey, Big Boy! Want a good time? C'mere."

We have minimarts on every block, beef jerky sticks and Mars bars in every gas station, vending machines stuffed with Ho-Ho's, cheese worms and ice cream sandwiches in every factory and office building. We even have pizzas chauffeured to our doorsteps.

And just in case our minds should drift away from food when we're not in its actual presence, we are relentlessly assailed by its striptease and siren song on television. (If you have ever been on a diet, you have no doubt become achingly aware of the number of food ads that bombard you every hour, no matter how hard you work the remote to dodge them.)

And speaking of working the remote . . .

"Almost by the day people get less physically active," says Kelly Brownell, Ph.D., co-director of the Yale University Eating and Weight Disorders Clinic. "Just look around at the number of things that conspire to save us exercise, with the lead probably being the remote control on the television. It doesn't sound like a big thing, but if you figure out the number of people who are watching television and the number of hours they watch it per day, and over the year the number of trips across the room that are now not made, it's an enormous change in exercise."

This may explain, he says, why in the past 15 years Americans have become the fattest people on the face of the Earth.

We were designed—genetically speaking—to live in a world where we had to get our bread by the sweat of our brow. But we have redesigned the world. Now we don't have to raise even a bead of sweat to get all the bread we want.

Depending on who you ask, the prevalence of obesity in this country has increased anywhere from 8 percent to 25 percent in the last 10 years. "There is no way that you can explain that increase by genetics," says Dr. Brownell. "The environment is getting worse."

By "environment" Brownell doesn't mean trees; he means the one that we have created for ourselves, replete with TVs and freezers filled with Tater Tots.

Nielsen Media Research, which monitors such things, says that the typical American guy glues himself to the tube for more than 3½ hours a day. The more TV you watch, the fatter you are likely to be. One study of more than 6,000 men found that those who viewed the tube more than 3 hours a day were twice as likely to be fat as those who viewed less than 1 hour.

Even your internal thermostat doesn't have to work that hard anymore. In the winter you move from one heated box to another; in the summer you have central air.

As you bask in your cozy home, just remember that the world you were designed for is the one you see the squirrels in your backyard living in: howling winds, freezing rain, and a lot of now-where-in-the-heck-did-I-put-that-nut?

Our bodies are still programmed that way. Genetically speaking, there is virtually no difference between us and our greatest of grandfathers. In fact, the difference between us and our Stone Age ancestors is "probably somewhere between three and five one-thousandths of 1 percent," says S. Boyd Eaton, M.D., associate clinical professor of radiology and adjunct associate professor of anthropology at Emory University in Atlanta and co-author of The Paleolithic Prescription.

And so our bodies are dutifully storing away all those extra calories that we are taking in for the hard winter that never comes.

Man as Man

Finally, there is the business of being a man.

Men store fat on their guts; women store it on their butts. That's just the way the two genetic packages work, says George L. Blackburn, M.D., Ph.D., director of the Center for the Study of Nutrition Medicine at Beth Israel Deaconess Medical Center West of the Harvard Medical School in Boston. If your package happens to include a penis, there's a gut waiting for you on layaway.

The why or wherefore of this is a matter of speculation.

"Who knows?" says Dr. Blackburn. "Maybe for hunting and gathering, it was better that men's leg or running muscles be thin. Whereas women need to have a very efficient store of fat, enough to carry a pregnancy to term, 120,000 calories, so they needed a special place for their fat: those saddlebags."

Which, says Dr. Blackburn, raises an interesting point. "Evolution is not interested beyond the period of propagation of species," he says. "And so our problems with obesity are just leftover consequences of what Mother Nature did to make sure that we didn't starve to death while we were propagating."

In other words, Mother Nature designed you to store up fat so that you would survive long enough to mate. After that, you're on your own.

WHO GETS A BELLY?
WHO DOESN'T?

In the end, after all their eye-glazing talk of "macronutrient balance" and "de novo lipogenesis," the researchers who make it their business to study this stuff come down to the same bottom line: If you take in more energy than you expend, you are going to get a bigger bottom line.

Period.

This is the first law of thermodynamics: "Energy can neither be created nor destroyed." It is a law of nature as old as the universe. It applies to the sun, the moon, the stars, and your belly.

What this means is that if you eat more calories than you burn, those leftover calories become a permanent part of your person. They do not magically disappear.

"We can't get away from the first law of thermodynamics. Energy in, energy out. That's really the bottom line," says John B. Allred, Ph.D., professor of nutrition in the Department of Food Science and Technology at Ohio State University in Columbus and co-author of *Taking the Fear Out of Eating: A Nutritionists' Guide to Sensible Food Choices.*

The answer to the question of "Who gets a belly?" then, is simply this: anyone who eats more calories than he burns.

Nothing Wasted, Everything Saved

Granted, some of us seem to be much more efficient energy burners than others, depending on such factors as our age, sex, weight, genetics, and physical activity levels. But over the long haul, when you take in more calories than you can burn, your body will save them up for you. It is sort of like your own personal energy conservation system.

For example, if you are an average-size guy (5-foot-9 and 172 pounds) who watches the average amount of television (more than 3½ hours) and does the average amount of exercise (not much) a day, you probably shouldn't be taking in more than 2,900 calories a day to maintain that average size.

Now let's say that you take in exactly that amount *plus* one carrot. ("Hey, what's one lousy carrot?") One carrot will give you 31 extra calories a day.

Multiply that carrot's calories by 365 days, and you'll see that you're taking in 11,315 extra calories a year, which, if your body stored them all as fat, would make you more than 3 pounds heavier a year from now.

ries, for example, but not at all good at storing excess calories from protein, carbohydrate, or alcohol.

In fact, there is a hierarchy to what gets burned first: "Alcohols burn first, then protein, then carbohydrate, and last fat," says George L. Blackburn, M.D., Ph.D., director of the Center for the Study of Nutrition Medicine at Beth Israel Deaconess Medical Center West of the Harvard Medical School in Boston. "And if there are no calories needed, the leftover calories are fat calories, and those are the ones that are stored. And that's where all the fat in humans comes from, 95 to 98 percent of it at least."

This fact, plus the first law of thermodynamics, could go a long way toward explaining how the average American managed to gain 8 extra pounds during this past low-fat/high-carbohydrate–diet decade.

According to Dr. Allred, this is because we are stuffing so much low-fat stuff into our faces, under the impression that we can eat as much as we want as long as it is low-fat.

It used to be that people counted calories, he says. Now they just count fat grams.

Big mistake.

"The problem is that even if you ate a low-fat diet and excess carbohydrate, the body uses that carbohydrate instead of using stored fat," says Dr. Allred.

So the bottom line is that if you eat 2,000 calories a day and you burn only 1,800, even on a low-fat diet you will gain weight.

Now, imagine that you're treating yourself to a daily Kit Kat candy bar instead of a carrot. That will add an extra 490 calories a day. If every one of those calories were stored as fat, in just a year you would be waddling around some 51 pounds heavier than you are right now.

Living Large

Obviously, we don't store every extra calorie that we take in (if we did, we would all look like dirigibles). Some calories get burned in the process of storing others, and some pass right through. In addition, your body does not treat every calorie the same. It is extremely efficient at storing extra fat calo-

Reversing the Equation

If this is news that makes you want to give up in despair, don't. The solution is simpler than you think: Obey the law, says Dr. Allred. The first law of thermodynamics, that is.

You need to "turn that equation around: Calories out need to exceed calories in, in order to lose weight," says Dr. Allred.

"Now, you can do that two ways," he says. "Decrease caloric intake, and I think what you do to stay on a reduced 'diet' is simply to reduce serving size. The second thing is that you want to increase calories out, and the best way to do that is to exercise."

Indeed, as you will see, these are the two keys to banishing your belly.

HUNGER VERSUS APPETITE
GETTING YOUR BEARINGS

If humans only ate when they were truly hungry, there wouldn't be much need for a book like this.

Except for the tiny fraction of us who actually have glandular problems, we'd all be as thin as whippets.

Unfortunately, though, for us and our bellies, we eat for all sorts of reasons that have nothing whatsoever to do with hunger.

We eat because we're happy, sad, angry, lonely, worried, nervous, frustrated, disappointed, tired, and bored.

We eat because our brains, like the brains of Skinnerian pigeons, have been shaped by conditioning. Regardless of whether we were hungry, our mothers always made us clean our plates. So to this day our brains command us: "Clean your plate."

We eat to reward ourselves. Whenever we were very good, Dad would buy us an ice cream cone. Now every time we think that we deserve a reward, the Dad in our heads says, "Have yourself some ice cream."

We eat to punish ourselves. "Look at yourself, you fat hog," we say in our darkest moments. "You fell off the wagon again by eating that bowl of ice cream. Might as well finish up the carton."

And we eat for no particular reason at all: simply because our mouths and something to put in them happen to find themselves in the same room at the same time.

A Hunger Primer

All of these reasons for eating can be lumped together under the heading "Appetite." They should not be, though they often are, confused with hunger. Hunger is pure physiology, the product of various (and mysterious) conversations between your brain and your gut.

Researchers still don't understand exactly how these conversations work, but they do know that your sense of hunger is less a product of an empty stomach than an empty small intestine.

We seem to be designed to eat every 3 to 4 hours, which is about how long it takes your stomach to slice, dice, chop, puree, and liquefy a meal and for your small intestine to absorb it. When there's nothing left to absorb, chemoreceptors in your small intestine put out the call for another delivery. And you get on the horn to the pizza shop.

Of course, we're simplifying the picture here, but the point is just that there is a physiological thing called hunger.

How to Shrink That Craving

"Please lie down on the couch. Good. Tissue? You're welcome. Now. What seems to be troubling you?"

"Doc, I have this compulsion to eat whole packages of Archway cookies in one sitting."

"Really? What kind?"

"The fruit-filled kind."

"Yes, yes, they are very tasty. But surely you know that a whole package contains 48 grams of fat and 1,320 calories?"

"I know, but I just can't help it."

"Hmmm. And why do you think this is?"

"I dunno, but I do know they're just like the cookies Grandma never used to make."

"Don't you mean 'always' used to make?"

"No. Grandma wasn't much of a cook. She always gave me Archway fruit-filled cookies."

"Aha! And you loved your Grandma, didn't you?"

"Yeah, she was cool."

"That's it. You're not just eating cookies; you're trying to eat your way back to the way you felt when you visited your beloved Grandma. And, of course, you cannot. Which is why you're eating whole packages."

No, you don't need to go to a shrink to figure out your cravings. Remember that cravings are rarely driven by physiological needs, says Kelly Brownell, Ph.D., co-director of the Yale University Eating and Weight Disorders Clinic. Instead, they most often satisfy psychological needs. And once you figure these needs out, you're going to be better equipped to deal with them in ways that don't involve food.

And hunger, as opposed to appetite, expresses itself in ways that are easy to recognize, says Nancy Clark, R.D., director of Nutrition Services at Sports-Medicine Brookline near Boston and author of *Nancy Clark's Sports Nutrition Guidebook*. "Sometimes people are physically hungry and their stomachs are growling. Other times they have low blood sugar and feel tired or irritable. Sometimes they feel sleepy."

You need to tune in to your body to figure out what your personal hunger signs are, Clark says, and to be able to distinguish them from the vagaries of appetite.

"There are many ways hunger gets expressed, and it varies from person to person," she says. "But it's important to learn your own body's clues for hunger, because appetite's just a desire to eat, and that doesn't always mean your body needs calories."

What's My Line?

Unfortunately, it's not always that easy to distinguish hunger from appetite. Appetite, as the poet Delmore Schwartz put it, is "the heavy bear who goes with" you, that "stumbles, flounders, and strives to be fed." And it's often tough to tell which of you is talking: you or the bear.

"It's not easy to distinguish one from another," says Kelly Brownell, Ph.D., co-director of the Yale University Eating and Weight Disorders Clinic. "And the reason is that people have had tens of thousands of times in their lives when they have practiced eating in response to appetite rather than hunger."

If, for example, you eat every time you watch TV, then watching TV can make you want to eat. "Think back to Pavlov's dog," says Dr. Brownell.

Perhaps the best way to distinguish hunger from appetite is to keep a diary, says Dr. Brownell. For a couple of weeks, keep track of what you eat, how much you eat, when you eat it, and where you eat it. Also, note what you were doing (if you were doing anything else while you were eating) and how you were feeling.

Do this, and you'll start to see patterns in your eating habits. You may discover, for example, that you have the habit of eating a Danish every morning at 10:00 while staring into your computer screen.

Chances are, says Dr. Brownell, you're not eating that Danish out of hunger so much as habit. And it's unlikely that you can even remember how that Danish tasted 5 minutes after the last bite went down.

By keeping a diary, you're going to become more conscious of the number of times each day that you eat for reasons other than hunger, and this is your first step to changing some of these habits.

We'll get into how to make those changes later in this book, but for now, it's important to keep the following things in mind, says Dr. Brownell.

- **You don't have to keep a diary of what you eat for the rest of your life, just for a couple of weeks. But while you're doing it, you must do it faithfully.**
- **Carry it with you everywhere so that you can write down everything you eat right after eating it. Otherwise, you'll forget stuff.**

Yeah, we know. It's a pain in the butt, but this is a key step in keeping your weight under control.

BELLY FAT
AND ENERGY
BODIES AT REST

"Well, who wants to be young anyhow, any idiot born in the last 40 years can be young, and besides 45 isn't really old, it's right on the border; At least, unless the elevator's out of order."

If Ogden Nash were writing these lines today (instead of more than 30 years ago), he might pick a younger age—35? 25? 15?—as the threshold of decrepitude.

Why?

Because Americans are deteriorating sooner than they used to. Big bellies have become the prerogative not only of us middle-aging men but of our children, too. In fact, the incidence of obesity among our kids has increased by more than 50 percent since the mid-1970s and is now estimated to affect one out of four of them.

Not only are we getting fatter younger, but we're suffering the consequences. Several studies have shown that kids are starting to develop the kinds of early-warning signs of heart disease— high blood pressure and high cholesterol—that were reserved for their parents in generations past.

Why is this happening? Perhaps it is simply that, as a nation, we have become too tired to get up.

And why are we tired? Because we are fat. And why are we fat? Because we don't get up. There is even a name for this depressing state of affairs. Researchers call it sedentary inertia.

A Nation at Rest

According to the U.S. Department of Health and Human Services, approximately one-quarter of the population is "essentially inactive." These are people who "have sedentary jobs, do no heavy house- or yard work, do not participate in any sports or fitness programs, have no active recreational pursuits, and avoid physical activity during routine daily activities by taking elevators and escalators, driving short distances instead of walking, and searching for the closest parking place to their destination."

These are people who go to such lengths to avoid doing anything that you might say that they are *actively* inactive.

Less than 20 percent of us, according to Health and Human Services, are "vigorously physically active." Many researchers believe that this is the root of the problem. The guy most likely to get a belly is the guy who sits on his behind. And the guy with the belly, as we have seen, is often the guy with low energy.

"The problem is not that we're eating more; it's just that we're exercising even less than we're

Between the medical expenses we incur from it and what we spend trying to lose it, our excess fat costs us some $100 billion a year, more than double the gross national product of Ireland.

Here's another way to measure the cost of being overweight: Count the lost seats at Yankee Stadium.

When they renovated Yankee Stadium in the 1970s, seating capacity shrunk by 8,000 seats, says S. Boyd Eaton, M.D., associate clinical professor of radiology and adjunct associate professor of anthropology at Emory University in Atlanta.

Why? Because the original seats, installed when the stadium was built in 1922, were 19 inches wide. The new seats had to be 3 inches wider to accommodate Americans' bigger butts.

Dr. Eaton admits that some of this widening may also have been for the purpose of making the stadium more posh. But chances are, they would lose a few thousand more seats if they renovated again today. After all, since the 1970s, American butts have only gotten bigger.

eating," says S. Boyd Eaton, M.D., associate clinical professor of radiology and adjunct associate professor of anthropology at Emory University in Atlanta.

Energy Begets Energy

If you remember what you learned in your high school physics class, you no doubt remember that business about inertia: "Bodies at rest tend to stay at rest." This principle applies to human bodies just as much as it applies to inanimate objects. It comes back to that thing called sedentary inertia that we mentioned earlier.

To exercise, you have to have energy. If you haven't been exercising, of course, you may already have a belly—and have probably discovered for yourself what some studies have shown: There is an inverse relationship between how fat you are and how much energy you feel that you have. Basically, the heavier you get, the harder it gets for you to get up and go.

This is not surprising, of course, given that there is so much more of you to move. In fact, because there is so much more work in hauling that excess weight around, you actually burn more calories even when doing the same activities as your skinnier peers.

Fortunately for you, the converse of that old physics principle is also true: "Bodies in motion tend to stay in motion."

This means that once you get yourself up and moving, you'll find it easier to keep moving. In fact, one thing every regular exerciser will tell you is that energy begets energy.

"That is the experience of many," says Ann Bolin, Ph.D., associate professor of anthropology at Elon College in Elon College, North Carolina, and a competitive bodybuilder. "And when you talk to someone who's had a layoff, that's exactly what they talk about: One of the things they lose is their endurance, their ability to last through a workout. And they also feel very sluggish. Working out definitely gives you a sense of energy."

You don't have to be a hard-core athlete to experience the surge of energy from exercise. Indeed, if you'll do even a small amount of exercise, just getting up and taking a 10-minute walk around the block, for example, you'll find that "you have a lot more energy, you feel a lot better, you think a lot clearer, and you move better," says Brian Wallace, Ph.D., chairman of sport fitness at the U.S. Sports Academy in Daphne, Alabama.

Bonus: More Sex

All of which raises an interesting question: What do you do with extra energy once you have it? There is some evidence that it gets translated into a more active sex life. Many respondents to a *Men's Health* magazine survey claimed that exercising and losing weight had liberated their libidos.

And when researchers at the University of California, San Diego, put a bunch of sedentary, middle-aged men on a program of aerobic exercise, the exercisers started having sex about 30 percent more often than they had before.

Good reason to take the stairs, whether or not the elevator's out of order.

BELLY FAT AND HEALTH
SCALING BACK THE DANGERS

Brian Wallace likes to tell the story of the guy in Utah who weighed 400 pounds.

"His blood pressure was 220 over 180, which is incredibly high; his blood sugar was 487, again, incredibly high; he actually was vision-impaired—blind—because of diabetes, which he didn't even know he had.

"Then he put himself on an exercise program, a pretty intense program. In eight months he had lost 200 pounds, his blood pressure was down to normal range, he was off all medications, his blood sugar was down to 67, and he could see."

For Brian Wallace, Ph.D., chairman of sport fitness at the U.S. Sports Academy in Daphne, Alabama, the guy from Utah is a perfect, if extreme, example of the kind of price we pay when we let our bellies take over our lives.

"It's as much a commentary on the negative effects of a sedentary lifestyle as it is on the benefits of exercise," Dr. Wallace says. "I think it's just amazing what people will let themselves do to themselves."

By the same token, it's a commentary on what you can do when you put your mind to it. Within 10 months of going on his exercise program, says Dr. Wallace, the guy from Utah was running in a marathon.

The Risks of Being Round

You might say that every one of us makes a bargain with his body, and regardless of which deal we make, we all pay a price. It's just a matter of which price you pay and whether you pay now or later. If you want to be svelte and healthy, you pay now with the sweat and effort needed to maintain your machine. If you choose instead to sit on your butt and cultivate a belly, you pay later with a plague of illnesses and an early grave.

If this seems like a strong statement, you should know that while excessive belly fat does not unconditionally guarantee that you will suffer a host of maladies and cut short your life span, it is, without question, a large step in a direction that you don't want to go.

Henry Kahn, M.D., an internist and associate professor of family and preventive medicine at Emory University School of Medicine in Atlanta, studied heart attack victims in six Atlanta hospitals. He found that a man may be the same in most respects to his next-door neighbor, but it was the guy with the bigger belly who ended up with a heart attack.

Asleep at the Wheel

Experts agree that the fatter you are, the more likely you are to suffer from high cholesterol and high blood pressure levels, both of which can lead to heart attack or stroke. In addition, there is ample be more tired most of the time—not only because it is extra work to move all that extra you around but also because one common affliction of the overweight is sleep apnea, a condition in which you stop breathing for short periods many times during the night. The overall result? You wake up repeatedly during the night and therefore feel like a zombie most of the day.

Fatigue, no less than heart disease, can be a killer. In one study, researchers at the Stanford University Sleep Disorders and Research Center found that fat truck-drivers are more likely to suffer breathing problems when they sleep and so are more likely to zone out at the wheel and run you over. As a matter of fact, the researchers showed that fat truck-drivers have more than twice as many accidents per mile as thin ones.

Think about that the next time some huge guy in a semi climbs your tail.

Mr. Unhappy

In addition to being linked to a mass of physical problems, obesity has been tied to a variety of psychological problems as well. Put simply, fat people are more likely to be unhappy and to suffer depression and anxiety than their thinner peers.

Here's the kicker: Anger, depression, heart disease, high blood pressure, and diabetes have all been linked with a higher probability of impotence.

The explanation is not hard to find: Fat bellies tend to be accompanied by cholesterol-clogged arteries (atherosclerosis). Cholesterol doesn't just plug up the arteries running to your heart; it plugs up the ones running to your penis as well. In other words, the more you line your belly and your arteries with fat, the harder it is for your heart—or your penis—to keep on pumping.

Reversal of Fortunes

Fortunately, there is a lot of evidence that a reduction in belly fat can alleviate a lot of health problems. You don't even have to lose all your belly to make significant improvements to your health. Even a 10 percent reduction in body fat can reduce the severity of high blood pressure, high cholesterol, and diabetes.

Studies show, for example, that symptoms of diabetes may improve within days of beginning a

evidence that the more ample your belly, the more likely you are to become a victim of diabetes, heart disease, sleep apnea, gout, and cancer of the prostate and colon.

This is serious business here. And the equation is fairly straightforward: The heavier you get around the middle, the more serious your risk of chronic disease.

It's difficult to find a part of your life that is not affected to some extent by being overweight. For example, if you are really heavy, you also tend to

It Ain't Over 'til the Fat Man Sings

There is certainly no profundity in suggesting that rotundity is an occupational hazard of the opera trade.

Pavarotti, wrapped in his scarves, and Jessye Norman, draped in her robes, are, well, really big. And, we might add, typical.

Now you may say that this is simply because they both ply a mean knife and fork.

But Angela N. Slover and Johanna T. Dwyer, in an article in <u>Nutrition Today</u>, sought a more scientific explanation. Calling it the diva syndrome, Slover and Dwyer said that the weight of opera singers tends to crescendo for the following reasons.

- They often have stage-frightened stomachs, causing them to fast before they perform and to dine after their last curtain call—by which time, of course, they are ravenous and (except for after matinees) the hour is late.
- They go to a lot of parties hosted by the glitterati, where they soothe their nerves with hors d'oeuvres and high-calorie social lubricants like martinis.

- They often devour huge amounts of food to console themselves after bad performances and huge amounts of food to reward themselves after good performances.

Nowhere have the perils of the profession been more dramatically illustrated than by Richard Versalle, a tenor with the New York Metropolitan Opera. On January 5, 1996, Versalle, 63, was singing the role of Vitek in the opera <u>The Makropulos Case</u>.

In the opening scene Versalle had to climb a 10-foot ladder. As he stood atop the ladder, he sang, "Too bad you can only live so long," then suddenly stopped and toppled backward onto the stage.

He was pronounced dead shortly after his arrival at St. Luke's–Roosevelt Hospital.

There's food for thought in this, given that a lot of us use food in a similar manner without the excuse of being opera singers. Which is to say that we, too, use food to cope with stress, which is not a healthy thing.

---

weight-loss program. Many of those who stick with the program can actually improve to the point where they don't need medication.

And there is overwhelming evidence that losing excess weight reduces blood pressure. In fact, obese patients can often bring their blood pressures down to normal by losing only half their excess weight.

Losing weight has beneficial effects on cholesterol as well. One, it helps reduce the amount of "bad" cholesterol that's flowing through your veins while increasing levels of "good" cholesterol. And two, the process of losing weight—as long as it involves an intense exercise like playing tennis or basketball or running faster than 5 miles per hour—can cause further decreases in total cholesterol.

Fat Ain't Fate

Your belly is not your destiny. We said earlier that every man makes a bargain with his body. Not only can you renegotiate it, but, like the 400-pound guy from Utah, you can turn back the clock.

So if you have yourself something of a belly already, and even some of the related health problems, don't despair. There are more than a few

ways to shed your past and redesign yourself. For starters, here are a few simple recommendations.

START SAFE. Since men with high levels of abdominal fat are at increased risk for so many serious conditions, it's important to get checked out by a doctor at least once a year, says David Levitsky, Ph.D., professor of nutritional sciences and psychology at Cornell University in Ithaca, New York. Catching weight-related health problems early gives you a much better chance of preventing them from getting serious later on.

TAKE A WALK. Even small changes in your habits can make a big difference in your health. Doctors recommend that you try to do a minimum of 30 minutes of moderate-intensity physical activity a day. This means taking a brisk (3 to 4 miles per hour) walk or doing something that requires a similar level of exertion, like biking or even vigorous yard work.

Even if this 30 minutes is broken up into smaller chunks of time during the course of the day—10 minutes in the morning, say, followed by 20 minutes after supper—the benefits will still accrue, says Dr. Levitsky, who gets his exercise by riding a bike to work, a 15-minute ride each way.

Are You Overweight?

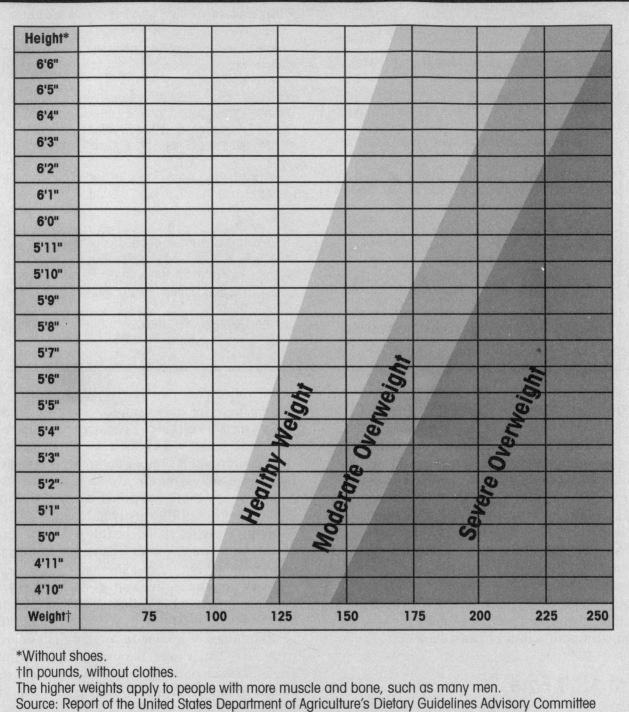

*Without shoes.
†In pounds, without clothes.
The higher weights apply to people with more muscle and bone, such as many men.
Source: Report of the United States Department of Agriculture's Dietary Guidelines Advisory Committee on the Dietary Guidelines for Americans, 1995, pages 23–24.

WATCH YOUR MOUTH. In particular, start tuning in to how much fat and salt you put in your mouth every day. You want to minimize fat because, well, it makes you fat. As for salt, most of us eat a lot more in a day than we really need, according to the U.S. Departments of Agriculture and Health and Human Services. And there is plenty of evidence linking a high salt intake to high blood pressure.

One easy way to curtail fat and salt? Eat more fresh fruits and vegetables.

BELLY FAT AND IMAGE
WHEN SIZE BRINGS YOU DOWN

It wasn't just that the guy was wearing a T-shirt. It was where he was wearing it: to his teenage daughter's high school music recital.

And stretched across that T-shirt was a message we couldn't forget: "This is NOT a beer gut!" it proudly proclaimed. "It's the fuel tank for a SEX machine!"

After our initial amusement, we shrank inside as we imagined his daughter's embarrassment, and we wondered whether there wasn't a fund we could contribute to for all the shrink bills she was going to have.

Sins of the Flesh

Fortunately for our children, most of us do not consider an ample middle something to advertise. If anything, it's something we would just as soon nobody noticed.

There is a reason for our embarrassment. We know that in our society our stomachs are much more than mere extra weight; they are a reflection of ourselves, our moral character writ in flesh—and by that flesh shall our neighbors judge us. A hefty gut is often perceived as a sign of spinelessness, slovenliness, and wanton indulgence.

A man's "stomach is sort of the messenger, if you will, of his adiposity," says Thomas Cash, Ph.D., clinical psychologist at Old Dominion University in Norfolk, Virginia. "We tend to blame people for the size of their bodies whether they're responsible or not."

Unfortunately for the overweight, this prejudice can be reflected in nearly every aspect of life: social status, self-esteem, income, and sexual satisfaction.

Pounds and Prejudice

There have been numerous studies demonstrating what we all know to be true: To be fat is to be an object of derision.

The attitude starts early. In one study, six-year-old children described their fat peers as "lazy, dirty, stupid, ugly, cheats, and liars."

We don't become any more enlightened as we grow up. In fact, even those of us who should know better, doctors and dietitians, have been shown to harbor intractable prejudices toward fat patients.

As a society, we make fat people feel so miserable that they would rather suffer just about any other kind of handicap. When 57 formerly obese people were asked whether they would rather be fat again or deaf, 100 percent of them said that they would rather be deaf. And 90 percent of them said that they would rather lose a leg or be legally blind than be fat again.

A History of Obesity

There have been times in the history of mankind when big bellies were social assets, even status symbols, says S. Boyd Eaton, M.D., associate clinical professor of radiology and adjunct associate professor of anthropology at Emory University in Atlanta and co-author of The Paleolithic Prescription.

Some of the art of our Stone Age ancestors suggests that obesity may well have been considered beautiful, which certainly made evolutionary sense since heavier people were better adapted to survive a famine, says Dr. Eaton.

More recently, says Anne Bolin, Ph.D., associate professor of anthropology at Elon College in Elon College, North Carolina, there was at least one time in American history when portliness was in.

"In the 1800s, there were two body styles that were prominent," Dr. Bolin says. "One of them that occurred throughout the first part of the 1800s was a style associated with the thin, pale intellectual. In the 1860s, another type emerged. This was the corpulent, prosperous type, the portly, round man, a man who wore his prosperity on his body."

Back then, portliness conveyed the message: "A fat bank account tends to make a fat man."

Since then, however, largeness has rarely been shown any largesse, Dr. Bolin says.

These days, Dr. Bolin says, when she asks students in her classes to select the male body images that they find most attractive, the most popular image is "a youthful figure (of course) muscled to about the degree that you find on the show Baywatch."

In the eyes of many, being fat signals a lack of class. "We know that people in lower socioeconomic groups tend to be more likely to be heavy, so it tends to convey issues of social status," says Dr. Cash.

All of which goes a long way toward explaining why "the stomach is probably the number one disliked area of the body," says Dr. Cash. When he did surveys to learn how people feel about different parts of their bodies, he found that "roughly half of men are dissatisfied with their stomachs."

Dr. Cash, author of *What Do You See When You Look in the Mirror?*, has spent 25 years looking at how people's looks affect their lives and, more recently, what people see when they look at themselves.

What we see, Dr. Cash says, often bears little resemblance to reality, but it can have a profound impact on our self-esteem. "About a fourth of our self-esteem is influenced by how we feel about our looks," he says. "It matters not so much what you look like but how you feel about what you look like."

Quantity over Quality

How you feel about your looks can have a lot to do with the quality of life you lead.

There's plenty of evidence, for example, that people who are obese and dislike their looks also have problems with depression, anxiety, and low self-esteem. And it's no secret that some people have a common coping method for depression, anxiety, and low self-esteem: They eat.

A questionnaire developed by Ronette Kolotkin, Ph.D., a clinical psychologist and director of behavioral programs at the Duke University Diet and Fitness Center in Durham, North Carolina, and Michael Hamilton, M.D., medical director of the center, has revealed that even the loss of a small amount of weight can result in big (and very positive) psychological changes.

Conversely, Drs. Kolotkin and Hamilton have found that as men (and women) got fatter, they generally felt worse. "The bigger they got, the greater the impact of weight on health, social and interpersonal life, mobility, self-esteem, sexual life, and the activities of daily living," Dr. Kolotkin says.

Incidentally, it seems that men are a little slower on the uptake when it comes to tuning in to how big they have become. "It seems that men need to get bigger to notice that it's time to do something," Dr. Kolotkin says.

On the other hand, she says she has seen a shift in men's fat-consciousness in the past few years. "We're seeing more and more men at the center. Today we have a 60/40 population of women and men. When I started working here, it was about 90/10 women to men."

Weight and Sex

Not surprisingly, our self-images have a lot to do with our sex lives. In one study of 83 seriously obese women who had gastric bypass surgery, the women reported that they had become more interested in sex, had sex more often, and enjoyed it

Is Your Belly Bringing You Down?

Do you sometimes wonder if your belly is stealing some of the gusto from your life? Try answering some of the questions from the "Impact of Weight Questionnaire," which was developed by Ronette Kolotkin, Ph.D., and Michael Hamilton, M.D., both of the Duke University Diet and Fitness Center in Durham, North Carolina.

We can't include all 74 questions from the original survey, but we can give you enough of a sampling to tell whether you feel your weight's an issue for you. You should answer "always true," "usually true," "sometimes true," "rarely true," or "never true" to the following statements.

"Because of my weight...

- "I am embarrassed to be seen in public places."
- "I experience ridicule, teasing, or unwanted attention."
- "I don't receive appropriate raises, promotions, or recognition at work."
- "I have trouble crossing my legs."
- "I have trouble tying my shoes."
- "I have trouble using stairs."
- "I have trouble picking up objects."
- "I feel the need to use handicapped spaces in parking lots or to park as close as possible."
- "I avoid recreational or social activities that involve physical activity."
- "I am self-conscious."
- "I avoid looking in mirrors or seeing myself in photographs."
- "I spend a lot of time worrying about my weight."
- "I do not feel sexually attractive."
- "I do not enjoy sexual activity."
- "I avoid activities where wearing a bathing suit or shorts is expected."
- "I worry about fitting into seats in public places (e.g. theaters, restaurants, cars, or airplanes)."

If you find yourself answering "always true," "usually true," or "sometimes true" to any of these questions, then your belly is clearly affecting the quality of your life.

The good news is that you can do something about it. With the loss of even a few pounds, researchers say, you'll probably start feeling a whole lot better about your life.

more than they had before the operation.

Men are less likely than women to let a little extra weight get in the way of their sex lives. "We have a sexuality workshop, and one thing that's been fascinating to me is that each time we've brought up the issue of weight and how that affects one's own sexuality, the women say, 'God, he might touch my stomach. I'd be so embarrassed. I have to hide under the covers,'" Dr. Kolotkin says.

"But the man who's 100 pounds overweight is saying, 'Everything's great. I'm attractive. I'm desirable. I'm still potent. Everything's super.'"

Still, both men and women reported feeling more sexual feelings and greater interest in sex as they lost weight in the program, Dr. Kolotkin says.

Money

Having extra poundage affects more than just the so-called touchy-feely stuff. We're talking hard-core stuff, too, like how much money you make, which schools you get into, and what kind of jobs you can get. Studies have shown, for example, that fat people have more difficulty getting hired than thinner folks.

Fortunately, as Dr. Kolotkin observes, even a small amount of weight loss can lead to big improvements in most aspects of a person's life. All of which probably comes as no surprise to you, but certainly, if you're looking for more reasons to lose that belly, the levels of discrimination experienced by the big-bellied at the hands of the bellyless is one.

How to Gauge Your Own Situation
Let the Scales Fall from Your Eyes

Forget about bathroom scales. Don't step on them. Don't look at them. What they have to tell you is almost completely meaningless.

This is because scales will only tell you what you weigh—not how fat you are.

Here's the deal: It's perfectly conceivable that you could weigh exactly what you weighed when you were a slender senior in high school and still be fatter than you were back then.

If you're an average-size guy (for example, 5 feet 9 inches tall and weighing 172 pounds), you're right on the borderline between being a "healthy weight" and "moderately overweight," according to guidelines issued by the U.S. Departments of Agriculture and Health and Human Services.

But chances are, if you have reached the ripe old age of 30-something, 40-something, or 50-something without being any more active than the average American, a lot of your weight has shifted around on your body. Moreover, a lot of what used to be muscle is now fat.

In other words, it's possible to be "overfat" without being overweight.

"I weigh less now than I did when I was 26, but my body doesn't look as good," says Charles T. Kuntzleman, Ed.D., adjunct associate professor of kinesiology and director of the Blue Cross/Blue Shield Fitness for Youth program at the University of Michigan in Ann Arbor. "My waist is larger and my chest is smaller, and my muscle mass isn't what it used to be. That's partly age, but it's also because I don't exercise as strenuously as I did back then. The scale never tells you that."

How Fat Are You?

If the scale lies, how do you get a realistic handle on your status? Dr. Kuntzleman offers several handy methods.

GET NAKED. Strip down to your birthday suit, stand in front of a full-length mirror, and take a look at yourself. Is it hard to look at what you see? Do you think you look fat? If so, then, let's face it, you probably are.

Sure, it's not a pleasant sight, but remember why you're doing this: You're going to be getting rid of this belly, and to do that you need to start by making a good, cold-blooded appraisal of your situation. Know thy enemy, as they say. So do your best to give an honest answer to these questions.

- **Does my gut stick out?**
- **Is my butt too big?**

Are You Too Fat?
Do a "Spot" Check

If your dog looks as though he has wolfed down a few too many Milk-Bones while watching <u>Lassie</u> reruns, then probably you do, too.

"If your dog is too big, there's a good chance you may look a little pudgy, too," says Karen J. Wolfsheimer, D.V.M., Ph.D., associate professor in the Department of Veterinary Physiology, Pharmacology, and Toxicology in the School of Veterinary Medicine at Louisiana State University in Baton Rouge.

This is because

    a. people and their dogs really do tend to look like each other. And at least part of the reason for this is . . .
    b. dogs share their masters' lifestyles, which means that . . .
    c. if you spend a lot of time sitting on the sofa noshing Zapp's Cajun Crawtators, then your dog probably does the same.

"We sit in front of the TV eating junk food, and our dogs are begging with big, brown, pitiful eyes," Dr. Wolfsheimer says. "It's easy to toss them a chip or two as we eat our way through a 12-ounce bag of chips over the course of an evening."

That sort of lifestyle makes humans—and their dogs—overweight. By some estimates, roughly the same percentage of American dogs (somewhere between 25 and 45 percent) as American masters (33 percent) are overweight.

To help both of you stay trim, Dr. Wolfsheimer suggests taking regular trips around the block—on foot, naturally. If you take your dog for even a leisurely stroll for 20 minutes a day, five days a week, you'll burn several hundred more calories each week than you would by sitting on your behind.

Here's a technique for telling whether your dog is really and truly overweight: Feel his ribs.

"You should be able to feel his ribs and maybe just a very light layer of subcutaneous fat overlying them," Dr. Wolfsheimer says. "If you can't easily feel his ribs, then he's too heavy. The other thing is that most breeds should have a nice waistline, tucked in to some extent behind the rib cage."

In other words, little or no belly.

- **Do I have love handles above my hips?**
- **Do the backs of my arms seem flabby?**
- **Do my thighs seem to have the texture of cottage cheese?**
- **Does my chest look flabby?**

If you have to answer yes to any of these questions, says Dr. Kuntzleman, you're too fat.

DO THE JIGGLE. No, it's not a new dance, though, come to think of it, you may find that you inadvertently do it whenever you do dance.

Still in front of that mirror? Good. Now, run in place for a few seconds. Do you see parts of your person jiggling up and down? Do your chest and belly bounce just a bit behind the beat?

If they do, you can bet that what you're seeing jumping there is fat, says Dr. Kuntzleman.

CHECK YOUR GIRTH. Stand up straight. Put your shoulders back, feet together, and arms at your sides. Now, run a tape measure around your hips. Write that number down.

Now, run that tape measure around your waist right at your belly button. Your stomach should be relaxed when you take this measurement—no sucking in your gut. Again, write that number down.

Divide your waist measurement by your hip measurement. If the number you get is .85 or greater, your belly's too big.

PINCH YOURSELF. With your thumb and forefinger, pinch the skin anywhere on your belly, arm, thigh, or hip. If the thickness of the skin held between your finger and thumb is more than ¾ inch, you have too much fat.

BUCKLE UP. And finally, the easiest measure of adiposity of all: Ask yourself what's happening to your belt buckle, suggests Dr. Kuntzleman. "If you notice that you're going to another hole—the wrong way—you can conclude that you're putting on more body fat. It's just that simple."

THE THEORY OF BELLY BANISHING
NEVER GO BACK TO YOUR OLD WEIGHS

If there's one thing that every researcher on the subject of belly banishing agrees on, it is this: The only way that you're ever going to tame that belly and keep it tamed is to make permanent changes in the way you live day by day.

You have to change the way you eat, and you have to make exercise a regular part of your life.

"Both those things have to change," says J. P. Wallace, Ph.D., associate professor of kinesiology and director of the adult fitness program at Indiana University in Bloomington. "It has to be a total change in lifestyle. You're not just doing it to lose weight, because once you stop, you're going to gain the weight back."

Indeed, this is your biggest challenge: keeping that belly at bay. It's a lot like quitting smoking. Any smoker will tell you that it's easy to quit; he's done it dozens of times. The hard part is quitting once and for all. Same thing with banishing a belly: The "easy" part is losing the pounds; the hard part is keeping them off.

Here are the basic principles of belly banishing.

Becoming Conscious

When you're trying to trim down, the first step you have to take is increasing awareness, says Kelly Brownell, Ph.D., co-director of the Yale University Eating and Weight Disorders Clinic.

Most of us are unconscious when it comes to our eating and exercise habits. We have in the course of our lives acquired whole sets of behaviors that we go through every day without giving them a moment's thought.

This is why Dr. Brownell and other researchers suggest that you start your belly banishing by keeping a diary of what you eat each day. More than likely, you're going to be surprised at how much you actually put away.

This is because most of us grossly underestimate how many calories we consume on any given day. And indeed, evidence suggests that the bigger your belly, the more you will underestimate your caloric intake, sometimes by as much as 30 to 40 percent.

Once you have a handle on how many calories you're taking in each day, what kind of calories they happen to be (carrot or Twinkie calories, for example), and where and when you're taking them in, you're going to have a good idea of what, where, and when you can cut back.

Don't worry. We're not going to have you counting calories for the rest of your life. Instead, you're going to focus on your "fat habits," unconscious eating habits that add excess fat to your diet (and your midsection) and which, because they are done unconsciously, really don't add all that much joy to your existence.

You also need to tune in to your level of physical activity. What kind of exercise, if any, are you getting every day? Again, a diary of your daily activities will help you get a better handle on this.

The Six Axioms of Belly Banishing

Any successful and lasting reduction in the size of your belly depends on diet and exercise. With the help of Charles T. Kuntzleman, Ed.D., adjunct associate professor of kinesiology and director of the Blue Cross/Blue Shield Fitness for Youth program at the University of Michigan in Ann Arbor, we've cooked up six axioms to guide you.

When it comes to exercise:

1. Anything is better than nothing.
2. More is better than less.
3. Faster is better than slower.

But when it comes to diet:

4. Nothing is better than anything.
5. Less is better than more.
6. Slower is better than faster.

Before you start starving yourself and running like a rat on a treadmill, let us explain.

1. If there's just one message researchers wish we would get, it's this: Get off your duff and do something. Take a walk. Play tennis. Do the hokey-pokey. Just do it. Anything you do will burn more fat than sitting still.
2. The greater the intensity of your workout, the more you'll burn. Simple enough.
3. Not only that, the faster you go, the more calories you'll use.

Now, on the diet side of the equation:

4. We're not suggesting that you fast. In fact, that won't banish your belly. What we are suggesting is that when the hors d'oeuvre tray comes around, there's no law that says you have to eat one.
5. Which brings us to our central diet axiom: You can carve away some of that belly by carving extra calories out of your diet. We'll be showing you how to do that without feeling like a martyr.
6. Finally, it is better both to eat slowly and to lose weight slowly. The slower you eat, the sooner you'll feel full, which means you'll eat less. And when it comes to losing pounds, research has shown that you're going to be much more likely to keep that belly off if you take it off slowly and steadily, like the tortoise in the race.

Becoming Someone New

Once you have a better sense of how you eat and what you do every day, you have to start retraining yourself with a whole new set of habits, says Dr. Brownell.

For example, instead of coming home every night and flopping down in front of the TV, you may start going out for a brisk 30-minute walk.

And instead of doing your daily Danish, you may switch to a plain bagel.

But losing weight for the long haul involves more than just doing a few things differently, says Anne Bolin, Ph.D., associate professor of anthropology at Elon College in Elon College, North Carolina.

"It can't be just, 'I'm going to change my diet, and I'm going to make myself exercise.' It has to be a life change," says Dr. Bolin. "Whatever you're doing on a routine basis has to be gradually changed so that you have something else that becomes part of who you are. This isn't just something you're doing; you're creating a new identity."

Do What You Like

Finding an activity or combination of activities that you like doing is a critical part of any weight-loss plan. A lot of people force themselves to do things that they don't really enjoy—stationary bicycling, say, or jogging before work—with predictable results: About half the people who get into an exercise program will drop out in the first six months, says Dr. Wallace.

When she studied exercisers, she found that the ones who were most successful at staying with the program were those who "did what excited them."

If running is fun, run. If swimming is it for you, swim. Find an activity that you enjoy, because then it will be something that you look forward to and can stick with, says Dr. Wallace. If, on the other hand, you hate it and are just doing it because you know it's good for you, you won't be doing it for long.

Once you've found something that you really like doing, make it a part of your new definition of yourself. Say to yourself (and to others), "I'm a runner." Or "I'm a swimmer." Or "I lift weights."

"What it means is finding the athlete in yourself so that you become that athlete," says Dr. Bolin. "Once you've become that athlete, that's who you are."

THE THREE TYPES OF EXERCISE
WHY YOU NEED ALL THREE

If you have ever spent any time at a gym, you have seen him. Perhaps (we hope not) you even are him.

We're talking about the guy who goes to the gym, suits up, and then hangs around making chin music to everybody else in the place.

Sometimes he'll do a couple of stretches, a few half-hearted lifts, or maybe take a desultory stroll on the treadmill. But most of the time, he beats his gums. And most important of all, he never—repeat, *never*—breaks a sweat.

Now you know the guy we're talking about? Yeah. He really honks you off, doesn't he? It's not just that he's not serious; it's the way he always gets in your way. Like when you're trying to work through a few sets of weights, and he's using the bench press as a La-Z-Boy recliner.

You wonder sometimes after you kick him off: What does he think? That he'll get fit by sitting there? Or maybe he thinks that he'll burn off his flab just by being around other people who are burning theirs, sort of an exercise-by-osmosis kind of thing.

Our point? Going to the gym and jawing with your friends is *not* one of the three types of exercise. Fact is, if you turn your workout into a kaffeeklatsch, you will burn only about 20 more calories an hour than you would burn watching TV.

Let's face it. If you're serious about getting in shape, you have to get serious about exercise. Sure, it's possible to lose weight just by cutting back on calories, but then you lose muscle mass as well as fat and end up weaker as well as skinnier. And, hey, do you really want to wind up looking two sizes too small for your birthday suit?

The three types of exercise that you should be doing, according to Charles T. Kuntzleman, Ed.D., adjunct associate professor of kinesiology and director of the Blue Cross/Blue Shield Fitness for Youth program at the University of Michigan in Ann Arbor, are aerobics, weight training, and stretching, and all of them require some real exertion on your part. We'll be talking about these exercises in more detail later (see "Aerobic Exercise" on page 28, "Weight Training" on page 29, and "Stretching" on page 30).

In this chapter, we're going to take a look at what each one has to offer in the way of belly banishing and why you really need all three to do the job.

Who Needs This?

Before we get into the nuts and bolts of the different types of exercise, you may find yourself asking, "Why do I need to exercise? Generations of humans before me lived long and prospered without having to resort to jogging and Butt-Masters."

True. But then, they didn't need to. If you'll think back to our example of a day in the life of

Remote Kid-trol

Not all exercise has to happen in a gym. In fact, there are daily opportunities to catch little bits of exercise that most of us pass up. And even the smallest of these, in themselves unimpressive, can carve large amounts of lard off your belly.

"I don't think people realize how much they sit, when they really could be moving more in a day," says Margery Lawrence, R.D., Ph.D., associate professor in the Department of Nutrition and Family Studies at St. Joseph College in West Hartford, Connecticut. "People are just very lazy. You know, you use your kids to get you things. I mean, before there were remote controls, come on, who changed the channels? For a while, I thought that's why my parents had kids."

And your kids don't waste any time in trying to be just like Daddy.

"When I see students, 20 years old, getting off the elevator in a three-story building, I could just scream," Dr. Lawrence says. "If that's a habit of yours, when you get to middle age, you're going to start puffing on the stairs."

Consider this: For every minute you spend climbing the stairs instead of taking the elevator, you will burn about 6½ extra calories. And if you take those steps two at a time, you will burn more than 16 extra calories a minute.

Let's say that you spend a total of 5 minutes a day, five days a week, climbing the stairs—two at a time—at your office. In just one week you'll burn 460 calories, and in one year (with a couple weeks off for vacation), you'll burn more than 23,000 calories, roughly 6 pounds of fat. And that's without counting the calories you burn going down the stairs.

Charles T. Kuntzleman, Ed.D., adjunct associate professor of kinesiology and director of the Blue Cross/Blue Shield Fitness for Youth program at the University of Michigan in Ann Arbor, codifies this principle as, "Never use a machine when you can use body power instead."

If you can get there by walking or biking, do that instead of driving. If you can rake those leaves or shovel that snow, do that instead of using a blower. And it's always better to push a lawn mower than to ride one.

The lesson is simply this: You can lose a lot of flab just by showing some signs of life. You burn more calories walking than you do standing still, you burn more calories standing still than you do sitting, and you burn more calories sitting than you do lying down. Hey, dead guys lie down a lot, and they don't burn a one.

---

your greatest of grandpas (see "Stone Age versus Phone Age" on page 5), you'll recall that his was a far more active and physically demanding life than yours.

And Stone Age life demanded that he be fit in more ways than one.

"These people were more like decathlon athletes than ultramarathoners or power lifters," says S. Boyd Eaton, M.D., associate clinical professor of radiology and adjunct associate professor of anthropology at Emory University in Atlanta and co-author of *The Paleolithic Prescription*. "Their daily activities required all sorts of exertion in different respects, and, as a result, they were like cross-trainers."

Grandpa, for example, had to be aerobically fit, able to outrun his breakfast (or anything that wanted to have him for breakfast); he had to be muscularly fit, able to hoist heavy hunks of mastodon meat and such; and he had to be flexible so that he wouldn't develop a paralyzing calf cramp at an inopportune moment. In short, he had to be able to run, jump, lift, and throw.

Life has gotten a lot easier since the Stone Age, of course, but only very recently. Even your grandfather or your great-grandfather, depending on how old you are, grew up in a primarily agrarian-industrial society where the mass of men earned their livings by their backs.

"People always say to me, 'Charlie, you're really active,'" says Dr. Kuntzleman. "And I say, 'I'm not active. I'm a sedentary person who's active 1 hour a day.' My grandfather was active. He was up in the morning, did 2 hours of farm chores, walked to the coal mines of Pennsylvania, did pick and shovel work in the coal mines for 8, 10, 12 hours, walked home 3 miles, did a few more chores, and collapsed into bed. Now there was an active human being."

By comparison, Dr. Kuntzleman says, most of us—even those of us who work out every day—are extremely sedentary, spending the bulk of our day sitting in a car, sitting at a desk, or sitting in front of a television.

The problem is that we weren't designed for this. And an estimated 250,000 of us die every year for lack of exercise.

Why? Because our bodies were designed to run, jump, lift, and throw. And when we don't use them, they rust. Just like a car when you park it for a few years in your backyard. Park your body on the couch for several years, and it will become the fleshy equivalent of a frozen mass of scrap metal.

Minimum Fitness: No Excuses

This isn't to say that you have to take that old Dodge Dart of a body out and "redline" it every day. Research has shown that you can make a big difference in your health—and inroads on your belly—just by regularly taking your body out for a pleasant drive.

Because of this, the Centers for Disease Control and Prevention in Atlanta and the American College of Sports Medicine, headquartered in Indianapolis, recommend a minimum of 30 minutes or more of moderate-intensity physical activity, preferably every day.

Moderate-intensity is defined as doing such things as taking a brisk walk at 3 to 4 miles an hour, bicycling at speeds up to 10 miles an hour, playing table tennis, fishing (when you're standing and casting), leisurely canoeing, or pushing a power mower around your lawn.

As you can see, we're not talking the Boston Marathon here; we're just talking about getting up and moving around.

Moreover, research has shown that you can derive major health benefits simply by racking up a total of 30 minutes of activity during the day, even if it is broken up into smaller increments of only 8 to 10 minutes here and there.

"Even that minimum amount has been demonstrated to be effective," says David Levitsky, Ph.D., professor of nutritional sciences and psychology at Cornell University in Ithaca, New York.

Not only is it effective, but if you go from 0 to 30 minutes of physical activity a day, you are going to derive a bigger benefit than will the guy who is already doing 30 minutes and increases that amount. Which is not to say that more exercise is not better for you; only that any exercise is a lot better than none.

Aerobic Exercise

Still, it doesn't hurt to stomp on your accelerator every now and then. Nothing is better for your heart—your engine, if you will—than to boost the rpms. And nothing does that better than aerobic exercise.

Aerobic exercise is anything you do that makes you breathe hard. If you run, walk, swim, or cycle, you are engaging in aerobic exercise. All of this is wonderfully good for your heart and lungs. The more aerobic exercise you do, the more efficient your heart and lungs will be. This is why a guy who hasn't done any running in years will be gasping within seconds of beginning a sprint, whereas a guy who has been running regularly can go on for miles while carrying on a normal conversation.

And if you did an EKG on those two guys, you would find that the runner's resting heart rate can be as little as half that of the slacker's. Again, this is because when you do a lot of running (or other aerobic exercise), your heart and lungs become so efficient at getting oxygen to your muscles that they don't have to work (and you don't have to breathe) nearly as hard.

"Okay, okay," you say. "Aerobic exercise is good for my heart. But what about my belly?"

We can tell you unequivocally that nothing burns fat faster than aerobic exercise. Nothing.

"But," you say, "wasn't there a study somewhere that showed that walkers burned more calories of fat than runners?"

Yes and no.

Walkers do burn a higher percentage of fat than runners, but they don't burn more calories, according to Brian Wallace, Ph.D., chairman of sport fitness at the U.S. Sports Academy in Daphne, Alabama. "When you're doing high-intensity exercise for the same duration, you're going to burn more calories of fat."

Let's say, for the sake of argument, that 70 percent of the calories you burn while walking are fat calories, compared to only 50 percent of those you burn while running. Now, if you took a half-hour walk, during which you traveled at 3 miles an hour, you would burn a total of 168 calories, 118 of them from fat. Meanwhile, if your next-door neighbor ran for a half-hour at 6 miles per hour, he would burn a total of 369 calories, 185 of them from fat. Yes, you burned a higher *percentage* of fat calories than your neighbor in that half-hour, but who burned the *most*?

So, if it's your belly that you want to be burning, and you can only undertake one kind of exercise, take up something aerobic.

Climbing the Plateau

Experts have long recognized that it's extremely difficult to lose weight by dieting alone. This is because your body has a cruel habit of slowing down its resting metabolic rate whenever you cut back on the calories.

Your resting metabolic rate is the rate at which your body burns calories just to maintain normal functions, and it accounts for 60 to 75 percent of the calories you burn in a day. When you decide to reduce the number of calories that you are taking in every day, your body responds by saying to itself, "Whoa, dude! Starvation City. Better conserve those calories," and it slows your resting metabolic rate way down.

This is why when you go on a diet, you will have the disheartening experience of dropping a few quick pounds and then plateauing. Your body—genetically programmed in a prehistoric time when fewer calories coming in was a signal of famine—is doing its bit to keep you alive.

Fortunately, studies show that if you do a half-hour to an hour of moderate-intensity aerobic exercise a day, four to five days a week, you can prevent some of that decrease in resting metabolic rate.

Which is one reason why researchers concur that combining diet with exercise is far more effective than simply going on a diet.

Weight Training

While aerobic exercise is good for you, you should know that you're not going to be your fittest unless you do weight training, too. Basically, weight training is any exercise that pits your muscles against the force of gravity. Sit-ups, push-ups, chin-ups, weights—these are all weight training.

When you do weight training in conjunction with cutting back on calories, you burn up more fat and less muscle tissue. Or, as Dr. Wallace puts it, "you become a metabolic machine."

This is because muscle tissue burns more calories than fat tissue, even when you're resting, says Dragomir Cioroslan, head coach of the U.S. Weightlifting Federation and the 1996 U.S. Olympic weightlifting team.

"Weight training is an excellent, effective tool in changing the composition of your body and replacing fat tissue with lean body mass," says Cioroslan.

And the higher your lean body mass, the higher your resting metabolic rate—which is to say that you burn more calories even when you're not working out.

"This is because you have increased protein synthesis," Dr. Wallace explains. "You're constantly burning those calories because you have to keep the protein moving into those muscle cells and out."

How much weight training do you need to do to convert your body into a metabolic machine?

While researchers generally recommend doing aerobic exercise of some kind at least five days a week, you can achieve the results you want with weight training by doing it just three days a week.

"Three times a week, and the number of exercises should be somewhere between 8 and 12 in a period of time of 45 to 60 minutes," adds Cioroslan.

Ideally, you might want to get into a pattern of doing aerobic exercise one day and doing weights the next, alternating so that different muscles get worked and rested, he says.

"For losing weight, you can expend the calories any way you want," says Dr. Eaton. "But for overall health, the best situation is to train for aerobic fitness and also for strength."

By the way, says Cioroslan, "stretching and warming up are absolutely necessary before the workout, and you also need to stretch and cool down after the workout. These have an impact on the entire exercise program."

Stretching

We know. It's hard to imagine anything more simple, but stretching is important nonetheless. True, it doesn't burn up many calories, but it does make it possible for you to do so. In brief, stretching is what you do so that you can do everything else.

Fortunately, you don't have to spend a lot of time doing it, and we're not going to make you spend a lot of time here reading about it. Here's the quick skinny, according to Dr. Wallace.

First of all, before you stretch you need to warm up your muscles a bit. Unless you're a masochist, the kind of guy who enjoys limping around in pain, you don't want to be stretching a cold muscle.

Second, don't bounce. Do your stretches slowly and gently so that you don't pop your sockets.

You see weekend runners doing this all the time. Before they take a step, they bounce the bejeezus out of their hamstrings. These same people wonder why they're always getting injured and why their hamstrings always seem to be so sore.

So warm up a little bit, and then stretch before you exercise. Stretching, done properly, prepares your joints and muscles for the exercise, making it easier to do while sparing you a lot of injuries. It's also a good idea to stretch after you exercise, this time to prevent your muscles from becoming stiff and sore.

In a word, stretching keeps you flexible. You want to be flexible "because as you become less flexible, you become more prone to injuries," says Dr. Wallace. "If you get tight around the joints, a movement could injure you."

You should focus your stretching on the muscles that you're going to be using, doing a couple of stretches for each. Dr. Wallace suggests that you just take the first stretch to "the point of a mild tension," and hold it for 10 to 15 seconds. With the second stretch, "you can hold that, as you become more fit and flexible, up to 30 to 90 seconds."

There. Done. Was that so bad?

Why All Three Are Important

If you have been reading along here, you already know the answer.

Aerobic exercise is important because it is the number one belly-burner in your exercise arsenal and because it makes a tremendous contribution to having a healthy heart and lungs.

Weight training is important because your body is more than just a set of heart and lungs and because, by strengthening your muscles, you're going to be a better runner, basketball player, or whatever else you want to be. You will be less prone to injury, and you will be burning more calories at rest than you would if you did aerobics alone.

Stretching is what keeps you flexible enough to do the other types of exercise without being laid up with pulled muscles and torn ligaments.

The final answer is that if you make doing these three types of exercise a part of your daily life, you're going to look and feel better than you have in years. Plus, you're likely to live longer than Mr. Kaffeeklatsch.

GETTING MOTIVATED
LIVING AN ALTERED LIFE

You should know up front that the hardest part of belly banishing is just getting started. Once you've begun, it gets easier and easier.

Remember what we said about inertia a few chapters back? How a body at rest tends to stay at rest? Even more powerful than inertia is the force of habit.

Every one of us is a collection of habits. Who we are and how we look are in many ways a product of that collection. If, for example, your particular collection of habits includes frequent trips to the icebox between innings on the idiot box, it's a pretty safe bet you have yourself a gut in progress.

The only way to redefine yourself—to start achieving leanness rather than merely worrying about being overweight—is to acquire a new set of habits. How do you do that? By doing things over and over again until they become habits.

Put succinctly, who you are is what you do. In other words, you can become someone else by doing something else.

Get Ready

How do you get yourself to take that first step? For starters, you need to decide whether you are really ready to do what it takes to banish that belly.

According to Kelly Brownell, Ph.D., co-director of the Yale University Eating and Weight Disorders Clinic, a good way to do this is to make a list of the pros and cons of changing your ways.

A pro, for example, may be "I will look skinnier in my Skivvies." A con may be "the pains of Big Mac withdrawal." After you make your lists, look at which is longer. Are you ready? If the cons outnumber the pros, you're probably not.

If, however, the pros win, your next step is to figure out what's going to be the best motivator for you. Is it that you'll look better? Feel better? Be healthier? Live longer? Be a babe magnet? Be able to shoot hoops with the kid without losing your wind?

"Motivation is probably the most important factor," says Dragomir Cioroslan, head coach of the U.S. Weightlifting Federation and the 1996 U.S. Olympic weightlifting team. "And understanding the benefits is a strong motivating factor."

This is because regardless of what your biggest motivator is—and we'll talk about what's realistic in the next chapter—it's something you're going to want to keep in the forefront of your mind for all those times when you just can't seem to shake off your inertia.

Believe in Yourself

Perhaps the hardest thing you have to do—harder than changing your eating habits, harder

Beware the Lapse Traps

If you're of a fatalistic frame of mind, fat will likely be your fate.

With that attitude, it's all but guaranteed, if for no other reason than we tend to fulfill the prophecies that we make for ourselves.

Nowhere is this more clearly demonstrated than in the matter of lapses. Everyone—no matter how virtuous or determined—has a lapse now and then. You've been running, working out, watching what you eat, the whole shtick, when suddenly you find yourself more than a little lit at an old friend's wedding banquet.

You wake up the next morning cursing the inventor of champagne and cursing yourself for having inhaled quadruple your daily quota of calories.

That is a lapse.

But it's not the lapse that's important; it's how you deal with it.

One way is to become a victim of "lightbulb thinking." According to Kelly Brownell, Ph.D., co-director of the Yale University Eating and Weight Disorders Clinic, this is where you view everything as black or white, on or off. This is where you say to yourself, "Damn, I blew it. Should have known I couldn't do it. I'm off my program now," and then proceed to eat a carton of rocky road ice cream.

The other way is to pick yourself up, dust yourself off, and get back on the track. Say to yourself, "Oh well, the wedding was a gas. But now I have to get it together and go work out."

The moral? Don't let lapses become final arbiters of what kind of life you live.

than working exercise into your life—is to change the way you talk to yourself.

Don't act innocent with us. Maybe you don't talk aloud, but if you're a human being, you do talk to yourself. Like cartoon characters who have an angel perched on one shoulder and a devil on the other, all of us carry on internal dialogues with ourselves.

Unfortunately for many of us, the devil often gives the angel the boot. And the devil is clever. Not only does he tempt us into sin ("Hey, you're fat already! What's another slice of cheesecake?"), he has an even more subtle tool for undercutting our self-confidence: the "if . . . then" way of thinking. "If you can just lose 20 pounds," he tells you, "then you'll feel great about yourself."

This kind of thinking will get you nowhere, says Daniel Kosich, Ph.D., a senior consultant for the International Association of Fitness Professionals and author of *Get Real: A Personal Guide to Real-Life Weight Management.*

"What happens when people go into a weight-loss program with an 'I'll-feel-better-about-my-self-when-I-get-there' sort of attitude is that it makes the program a punishment," Dr. Kosich says. "It's like they're a bad person now, but if they can get to a certain place, then they can be a good person. I think that really makes it difficult

to achieve the long-term goal."

If you're going to stay motivated, Dr. Kosich says, you have to learn to like yourself first. Don't undertake this program because you can't stand the way you look right now. Do it because you like yourself for who you are and because you want to improve the quality of your life.

Dr. Kosich argues that this self-acceptance is key to any successful weight-maintenance program.

Accentuate the Positive

One of the most important things that you can do—indeed, you must do—is to keep reminding yourself of your accomplishments. Nothing will short-circuit your efforts more quickly than focusing on all the weight you haven't lost. Focus instead on the weight you've shed, and you'll find encouragement in each small victory.

People often overlook the benefits of even a small amount of weight loss, says Ronette Kolotkin, Ph.D., a clinical psychologist and director of behavioral programs at the Duke University Diet and Fitness Center in Durham, North Carolina.

So if, to invert the cliché, you can look at your gut as half empty instead of half full (and remember when it was all full), you'll keep yourself psyched to keep going.

SETTING REALISTIC EXPECTATIONS
FACT: YOU ARE NOT STALLONE

Let's be brutally frank. Unless you're willing to devote enormous time and effort to working out, and unless you have just the right genetic makeup, you are probably never going to have abs like the washboards you see on male fashion models.

We'll say it again another way: You'll never have the "shredded" look of a bodybuilder unless you subject yourself to the regimen of a bodybuilder. And even then, you won't succeed unless you were born with the right type of muscular structure.

Why? The length of your muscle fibers is the single most important factor in determining potential muscle size. And muscle-fiber length is genetically predetermined. Sure, intense exercise can grow muscle significantly—but there is a limit. In other words, if you were born with average-length muscle fibers, you will never look like Stallone, who was blessed with unusually long muscle fibers.

In addition, you have two types of muscle fibers: fast-twitch and slow-twitch. Fast-twitch fibers provide tremendous force, the kind you need for sprints or lifting weights. Slow-twitch fibers provide endurance. Like muscle-fiber length, the ratio of fast-twitch to slow-twitch muscle in your body is genetically predetermined. Men with a greater proportion of fast-twitch fibers make better bodybuilders; guys with more slow-twitchers make better marathoners. So if you are a slow-twitcher, you are pretty much destined to a life of slow-twitching (of course, that means a fast-twitcher will rarely beat you in a mile run).

We don't mean to give you an excuse to stop working on your physique. Our point merely is that it is awfully tough to achieve the look of a bodybuilder. It is perfectly within your capacity, however, to add significant strength and definition to your body, and specifically, your belly, no matter what your genetics are.

"A flat stomach is very achievable for everyone," says Dragomir Cioroslan, head coach of the U.S. Weightlifting Federation and the 1996 U.S. Olympic weightlifting team.

How Much, How Soon?

Another question to ask yourself is how quickly can you realistically expect to lose all that flab that you have spent so many years collecting?

If you're thinking that you can drop 20 pounds in a month, we have bad news for you. While it may be possible to lose that kind of weight that

Beware the Flimflam Men

Every week in every supermarket checkout line, Americans wait with carts full of Lard-Dogs and Glutto-Chips, perusing the news about Elvis (who, by the way, has more lives than a cat), space aliens, and the newest miracle diets.

And every week they get a little fatter.

The truth is, we're all waiting for a magic bullet, the food or drug or diet that will melt away our pounds for good, says John B. Allred, Ph.D., professor of nutrition in the Department of Food Science and Technology at Ohio State University in Columbus.

Don't hold your breath, says Dr. Allred, co-author of Taking the Fear Out of Eating: A Nutritionists' Guide to Sensible Food Choices. While miracles are frequently advertised, they're rarely realized. If you are even thinking of embarking on one of those miracle food/drug/diet plans, first take this handy quiz to tell if it is a waste of time. If the answer to even one of these questions is yes, says Dr. Allred, it is.

1. **Does this diet promise that you can EAT AS MUCH AS YOU WANT! and still LOSE WEIGHT INSTANTLY!?**
2. **Will it "burn up" or "melt" your fat with no effort on your part?**
3. **Does it require you to eat a food or foods with "magical properties"?**
4. **Does it require you to take expensive dietary supplements?**
5. **Was it accidentally discovered by an unknown scientist in an obscure former Soviet republic?**

---

fast, it is certainly not healthy to do so. Moreover, when you lose it that quickly, you're not likely to keep it off.

"Don't try to change everything overnight," says Michele Trankina, Ph.D., professor of biological sciences at St. Mary's University and adjunct associate professor of physiology at the University of Texas Health Science Center, both in San Antonio. "Gaining the weight didn't happen overnight, so you need to lose it in a systematic way that takes a lot of patience."

What, then, is a reasonable amount of weight to aim to lose each week?

"I would say 2 pounds at the most," says Dr. Trankina. "It depends on the person and it depends on how much water weight he is carrying. A

person may lose weight, and it may be mostly water at first. If you lose 5 to 8 pounds a month, I think that's good. I think that's a healthy weight loss. For larger people, maybe 10 pounds."

And you're going to be healthier than if you followed a crash plan. Any program that promises you can lose 10 or more pounds a week, says Dr. Trankina, is going to require you to shun the nutrients that you need, which will "wreak havoc on the metabolic systems of the human body. Anytime you simulate starvation, that's an abnormal metabolic situation, and it should be avoided."

When you are losing weight at that rate, she says, you are most likely doing so at the expense of muscle mass (your body will burn it to give the brain the glucose it needs to keep running). Needless to say, if your goal is a lean, mean, muscular body, this is clearly the last thing you want to do.

Redefining "Comfort"

One fact you must face at the outset is that in order to lose weight, you're going to have to get comfortable with being uncomfortable.

More precisely, you're going to be redefining what feels comfortable to you.

"A lot of people don't have the heart to take some of the hard work that comes with it," says Cioroslan. "That's why you have procrastination. They don't want to get out of their comfort zones. But you must put yourself through some uncomfortable positions, spend time, work hard, sweat a little bit, control your diet. It takes a change in lifestyle. And that is the most difficult barrier to reaching consistent fitness: lifestyle."

So you must expect some initial difficulty in getting used to doing things that you didn't used to do. This is in part because you are redefining yourself and, in the process, redefining what feels good to you.

Stick with it, and you will discover that what seemed uncomfortable to you at the outset will become comfortable to you later on. In fact, it will be more than comfortable; after 6 to 12 weeks or so, says Cioroslan, you are likely to wonder how you got through a day without exercising.

Indeed, when you hit a day where you just can't make it to the gym, you may be surprised to discover that you feel frustrated, says Cioroslan. "You'll feel that something was taken away from you."

How to Start
Caution Pays

Don't be a statistic.

If you're a person who has spent the past few years impersonating Plymouth Rock, and the last time you had a checkup was when you went out for junior varsity football in ninth grade, don't—whatever you do—rush out in your sneaks and go tearing down the street. We don't want to be responsible for any cardiac arrests.

Now, we know that you hate being told to go to the doctor (particularly when there is nothing wrong with you). But if you're a sedentary guy over age 40 who is contemplating undertaking a vigorous exercise program, then you really ought to see a doctor to get checked out before you start. Or so say the researchers at the Centers for Disease Control and Prevention in Atlanta and the American College of Sports Medicine, which is headquartered in Indianapolis.

There are two reasons to do this: First, your doctor will make sure everything is in working order (remember, many big health problems are symptomless, such as high blood pressure, so you have no way of knowing without a doctor's inspection whether you have a problem); second, he'll give you accurate measurements that you can use as benchmarks.

Tell your doctor what you're planning to do and ask him for a routine physical, says Brian Wallace, Ph.D., chairman of sport fitness at the U.S. Sports Academy in Daphne, Alabama. He should check out your heart, blood pressure, blood sugar and cholesterol levels as well as any joints that might be aggravated by exercise. Also have him get an accurate measure of your body fat. He might also be able to test your heart rate at various levels of exertion to see how much cardiovascular exercise you are ready to take on.

Let's assume that your ventilation and plumbing get the nod of approval and you're ready to go. The first thing that we're going to tell you is this: Take it easy. If you don't—if, for example, you decide to pretend that you're 18 again and master of the track team—we can almost guarantee that you're going to do something you will regret.

At the very least, you'll end up sore, injured, and discouraged—and less inclined than ever to get on and stay on an exercise program.

"Most of the people that I come across will wait forever, but when they finally start a program, they'll want to be fit that day or that week, and they'll just overdo it," says Dr. Wallace.

The result?

"They're in and out of programs. They get too sore, or they get hurt."

As with diets, careers, or other long-term efforts, a workout plan isn't something that you start on Friday and finish on Sunday. It involves fundamental lifestyle changes, says Dr. Wallace. "Anybody can reach their goals within 6 to 12 months, really. It doesn't matter if it's 3 months, 6, 9, 12; I mean this is for your life. You're going to reach those goals, so the key is to stay with it."

And remember, though it may seem hard at first, it's going to get easier the longer you stay with it. In fact, after a few months, you will find yourself looking forward to it, Dr. Wallace says.

Getting Started

Let's say that you're a guy between 35 and 55 who has basically been an inanimate object for a goodly number of years. Now, you're looking in the mirror and saying, "I have to get my act together. How should I start?"

For starters, of course, you'll want to begin burning more calories than you're taking in, and that means you should eat a sensible diet. We won't dwell on it here, but let's just say that cutting back on red meat and other fatty foods and increasing the amount of fruits, vegetables, and grains in your diet are essential if you are ever

going to get your body into decent trim.

On the exercise front, Dr. Wallace recommends beginning with a light, interval-exercise aerobic program. For example, alternate brief (say, 6-minute) aerobic sessions—using a treadmill, bicycle, in-line skates, or anything else that gets your heart pumping—with a minute of walking around and stretching time. Repeat the cycle four times, for a total Day One workout of 24 minutes.

"The main thing in the first couple of weeks is to get your neuromuscular conditioning going, your joints, all of that," Dr. Wallace says. "You have to slowly let them adapt, too, as well as the heart and lungs."

Each time you exercise, you should increase the intensity and duration of the exercise by a small amount, whatever feels comfortable to you. Within three months, he says, you can be up to 20 to 30 minutes without a break on the bike and the same on the treadmill—or whatever else is your aerobic activity of choice.

About three weeks into it, you can also start doing weight training. Again, you should begin with very light weights because you want to learn the proper way to lift before you start straining. Dr. Wallace recommends that you find a qualified trainer to show you how to do it right. Once you have the technique down, you can do it on your own.

Staying Interested

Now, obviously, this kind of workout could get pretty boring in a hurry. That's why you need to change your routines as often as you get tired of them. On a nice day, get outside and run or walk or both and take in the scenery. Vary your weightlifting routine to challenge different muscles. And take up a sport or form of exercise that really is fun for you like bicycling, in-line skating, playing pickup basketball games, or competing in matches on your local tennis ladder.

But again, before you get competitive, remember to get in shape.

"After three to six months, you can do tennis, basketball, whatever you want to, really," says Dr. Wallace. "But you really need to get that underlying fitness first, you know, strengthen up the ligaments, the tendons, and joints as well as the heart and lungs. Otherwise, you could really be predisposing yourself to injury."

Make It Fun

Number one on the exercise excuse hit parade is: "I don't have time to exercise." What this really means, however, is that exercise isn't exciting you. (When was the last time you said, "I don't have time for sex"?) The only way to keep up with exercise is to make it a habit, and moreover, a habit you enjoy. Here are some things you may want to try.

ENLIST A FRIEND. A lot of people find it easier to start and stick with an exercise program if they enlist a friend to do it with them. It's more fun when you have someone with whom to share the trials and tribulations. And if you have a day when you're just not into exercising, your partner will help you stick with it.

"The buddy system is very effective," says Melinda Hemmelgarn, R.D., associate state nutrition specialist for the Department of Food Science and Human Nutrition Extension at the University of Missouri in Columbia. "So we encourage people to find someone to work out with."

DO LUNCH. If you're one of those people who can't even conceive of doing anything that requires you to get your blood pumping first thing in the morning, and you're always too whipped to exercise at the end of the day, your optimum workout time may be lunchtime.

"Eat during part of your lunch break and walk briskly for the rest of the time," suggests Hemmelgarn. "Or use your entire lunch break to walk or visit the gym, then eat at your desk later if you can."

APPEASE THE BOSS. Your boss looks askance at these longer lunches? Come in to work an hour earlier in the morning. Then nobody can give you a hard time, and you can work out with a clear conscience.

BREAK IT UP. As we've discussed in earlier chapters, you don't have to stuff all your exercise into a single session. There is nothing wrong with exercising for 8 to 10 minutes at a time, taking a rest, and then doing more later on. You will still reap real health benefits if you accumulate at least 30 minutes a day.

For example, do a brisk 10-minute walk before

Food for Thought

Dan is an old friend of ours who, in his mid-fifties, is in better shape than most guys in their twenties. He's the kind of guy who gets up at 5:00 every morning and runs 8 to 10 miles before breakfast. And he's a serious hockey-head. So serious that he routinely drives halfway across New England to play. So serious that he delayed his honeymoon so that he wouldn't miss a game the day after he was married.

But Dan is also the kind of guy who likes his steaks, likes his chips, and likes his scotch. (Nothing fancy. He's a Teacher's man.) And you can always count on Dan to have half a dozen quarts of vanilla ice cream stuffed in his freezer. What we're trying to say is that Dan eats pretty much whatever he wants.

"I exercise," he says, "so I can eat."

Most nutritionists agree that when it comes to losing weight, men and women tend to take opposite approaches. Women tend to think diet; guys tend to think exercise.

But can you really banish your belly and keep it off just by upping your exercise?

Not likely.

"One of the things you see is if people increase their exercise patterns without controlling their caloric intake, they simply tend to eat more calories to make up for the calories they're burning during exercise," says John B. Allred, Ph.D., professor of nutrition in the Department of Food Science and Technology at Ohio State University in Columbus. "So if you want to control weight, you really have to do both at the same time. Dieting without exercise is not very efficient; exercise without dieting is not going to work. What you really need to do is a combination of the two."

True, you can get away with eating a lot more junk if you work out than you can if you sit on your butt. But don't kid yourself. If you're taking in more fuel than you burn, you're still going to build yourself a belly.

Our friend Dan's secret is no secret, really. Fact is, while he can eat whatever he wants, he's not a big eater, and he burns up way more calories on a daily basis than your average weekend walker.

you head for the office, then slip in 10 minutes at lunch and another 10 at the end of your day. While this basic plan won't burn maximum fat, you're still going to start feeling a heck of a lot better. And the better you feel, the more likely you are to keep doing it.

RECRUIT THE OFFICE. Some companies promote a culture of fitness, which makes it easier for everyone to get fit and stay that way. "If your peers don't put a lot of emphasis on health and fitness, it's very difficult for you to be the odd person out," says Hemmelgarn. "That's why work-site programs can be very helpful."

See if you can't get something going in your company: a 5-K run for charity, for example. Stress to your employer that healthy employees miss fewer days of work and tend to be more productive. Even if the company won't invest a lot of money in setting up work-site programs, at least they may help support the effort by offering flextime, showers, casual days, and other exercise-friendly perks.

STICK WITH THE PLAN. Perhaps the main reason that it's so hard to get in shape is that it's so hard to start. The important thing here is just to get in motion. If you can do that and keep doing it for six months, chances are that you can make it a permanent part of your life.

"You can reach so many of your goals within that period of time that you're going to want to stick with it," says Dr. Wallace, "because you feel better, you've lost some weight, and you look better—and you worked so hard to get there."

PART II
EATING FOR LEAN

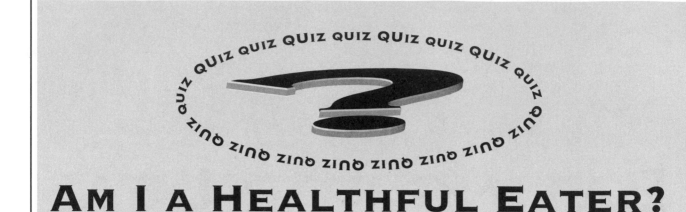

Am I a Healthful Eater?

How do you relate to food? Are you a mature, responsible adult? Or are you just a kid at Ice Cream World with a sawbuck smoking in your pocket?

Not sure? Maybe a bit of both? Take this quiz to see whether you're a healthful eater, a mere pretender, or a total funhog.

1. Like former President Ronald Reagan, I believe ketchup is a vegetable.

Yes   No

2. Like former President George Bush, I believe broccoli is a vegetable, and I would rather lose the support of the broccoli lobby than eat it.

Yes   No

3. Like President Bill Clinton, I believe Big Macs are a vegetable.

Yes   No

4. I actually make it a point to eat at least three to five servings of vegetables a day.

Yes   No

5. I make it a point to eat two to four servings of fruit a day.

Yes   No

6. Most of the food I eat in a day is food made from grains like barley, corn, and wheat—such things as bread, cereal, and pasta.

Yes   No

7. I try to eat fish at least twice a week.

Yes   No

8. Their gassy side effects aside, I recognize that beans are an extremely healthful substitute for meat and try to eat them a few times a week.

Yes   No

9. I try to eat some high-fiber foods every day, especially cereal fiber, because putting fiber in your diet can lower cholesterol and keep digestion regular.

Yes   No

10. In general, I try to limit fat in my food and look to buy low-fat foods whenever I can.

Yes   No

11. Because, after all, if it's low-fat, you can eat all you want.

Yes   No

12. I eat three squares a day, without snacking.

Yes   No

13. Breakfast is not a meal that I can deal with. Just give me a cup of coffee. But I always make sure to eat a big dinner.

Yes   No

14. I always was (and still am) a good boy, so I always clean my plate.

Yes   No

15. Maybe I'm in a rut, but I tend to eat pretty much the same things week after week.

Yes   No

16. Because I am so busy, I have a hard time eating on any kind of schedule, so I tend to eat pretty much anytime and anyplace that the opportunity presents itself.

    Yes   No

17. The worst way to cook a chicken (and just about anything else) is to fry it.

    Yes   No

18. When I eat meat, I try to get the leanest cuts of beef and cut off any excess fat. Also, when I eat poultry, I take off the skin.

    Yes   No

19. When I sauté anything, I use a no-stick spray rather than butter, oil, or margarine.

    Yes   No

20. The best way to lose weight is to go on a diet.

    Yes   No

ANSWERS

If indeed you are a healthful eater, here's what your answers to the questions should be.

1–3. No. Big Macs and ketchup are not vegetables, and the pickles on the Big Macs are at best former vegetables. But broccoli is a vegetable, and a darned good one, loaded with nutrients. Which is why, unlike the Bushman, you should be eating it.

4–10. Yes. If you're trying to eat a healthful diet, it's essential to eat less fat and more beans, grains, fruits, and vegetables.

11. No. Some experts say that this particular belief is a major cause of obesity in our society. Americans often take low-fat or nonfat to mean "calorie-free," and that's not always the case. Even if a food is low in calories and fat, that doesn't mean it has any particular nutritional value. Frozen ice pops are fat-free, but you can't live on them.

12–16. No. These questions deal less with what you eat than with your particular eating habits. The circumstances under which you eat can have a lot to do with whether you are eating a healthful diet. For example, if you always seem to be eating on the run, chances are you're eating a lot more fast food than is good for you. (And how much fast food is good for you? Do we really need to tell you?) Or if you're limiting yourself to only three meals a day, you're probably starving by the time supper comes around—and so are more likely to stuff the food down. It's better to eat less food more often—assuming, of course, it's healthful food.

17–19. Yes. What you should be eating the least of is sweets and fats, and that means cutting out those fats that seem to creep onto your plate at every opportunity.

20. No. There is not a bigger snake-oil approach to weight loss than the old concept of going on a diet. We'll be explaining to you why diets don't work and what does work in upcoming chapters.

Scoring

If you got 15 to 20 questions right, you're way ahead of us here. If the ones you happened to miss had less to do with what you eat and more to do with the circumstances under which you eat it, we'll be showing you how those circumstances can be an important part of nutrition.

If you got 10 to 14 right, you may need to brush up on your nutrition fundamentals. (See page 42.) This is not hard stuff, and we're going to keep it as simple as possible. After all, you're not interested in the minutiae here; you just want to know what's best for you to eat.

If your score was somewhere in the single digits, you may want to start saving up now for that coronary bypass you're going to be needing. Or change your ways while you still have time to change them.

NUTRITION FUNDAMENTALS
HOW TO STAY STOKED AND SATISFIED

"If you're eating dog food, you're gonna look like dog food." So says David Janicello, trainer and owner of Winners' Gym in Burlington, North Carolina.

Experts—though less colloquially—agree: What you eat affects how you look and feel.

What's their prescription for looking and feeling good? It would almost fit in a fortune cookie: Cut back on fats, meats, and sweets and eat more grains, beans, fish, fruits, and vegetables.

Unless you have been in a coma for the past 20 years, you already know this. We all know this. Still, most of us don't do it. Surveys show pretty much the same thing: We eat way too much of the former and way too little of the latter.

One survey found that, while we're supposed to be eating 5 to 9 servings of fruits and vegetables a day, we're eating closer to 3½ servings. And when you get women out of the picture (they tend to eat more of the good stuff than men do), only about one in five of us is eating as many servings as he should.

Meanwhile, we're eating a lot more meat than we need to eat. This is serious stuff. Not only because these eating habits tend to make us fat but also because they predispose us to the chronic diseases—including diabetes, heart disease, osteoporosis, stroke, and a variety of cancers—that are the leading causes of death and disability among Americans.

In other words, the way most of us eat is—quite literally—killing us.

So what can you do about it?

Simple Changes

It's almost absurdly easy to eat a healthful diet that will keep you lean, stoked, and satisfied. Forget about learning the minutia of vitamins, minerals, and trace elements. You don't have to become an expert in nutrition. You certainly don't have to turn your eating habits into some kind of religion.

You can make it as complicated as you like, of course, but the truth is, you're better off (and you're going to be more likely to burn off that belly and keep it off) if you just eat a good, healthful, sensible diet. And we're going to show you how to do that.

GO FOR VARIETY. The number one principle of good nutrition is to eat a wide variety of foods. This doesn't mean staggering your weekly stops at Mickey D's with trips to Taco Bell. What it means is working more grains, fruits, vegetables, low-fat dairy products, lean meats, fish, poultry, and dried beans into your diet—foods that, let's face it, you won't find in profusion at the fast-food emporia.

The reason it's important to go for variety and to eat more of these foods is that they supply you with much more of the essential vitamins, minerals, and fiber than do those burgers and burritos. And research suggests that those who eat a diverse diet are less likely to die of heart disease or cancer.

A tremendous amount of research has been done to determine exactly which nutrients do what, and much has been learned, but there is still a lot that experts don't understand. We know, for example, that oranges are good for us because they are loaded with vitamin C, and that if we don't get enough C, we can get scurvy. We also know that in every orange there is a host of other compounds that do *something*—but what that something is hasn't yet been determined, says Margery Lawrence, R.D., Ph.D., associate professor in the Department of Nutrition and Family Studies at St. Joseph College in West Hartford, Connecticut. "Researchers don't know specifically what it is in those foods that causes these decreases in the incidence of disease," Dr. Lawrence says. "So they really can't responsibly recommend one compound over another. But they can recommend a wide variety."

As you know, different foods supply different nutrients. An orange will give you a dose of vitamin C but no vitamin B_{12}; a hunk of cheese will give you vitamin B_{12} but no vitamin C. Which is why, says Dr. Lawrence, the first principle of good nutrition is to "try to maximize the variety of nutrients you get."

FOLLOW THE PYRAMID. How do you know how much of certain foods to eat? A fairly simple guide is the Food Guide Pyramid. Promoted by the U.S. Departments of Agriculture and Health and Human Services, the pyramid divides foods into five groups and specifies how many servings a day you should have from each of the groups.

At the base of the pyramid are grains, which include breads, cereals, pasta, rice, and whole grains. The pyramid recommends eating between 6 and 11 servings a day from this group.

"Wait a minute," you say. "Between 6 and 11? Which is it?" It depends on how big and active you are. If you're a small, sedentary fellow, the number should be around 8; if you're a large, active guy, it should be around 11.

The next level on the pyramid consists of vegetables; you should be eating three to five servings a day. Next up is the fruit group—shoot for two to four servings a day. Of dairy products—milk, yogurt, cheese—you should have two to three servings a day. And from the meats group, which also includes dry beans, nuts, eggs, and fish, you should be eating two to three servings. Finally, at the top of the pyramid are the fats, oils, and sweets. These

Essential Utensils

One of the great conundrums of life is the question "What is a serving?"

To answer this question (and help you keep track of what you're eating), Pat Harper, R.D., a nutrition consultant in the Pittsburgh area, suggests that there are three items that no man's kitchen should be without: a lightbulb, a deck of cards, and a tennis ball.

Let's start with what constitutes a serving.

One-half cup of cooked cereal, rice, or pasta is a serving. One-half cup of chopped fruit or vegetables is a serving. And 2 to 3 ounces of cooked lean meat, fish, or poultry is a serving.

Okay, you say, but what does half a cup—or a full cup, for that matter—look like? And how much is 3 ounces?

"A tennis ball is about a cup," says Harper. "And a 3-ounce portion is the size of a deck of cards."

What about the lightbulb? And is that a standard 75-watter?

"A lightbulb is the size of a serving of broccoli," Harper says. "And yes."

There are other ways to gauge how much you're eating. Something the size of the palm of your hand, for example, is about 4 ounces.

"Picture in your mind the amount you get in a cafeteria—that's usually a standard serving," Harper says.

"But the important message here is not that that's all you're allowed to eat," she adds. "That's just how you can tally what you eat compared to what's considered the standard portion. If you are eating a lot of servings and having trouble with your weight, that might be a clue to the problem."

don't count as a group, for the simple reason that you should be eating as little of them as possible.

EAT LESS MEAT. One huge way to cut back on the amount of fat in your diet (and therefore the amount of fat that ends up on your stomach) is to eat less of the cow and more of what the cow eats.

"We're one of the few countries in the world that eats so much animal protein," says Dr. Lawrence. And there's a strong correlation between eating a lot of meat and being beefy.

"The more meat you eat, the higher the chance of gaining weight and of gaining abdominal obesity," says Henry Kahn, M.D., an internist and asso-

How to Eat a Pyramid

According to the government's Food Guide Pyramid, you're supposed to eat between 15 and 26 servings of milk, meat, fruits, vegetables, and grains every day.

How on Earth do you do that? It sounds as though you would need to have your face in a permanent feed bag.

It's not as tough as it looks. What counts as a serving is actually pretty small. If you're an average-size guy eating average-size meals, you're already eating several servings at a sitting. Multiply that by two, three, or four—or however many times you eat each day—and you're probably already in the ballpark.

So let's say you are that average-size guy, and let's say you want to stay that average size. Here's what your day might look like if you worked your way through the pyramid—with a few extra add-ons for flavor.

Breakfast

1 cup of oatmeal = 2 servings from the grain group
1 cup of milk = 1 serving from the dairy group
2 teaspoons of brown sugar = sweets
1 orange = 1 serving from the fruit group
1 cup of coffee = 1 cup of coffee

Midmorning snack

1 bagel = 2 servings from the grain group
With 1 teaspoon of jam = more sweets

Lunch

A roast beef sandwich made with 3 ounces of meat = 1 serving of meat and 2 servings of grain (each slice of bread—whole grain, hopefully—counts as a serving)
½ cup of carrots = 1 serving from the vegetable group
¾ cup of cranberry juice cocktail = 1 serving from the fruit group
1 medium apple = 1 serving from the fruit group

Afternoon snack

1 granola bar = 1 serving from the grain group (plus the fat equivalent of ½ pat of butter)

Dinner

1½ cups of garden salad, made with leafy green lettuce, green peppers, and tomatoes = 2 servings from the vegetable group
With 1 ounce of blue cheese = 1 serving from the dairy group
1 chicken breast = 1 serving from the meat group
1 cup of broccoli = 2 servings from the vegetable group
1 cup of brown rice = 2 servings from the grain group

Total servings for the day:

From the grain group: 9
From the fruit group: 3
From the vegetable group: 5
From the dairy group: 2
From the meat group: 2

---

ciate professor of family and preventive medicine at Emory University School of Medicine in Atlanta.

For that reason, "you should eat less fats and meats," says Dr. Lawrence. "Fats, because you just don't need the calories and they're low, generally, in nutrients; and the proteins, because we don't need that much."

EAT MORE GRAINS. Most of the calories in your diet should come not from meats but from grains (and grain products like whole-wheat bread) as well as from fruits and vegetables. Grains include wheat, rice, oats, corn, and barley. (Just because it's made from grain, however, doesn't make it good; you should go for the whole grains here, not the "air bread.")

Besides providing you with a lot of essential nutrients, grains (and other plant foods) are your source for fiber. Fiber keeps your digestive system working properly and lowers the risk for heart disease and some cancers.

In a six-year study of 43,757 men ages 40 to 75, researchers found that those most likely to have heart attacks were the ones least likely to eat a good amount of fiber (particularly cereal fiber) on a regular basis.

EAT FROM THE GARDEN. Vegetables—whether fresh, frozen, or canned—are loaded with fiber, vitamins, minerals, and "hundreds of compounds that, when teased out in the laboratory, may have a variety of health-promoting qualities," says Dr. Lawrence. "If you eat a wide variety of fruits and vegetables, you're getting a wider variety of these compounds."

It's important to eat all kinds of vegetables, not just peas and potatoes. As a rule, fresh is better than cooked (because vitamins are lost in cooking), and frozen is generally better than canned (because manufacturers tend to add a lot of salt to canned vegetables).

The more vegetables you eat, says Dr. Kahn, the less likely you are to gain girth. In fact, he advises that you eat even more vegetables than recommended by the pyramid: "Eat a wide variety of vegetables, at least five vegetables a day, prepared without the addition of saturated fat," he says.

EAT MORE BEANS. We eat far too much meat and far too few beans, and that's too bad. Because in addition to being high in protein and high in fiber, beans are low in fat.

Which means that beans can make a real contribution to your belly-banishing campaign. Substitute a bean dish for your meat dish a couple times a week, and you'll be lopping a lot of fat out of your diet and replacing it with a lot of fiber.

Not to harp on this, but that fiber will do wonders for your cholesterol and your digestive system. The American Heart Association recommends that we get 25 to 30 grams of fiber a day. And, as we've said before, most of us are only getting about half that amount.

EAT MORE FISH. We also eat a heck of a lot less fish than we ought to. Ideally, Dr. Lawrence says, we should be eating fish two or three times a week. In addition to being a good source of protein, fish contains omega-3 fatty acids, types of fat that seem to be good for the heart. A diet rich in fish can help lower cholesterol, prevent blood clots, and possibly lower blood pressure.

While all fish have some omega-3's, the ones with the most include salmon, mackerel, sardines, herring, and tuna.

Don't fry that fish, though. Deep-frying not only destroys the omega-3's but turns that turbot into a fat torpedo—one aimed directly at your gut.

Better Living through Chemistry

Just how does food work, anyway? If you think of food as fuel for your engine, you're not far wrong. But food is also, to wring the metaphor, the mechanic who tunes it.

Take, for example, your basic large baked potato. Shovel one down your maw, and you give your body 51 grams of carbohydrates, which are your body's principle source of energy. Like an oil refinery, your digestive system uses enzymes, acids, and salts to convert these crude carbohydrates into simple sugars to fuel your tank.

But then there's all the mechanical stuff. That tater also contains 4.7 grams of protein, an essential material for refurbishing and replacing worn-out cells; 2.2 grams of fiber, good for scrubbing out and keeping things moving in your digestive tract; and about 26 milligrams of vitamin C, which, among other things, helps build your bones, teeth, gums, ligaments, and blood vessels and helps your body resist infections and heal its wounds.

That spud also contains vitamin B_6, very little sodium (16 milligrams), a great deal of potassium (844 milligrams), magnesium, niacin, thiamin, iron, and folate, none of which are fuel but all of which are essential to keeping you up and running. The way each of these compounds works is too complex to go into here. Our point is simply that this is why you should eat a wide variety of foods: Your body needs all sorts of nutrients to function, and every food has different mixes of these essential nutrients. No one food contains them all.

THE BANISH PLAN

AND WE'LL HAVE FUN, FUN, FUN 'TIL OUR DIET TAKES THE T-BONE AWA-A-A-A-AY!

Actually, that last bit isn't true. There is no diet, and nobody's going to take that T-bone away. Because the *Banish Your Belly* Eating Theory is this: If you take the fun out of eating, you take a lot of fun out of living, and nobody except monastic types—those kneecaps-to-the-granite penitents—are going to stick to any program that takes the fun out of living.

"Many people are not willing to give up all their favorite foods, and you have to figure out some way to try to accommodate them," says Pat Harper, R.D., a nutrition consultant in the Pittsburgh area.

Hence, no diet. No diet because diets do not work. Why? Because sooner or later, the long-suffering dieter realizes that there is no good answer to the question, "What's the point?" What's the point, indeed, if your life has become one long series of deprivations?

The *Banish Your Belly* Eating Theory is not a theory at all, really. It's a simple, practical approach to the dining life. On one level it is as simple as the principle "moderation in all things."

Lest you think moderation is another name for denial, let us stress that, to the contrary, in the practice of moderation, you will find deeper pleasures. Have you been eating more and enjoying it less? If so, we'll show you how—by eating differently—you'll enjoy eating more.

Deny Yourself Nothing

The most important part of the *Banish Your Belly* Eating Theory is that nothing is denied you. You want a Double Whopper with cheese? Eat it. Enjoy it. You say that you want a fistful of Oreos? Eat them. Enjoy.

Indeed, if you make regular exercise a part of your life, you'll be able to eat moderate amounts of these sorts of things without gaining weight. (Though we're banking on the fact that most people, once they really get into exercising, start to lose some of their taste for all those fatty foods.)

At the same time, of course, you're going to be changing your eating habits, especially those that you might call your fat habits. These are the hundreds of unconscious behaviors that you have adopted over the years that put poundage on your gut: the automatic glop of butter on your baked potato, the nightly bag of chips in front of the TV, those afternoon visits to the vending machines.

We're going to show you how to become aware of all the occasions on which you inject yourself with excess calories that you don't even taste. And given that you don't even taste them, you're certainly not going to miss those calories when you cut them out of your life or replace them with healthier ones.

The Five Ws

By paying attention to the who, what, where, when, why, and how of your eating habits, you can take control of what's going down your gullet; and when you take control, you're on the way to banishing your belly.

Who are you dining with? Believe it or not, how much you eat at a sitting can vary tremendously, depending on whom you happen to be eating with. Researchers have noted that we tend to eat more food when we eat with friends than we do when we eat alone or with strangers. We also tend to eat bigger meals if our tablemates are big eaters.

We're not suggesting that you start making dinner dates with strangers, but we are suggesting that if a lot of your social life consists of eating large with your large friends, you may want to get together with them in some other venue.

What are you eating? Needless to say, this is the biggest (and most obvious) question of them all. As we said in the last chapter, what you eat has everything to do with how you feel and what you look like. We have already given you some indication of what you should eat and what you should shy away from. (Hint: The number one thing to avoid is the fatty stuff.)

Where are you eating it? If you're eating anywhere and everywhere—in the kitchen, your car, or the basement—you're turning these places into your table. You can make real progress here just by restricting your eating to the cafeteria at work or your dining room table, explains Joanne Curran-Celentano, R.D., Ph.D., associate professor of nutritional sciences at the University of New Hampshire in Durham and nutrition research coordinator at the Center for Eating Disorders Management in Dover, New Hampshire.

When are you eating? If you eat whenever the opportunity presents itself (and in our culture that's just about always), you will often be eating not because you are hungry but simply because food has made itself available: for example, those little ice cream get-togethers in the office coffee room. This is why it's a good idea to set up a fairly regular schedule for yourself and to avoid opportunistic eating.

Perhaps even more important than when you eat is the question of when you stop eating. One study showed that a lot of men tend to eat until there is nothing left in front of them, which may be long after the stomach has had enough.

Why are you eating? If you have read this far, you already know that we eat for all sorts of reasons

Stop! In the Name of Glut!

Who says men and women aren't different animals?

Kathleen D. Zylan, Ph.D., former assistant professor in the Department of Psychology at Lynchburg College in Virginia, conducted a survey to see whether men and women have different reasons for saying "enough" at the dinner table. Not surprisingly, she discovered something of a gender gap.

She and her students passed out a questionnaire in which the respondents were asked to complete the sentence, "I usually stop eating a meal when . . ."

There were multiple answers to choose from as well as a blank space to write in an answer of their own. Most people, male and female, answered "when I feel full" when that answer was on the questionnaire.

But there were two versions of the questionnaire. The second version did not include that answer.

When women filled out this second version, they were more inclined to say that they usually stop eating "when the food stops tasting good" or "when everyone else is finished" or "when I've had all I'm allowed."

When do the men stop eating?

"When the food is all gone."

that have nothing whatsoever to do with hunger: rage, sorrow, boredom, and angst, to name a few. You can head off many unnecessary calories simply by stopping to ask yourself, "Am I really hungry?" before you take a bite, says Dr. Curran-Celentano.

How are you eating? Are you paying any attention to what and how much you're eating when you eat? Or are you eating on automatic pilot? If you're on automatic pilot, you're probably eating more than you need to and enjoying it only about half as much as you should.

And while we're on that subject, are you in an eating rut? There's a whole world of amazingly delicious low-fat food out there, everything from pho (Vietnamese soup) to frozen yogurt. If your idea of haute cuisine is limited to slab-o'-cow on a plate, you really should expand your food horizons. Make an Indiana Jones of your palate and send him off on some of our low-fat food adventures. Put more flavors into your life.

MAN IN THE KITCHEN
THE POWER OF GOOD COOKING

"The attitude of a gentleman toward animals is this: Once having seen them alive, he cannot bear to see them die, and once having heard their cry, he cannot bear to eat their flesh. That is why the gentleman keeps his distance from the kitchen," wrote the Chinese philosopher Mencius.

For millennia, men have cooked up excuses not to do the cooking. But two dozen centuries after Mencius, most of those excuses have grown pretty old. Now, a lot of us not only carve the occasional bird but stuff and truss it as well. And we whip up the gravy, sauce the cranberries, and convert actual pumpkins into pie.

In fact, many men have discovered that they can get their kicks in the kitchen. Cooking turns out to be a lot like fooling around with your kiddy chemistry set, but better. Because when you finish an experiment, you get to eat it. (And if it's a total bomb, you get to go out to dinner.)

When you take charge in the kitchen, you take control of what you eat. And by taking control of what ends up on your plate, says Colleen Pierre, R.D., a nutrition consultant in Baltimore, you put yourself in a stronger position to whittle down your gut and keep it there.

In the battle of the bulge, the kitchen is your battlefield and you are its commander. Remember the words of Sun-tzu, the great Chinese philosopher of war: "Because the able commander plans and calculates like a hungry man, he is invincible in battle and unconquerable in the attack."

The Lean Larder

It's up to you, the hungry man, to plan and calculate in order not to fall before the fatty foe. That stick of butter, the tub of sour cream, those hot dogs and cheese and peanut butter in your icebox and pantry—those are the arms of the enemy. Your larder should be your arsenal, not his. When you stock it lean, you're going to be cooking from a position of strength.

You want ingredients that are lean, versatile, and easy to use. Apart from that, the actual contents are entirely up to you. A man's pantry is a personal thing. You, for example, may feel that no kitchen is complete without a bottle of barbecue sauce, and no cupboard should lack graham crackers. That's cool. This list is not meant to exclude them. This is just a basic list of staples that, if you have them, can be used to produce all sorts of easy, healthful, low-fat meals and snacks. The point, really, is that when you provision yourself, you should go as low-fat, whole-grain, low-sodium, and high-fiber as you can.

Perhaps our point would be better made if we were to make a list of what your pantry is better off without: lard and marshmallow cookies, for example. Or frozen fish sticks.

On the other hand, we also include some things on our list that aren't necessarily good for you. Sugar, for example. Sure, it doesn't offer much in the way of nutrition, but you'll need it for some recipes that are nutritious. Or maybe you just need a spoonful to make those Breakfast Bran Buds go down. Either way, you don't have to give up sugar—or butter, mayonnaise, or other less-than-healthful foods—as long as you use them sparingly.

You can use this list to stock your pantry lean, to restock, and to fill in some gaps. But down the road, you're going to add to it when you buy those extra things that you'll need for various recipes. If you're planning to make pumpkin pie, for example, you'll need ginger and cloves in addition to cinnamon (not to mention pumpkins).

While we're on the topic of planning, that's a good way to build up your stores. Before you go to the supermarket, spend a few minutes thinking about what recipes you might be whipping up in the next week. Then build your shopping list around those recipes.

That said, your lean larder should contain the following, according to Pierre.

- Beans, canned or dried
- Bread, whole-grain
- Chicken breast, boneless
- Chicken broth, nonfat
- Eggs
- Fish, fresh or canned
- Flour, whole-wheat and white
- Fruits and vegetables, fresh
- Garlic, fresh or paste
- Honey and molasses
- Jam, all-fruit
- Ketchup and mustard
- Mayonnaise, low-fat
- Milk, 1 percent or skim
- No-stick spray
- Olive and canola oils
- Onions
- Parmesan cheese
- Pasta, dried or fresh
- Potatoes and yams
- Pretzels or other low-fat snacks
- Rice, white and brown
- Salsa
- Soups, canned or dried
- Sour cream, nonfat
- Soy sauce, reduced-sodium
- Spices (including blends)
- Steak sauce
- Sugar, white and brown
- Tomatoes, canned (either puree or paste)

- Vegetables, canned or frozen
- Vinegar
- Whole-grain crackers, low-fat
- Wine for cooking
- Worcestershire sauce
- Yogurt, low-fat or nonfat

Gearing Up

Once you have your larder stocked, it's time to buy some tools. Good kitchen tools aren't cheap, but it's better to spend a little more and have it for life than to buy cheap gear that you'll throw out a year later. Besides, choosing the right equipment can go a long way toward keeping fat out of your diet.

No-stick cookware. You can cut a lot of fat out of your diet just by acquiring a couple no-stick skillets with tight-fitting lids. Not only will they allow you to cook with little or no added fat but they're also easy to clean. What's better than that?

This is definitely not the time to go cheap. Cooking with good equipment is a pleasure; cooking with cheap junk is not. A well-made skillet, for example, will distribute the heat evenly and cook food better than a cheap one. If you don't believe it, try this: Buy a really nice professional-quality skillet and a really cheap aluminum pan. A month later, see which pan you always seem to reach for.

Stirring spoons. You'll use these nearly every time you cook. Just be sure to buy wooden or plastic rather than metal, which will scrape the surface of no-stick pans.

Blender or food processor. While it's not essential to have these high-power kitchen tools, they're incredibly handy for making your own low-fat soups, salad dressings, milk shakes, and such.

Wok. No man should be without one of these babies. If you could have only one pan in your kitchen, you might make it a wok because you can cook just about anything in one. Also, because of the high heats used in wok cookery, you only need to use tiny amounts of oil.

Broiling pan. This is essential for keeping your meats from swimming in a lake of liquid fat. All it is is a pan with a rack on top that allows fat to drain away during broiling or roasting.

Gravy separator. This gadget "looks like a measuring cup with a spout on it, but the spout is attached at the very bottom of the cup," says Pierre.

The New Fat

We know. It sounds like something you would find on the fabric label of a pair of edible underwear. But sucrose polyester is actually the technical name for olestra, a fake fat designed by Procter & Gamble to let you inhale potato chips without remorse.

The sucrose polyester molecule, which has a similar "mouth-feel" to fat, is undigestible, meaning it passes right through you without adding any padding to your pillow.

Unfortunately, this new "designer" fat isn't without problems. Some people using it have experienced digestive complaints, like cramps, bloating, and loose stools. In addition, as the fat moves through the small intestine, it may remove a variety of fat-soluble vitamins from the body. That's why the Food and Drug Administration ordered the company to add vitamins A, D, E, and K to products containing olestra.

The point of this isn't to slam a particular product. It's simply that, when you're trying to lose weight, it's not such a great idea to wait for science to come to the rescue. If you're waiting for a fat substitute as a substitute for willpower, you're just going to grow older and fatter while you wait.

Even if science eventually does find a perfect fake fat, we already know that it's mighty unlikely to help most of us lose much weight. Just look at how many Americans have already failed to lose weight because they eat mass quantities of "low-fat" foods.

Ah well, there are always plastic foam packing peanuts . . .

"You pour the liquid into this cup, and the fat rises to the top. Since it pours from the bottom, it allows you to pour the juices back into the pot, and the fat stays in the cup. It's the best."

Steamer. This is a great thing to have around for steaming fish and vegetables—and steaming is one of the best ways to cook these foods because the moist heat requires no added fat. In addition, steaming causes food to lose fewer nutrients than boiling does.

There are several types of steamers. The least expensive is the collapsible-basket type, which simply drops into any saucepan or skillet. Or you can get a freestanding metal or bamboo steamer, which typically has two or more levels for cooking a variety of foods at once.

Sharp knives. One of the great pleasures of cooking is having knives that simply slip through the food; one of the great pains is having a knife you have to saw with. Besides, you need them sharp to be able to trim that fat off your London broil.

You need at least three knives: a heavy-duty chef's knife (an 8-inch knife is ideal) for chopping vegetables, a good-size serrated knife for cutting meat, and a smaller paring knife for, well, paring.

Microwave oven. The microwave may be usurping the place of the dog as modern man's best friend. It's a great way to get cooking done fast without cooking badly. You can, for example, bake a potato in 8 minutes without adding a drop of fat or losing a vitamin.

Salad spinner. This is one of those gadgets that takes the drudgery out of washing lettuce or spinach for a salad. Simply rinse the greens, toss them in, and give them a spin. They come out ready to eat. Just be sure that when you go to buy it, you ask for a "salad spinner." Don't do like a friend of ours, who baffled many a salesclerk by asking for a "lettuce centrifuge."

Winning Strategies

Once you're properly provisioned, it's time to do battle. What are the cooking strategies of the general in the kitchen?

The ultimate goal is to cook lean so that you can eat lean, while filling your life with so much good flavor that you may never leave the kitchen again. Here are more than 30 strategies for cutting the fat (but not the taste) from your cooking.

USE NO (OR LITTLE) OIL OR BUTTER. That's the purpose of no-stick pans and no-stick spray: You can cook just about anything using little added fat. When frying an egg, for example, spritzing the pan with no-stick spray instead of using a pat of butter will save about 100 calories and 11 grams of fat. Or you can simply put a drop of oil in the pan and wipe it around with a paper towel.

FORGET ABOUT FRYING. No other cooking method will dump as much fat into your diet as frying will. Steam, bake, poach, broil, or boil it—or sauté it in a little oil—but don't fry it.

When cooking fish, for example, put away the skillet and put the fish in the oven, basting it with a bit of lemon or orange juice. Or poach it in a pan half filled with water and sprinkled with crab boil or any other blend of spices that appeals to you.

(There are some nice Cajun blends that can really jazz up your mackerel.)

HOLD THE MAYO. Unless it's low-fat, that is. And be aware of how much mayo is mixed in with sandwiches such as the lean-lunch staple, a good old tuna sandwich.

"Most people would think that's good for dieters," says Bonnie Liebman, a licensed nutritionist and director of nutrition for the Center for Science in the Public Interest in Washington, D.C. "But the smallest restaurant tuna sandwich we analyzed had 720 calories and 43 grams of fat."

Why? Restaurants and delis mix in so much mayonnaise that they turn tuna into a fat stealth bomb. So make that tuna salad with just a touch of low-fat mayonnaise or salad dressing, and don't put any mayonnaise on the bread.

SAUTÉ WITH FLUIDS. The traditional sauté, done with oil or butter, will transform the healthiest food into a high-fat (or at least higher-fat) meal. A good alternative is to sauté using broth or wine—or broth *and* wine. It will taste just as good, if not better, and you'll get a fraction of the fat.

MAKE AN EXCEPTION FOR VEGETABLES. When sautéing vegetables, you don't want to bury their distinctive natural flavors in broth or wine. Instead, use a low heat and add a little oil and water. The slower cooking time will cause the vegetables to release some of their natural juices, keeping the food from drying out.

ENJOY AN INSTANT STOCK. When you don't have broth ready-made for sautéing or anything else, you can make a quick stock by pouring boiling water over shiitake, porcini, or other dried mushrooms. Soak them for about 15 minutes, then strain out the mushrooms. It adds a hearty, meatlike flavor to sautés, stews, sauces, and pilafs.

PREPARE A VEGETABLE BROTH. This is one of the easiest ways to prepare a low-fat, flavorful cooking liquid. No slicing, dicing, or peeling required. Just toss onions, carrots, peppers, celery, and whatever other scraps you need to clean out of your vegetable drawer into a pot of water, Pierre suggests. Let it simmer until the vegetables are reduced to mush. Strain out the mush and—voilà—vegetable broth.

PUT COLD TO WORK. When you're making your own stocks and soups, particularly when using meat bones or scraps, it's a good idea to make them ahead of time, then put them in the refrigerator to chill overnight. This causes fat to rise and congeal on the surface, making it easy to skim off.

You can do this with canned broth, too. Just keep a couple cans in the refrigerator instead of the cupboard, and they'll be ready to skim whenever you're ready to use them.

MAKE LEAN SAUCES. Many traditional sauces call for large amounts of milk or cream as well as butter. It doesn't have to be that way. When making a white sauce, you can get the creamy texture without all the fat by replacing whole milk (or cream) with nonfat powdered milk, evaporated skim milk, or pureed mashed potatoes. For a red sauce, use pureed carrots or other vegetables as the fat substitute. You'll get the same nice texture, and you probably won't taste the difference.

BUY LEAN. When you're stocking up on beef, always look for the leanest cuts that you can find. One way to do this, of course, is simply to look for meats that appear to have the least fat. Or read the label: "Select" is the leanest grade cut, "choice" is a bit fattier, and "prime" will clog up your arteries before you can say "rib roast."

"Your best bet is to stick with round steak," Liebman says. "You'll get the least fat from eye of round, followed by top, bottom, and tip." A 4-ounce serving of select eye of round, for example, contains 5 grams of fat; a choice porterhouse steak contains 25.

GIVE IT A TRIM. Even the leanest cuts often require some trimming to remove excess fat. An easy way to do this is to put the meat in the freezer for 20 minutes. The fat will turn white, making it easier to see. Plus, the meat will firm up a bit, making it easier to trim.

GO EASY ON THE PORK. In spite of what the advertising suggests, pork is not an extremely lean meat. It has one-third more fat than skinless chicken and twice as much as skinless turkey. Still, the leanest cut of pork—pork tenderloin—is leaner than most popular cuts of beef.

PEEL YOUR POULTRY. You should skin your chicken or turkey before you eat it. That skin is loaded with fat, and you're better off without it. Don't peel poultry before cooking, however, since juices in the skin will help keep the bird moist.

GIVE THANKS EARLY AND OFTEN. If you only dine on turkey once a year in memory of the Pilgrims, you're missing out on one great food. Consider this: Mr. Turkey is less fatty than Mr.

Chicken. So why not eat more of the former and less of the latter?

DON'T GET SKINNED. Ground turkey can be a great substitute for ground beef—in burgers, meat loaf, and spaghetti sauce—but only if it's ground turkey breast *without* the skin. Ground turkey that is made with the skin can be 10 times as fatty as ground skinless breast meat, Liebman says.

USE STEALTH VEGETABLES. You can cut the fat in meat loaf and hamburgers by replacing some of the meat with shredded carrots, onions, and green peppers. No one's tongue, not even yours, will be the wiser.

MAKE A SLIM MARINADE. "Use a fat-free salad dressing for marinades," says Pierre. "In a marinade, what works as a tenderizer is the acid ingredient, so whether it's lemon or vinegar or wine, it's not the oil that you need. Fat-free Italian dressing is great for marinades. Five minutes for fish, 30 minutes for chicken, and an hour for meat."

MAKE THE MOST OF BEANS. It would be hard to think of a cheaper, easier way to reduce the fat in your diet than this. "Dry beans, peas, and lentils come with a recipe on the bag," Pierre says. "And lentils, in particular, don't require the soaking that beans do. You can make a pot of lentil soup in 20 to 25 minutes and have enough food to eat for the week or to freeze for other times. That's a real high-nutrition, low-cost food, but it can be very savory depending on how you season it."

STOCK UP ON RICE. To complement beans, buy some rice. "Long-grain rice in big bags is practically free, and, of course, it's relatively easy to cook, and the rice-bean combination gives you a nice complete protein," says Pierre.

Incidentally, you can get more fiber, vitamins, and minerals by using brown rice instead of white. Traditional brown rice is very slow cooking, but you can also get a 10-minute brown rice that makes cooking quick and easy.

SPICE UP YOUR LIFE. For a lot of guys, there are only three seasonings: butter, salt, and pepper. Don't cheat your taste buds (and expand your belly) by ignoring life's rich tapestry. There's a whole universe of spices out there that can make you forget about salt and butter. You don't have to spend a fortune in the spice aisle either. An economical way to add flavor to your foods is to buy a few spice blends.

To keep things simple, you may want to start off with just four blends: one each for meat, chicken, fish, and vegetables. Then you can slowly start adding individual spices as you need them.

TRY FRESH HERBS. While dried herbs have the advantage of always being there when you need them, they can't match the clean, bright taste of fresh. Simply adding a few shavings of fresh ginger to your next stir-fry or whipping up a batch of pesto with fresh basil will add depth and clarity to your meals that you simply can't get with dried.

GET LEAN CHEESES. Just as a smart chef wouldn't think of using his best wine to make a turkey gravy, there's absolutely no reason to cook with full-fat cheeses. If your recipe calls for grated cheese, for example, use a light sprinkling of Parmesan or another low-fat cheese to replace the fatty, whole-milk kind. The reduction in fat can be dramatic. For example, for every cup of 1 percent cottage cheese you use instead of whole-milk ricotta, your lasagna will be 30 grams of fat lighter.

USE LOW-FAT MILK. Recipes made with skim or 1 percent milk are virtually indistinguishable from those made with whole milk. Again, the reductions in fat are significant. If your recipe calls for a cup of cream and you use a cup of evaporated skim milk instead, you'll eliminate 60 grams of fat.

The one drawback to using skim milk is that it doesn't thicken as readily as the full-fat kind. So when you're making a sauce, you may want to thicken it a bit by adding nonfat milk powder.

PUT YOGURT TO WORK. Rather than larding up your meals with sour cream or mayonnaise, use a little nonfat or low-fat plain yogurt. Substituting a cup of nonfat yogurt for a cup of sour cream will save you 40 grams of fat. If it just has to be sour cream, try one of the nonfat versions that are out there. You'll achieve virtually the same fat savings, and you'll be pleasantly surprised at how good they taste.

SEPARATE YOUR EGGS. Even though egg yolks aren't the cholesterol demons that people once thought they were, they're still fairly high in fat. Most recipes don't need them, in any event. To get the binding power of eggs without the fat, all you have to do is substitute two egg whites for every whole egg. Give the yolks to Rover. They're good for his coat.

MAKE USE OF APPLESAUCE. When you're showing off your kitchen prowess by baking up muffins or a cake, you can cut a lot of fat by replacing some of the oil, butter, or margarine in the recipe with an equal measure of applesauce.

BAKE WITH BANANAS. Here's another way to cut fat from your baking recipes: Replace some of the butter or oil with mashed bananas. They add moisture with just a hint of extra flavor.

SUBSTITUTE PUREED PRUNES. "The other thing that you can use is pureed prunes in chocolate stuff, like brownies," says Pierre. Use it in place of the oil, she says, and "it tastes pretty good. People never guess that there are prunes in there."

CHANGE THE CHOCOLATE. You can save a little more fat if you replace the baking chocolate with cocoa powder and vegetable oil. Substitute 3 tablespoons of cocoa powder and 2 teaspoons of vegetable oil for 1 ounce of unsweetened baking chocolate.

BULK UP YOUR FLOUR. There's no reason for desserts to be devoid of nutrients. An easy way to get more fiber and vitamins in the mix is to replace half the white flour with whole-wheat flour. The resulting recipe will be just a little heavier, but not so much that you'll really notice it. An exception might be if you're making something airy and light, like angel food cake. In that case, you'll want to stick with the straight white flour.

MAKE LIKE A VIRGIN. There are dozens of olive oils, and knowing which one to buy can be a challenge. A rule of thumb is to buy a cheaper oil for cooking, since high heats will dispel much of the flavor. But when you want an oil to drizzle on your salad, spend a little extra to get extra-virgin oil. The taste is deeper and richer, which means that you can use less oil to get the same flavor.

CHECK YOUR OIL. There's no law that says you have to dump a lot of oil into salads. The next time you're tossing the greens, splash on a little balsamic vinegar. You may decide that you don't need the oil at all.

Incidentally, there are any number of great vinegars out there, including those that are infused with herbs and spices. Try using one of these when making your next oil-and-vinegar salad dressing—and cut back a bit on the oil. You may find that you prefer the lighter taste.

MAKE YOUR PIZZA LEAN. When making homemade pizza, use a thick whole-wheat flour crust, top it with tomato sauce and part-skim rather than whole-milk mozzarella, and add lots of onions, peppers, mushrooms, and other vegetables. (Try adding spinach.)

MAKE HEALTH EASY. One very elemental way in which you can reduce fat by replacing it with something else is to get into the habit of placing a couple of dishes of fresh fruits and vegetables in front of you (and your family) at every meal. Slice up a cantaloupe into bite-size cubes, add some apple slices and some baby carrots, celery sticks, and broccoli florets, and put them in the center of your dinner table. The variety of fruits and vegetables that you might do this with is limited only by your imagination. You'll be surprised at how these finger foods disappear. They will be eaten just because they are there. And for every bite of fresh fruit and vegetable that you eat, there's that much less room for what you're trying to avoid.

Great Books

There's no end to the cookbooks out there, but as anyone who is at all serious about cooking will tell you, a lot of them are not so hot. What you want are a few good cookbooks containing recipes that are both healthful and tasty. Here are five of the best, both from your belly's and your palate's point of view.

- **Joy of Cooking** by Irma S. Rombauer and Marion Rombauer Becker. If you can have only one cookbook in your kitchen, this is the one to have. It is the classic cookbook, an encyclopedic tome of great recipes and cooking techniques. It's not a book of low-fat recipes, though, so there will be times that you'll want to modify the recipes accordingly.
- **Jane Brody's Good Food Book**, by Jane E. Brody. One of the best cookbooks ever, loaded with healthful, low-fat, and delicious recipes.
- **Moosewood Cookbook**, by Mollie Katzen. Vegetarian recipes that—gasp!—actually taste like real food.
- **Jacques Pépin's Simple and Healthy Cooking** by Jacques Pépin. Gourmet food that is good for you, too.
- **Prevention's The Healthy Cook** by the food editors of **Prevention** Magazine Health Books. This book explains all the principles of healthy cooking and contains hundreds of recipes for making low-fat, high-flavor food.

How to Play the Calorie Game

Keeping the Numbers Down

Yeah, yeah, we know. The last thing on Earth you want to do—well, maybe after changing the darn cat litter—is to spend one minute of your precious time counting calories.

So before you hurl this book across the room, let us assure you: You won't have to. Uh, well, maybe you'll have to a little bit just at the beginning, but no, you will definitely *not* have to spend the rest of your life keeping track of the little buggers.

With the help of our experts, we'll show you a way to keep your calories under control without obsessing about them.

The important thing here is the big picture: Your goal is simply to take in fewer calories a day than you burn. And then, once you've slimmed down, to achieve what researchers call energy balance—that is, to keep your svelte form simply by keeping your daily calorie intake equal to your daily expenditure.

"Why should I watch calories?" you ask. "Can't I just eat low-fat foods?"

Nyet.

"People will say, 'I'm going to eat that food because it's a low-fat food,' because the assumption is that it should have fewer calories," says Charles T. Kuntzleman, Ed.D., adjunct associate professor of kinesiology and director of the Blue Cross/Blue Shield Fitness for Youth program at the University of Michigan in Ann Arbor. "And it should have fewer calories. But because of what we do with food to make it tasty so that people will buy it, we put certain things in it, and so the fat may be low but the calories are the same. So it's dangerous to just stay on the fat side of the equation."

One of the most common additives is sugar, and manufacturers often add enough sugar to bring the calorie count of a low-fat food to the same level as one high in fat.

How Many Do You Need?

"If you want to lose weight, calories out need to exceed calories in," says John B. Allred, Ph.D., professor of nutrition in the Department of Food Science and Technology at Ohio State University in Columbus and co-author of *Taking the Fear Out of Eating: A Nutritionists' Guide to Sensible Food Choices.*

So the first thing that you need to do is figure out how many calories you really need every day. Here's a formula dietitians use.

Multiply your weight by 10. Let's say you weigh 172 pounds. So, times 10, that would be 1,720. Now, honestly determine your level of activity. Are you a 3 (totally sedentary), a 5 (moderately active), or a 7 (very active)?

Take your number and multiply by 100. Let's say that you're a 3, so that's 300. Finally, add the 300 and 1,720, and your total calories per day should be no more than 2,020.

Obviously, everyone has a different metabolism, so this is just a rough guide. The real measure is what happens to your weight. If you find it creeping upward, you may want to try a more hands-on approach.

Keep a food diary for about a week to get a handle on how many calories you're actually taking in, recommends Dr. Allred. In the diary you'll note what you eat each day, and what the calorie content of each item is.

- **Write down everything.** Many of us grossly underestimate the numbers of calories that cross our lips in a day, researchers say. If you're going to get a real picture of where you're at, you need to include every stray chip.
- **Calculate the calories.** Most foods these days have labels that list the number of calories per serving. Or you can pick up a calorie guide at the supermarket or in a bookstore.
- **Figure your daily average.** After keeping your diary for a week, figure out what your average daily caloric intake is.
- **Reduce your daily intake by 500 calories.** "If you reduce it by 500 per day, what you should see is very effective weight loss," Dr. Allred says. "If you don't, then you have underestimated your normal caloric intake or the amount of calories you need to cut back on."
- **Don't weigh too often.** If you do lose a few pounds in the first week or two, you have found your benchmark. Don't, however, expect to continue losing weight as fast as you do in the beginning. Your weight loss will level off and be slow and steady.

Keeping Lean for the Long Run

If calorie counting isn't your game, Dr. Kuntzleman offers an even simpler approach.

"I tell people, 'Just tell me how many pounds you've gained in the last year.' If the person says 5 pounds, I know that person is out of calorie balance by 50 calories a day. If they tell me it's 10

Checking Your Burn Rate

Remember how, in our first chapter, we compared the calories that you might burn in a day with the number that your Stone Age grandfather might burn?

Now let's look at the other side of the equation: Who do you suppose is taking in the most?

Grandpa's breakfast was most likely a fairly lean beast (wild game is leaner than the meats we eat today) like wild boar, which he ate in great hunks accompanied by a root or two and a handful of nuts or berries.

So if Grandpa stuffed his gut, say, with 6 pounds of boar meat, (4,352 calories), a couple of sweet potatoes (234 calories), a fistful of blueberries (40 calories), and another of filberts (352 calories), he would have eaten just about enough to make up for the 5,199 calories he burned that day.

You, on the other hand, are burning less than half as many calories, but, we suspect, taking in even more. Let's take a look.

1 Egg McMuffin: 290 calories
½ pound spareribs: 899 calories
1 candy bar: 700 calories
1 small pepperoni pizza: 637 calories
½ of a 1-pound bag of tortilla chips: 1,200 calories
3 beers: 438 calories

Your total intake for the day is 4,164 calories, twice as much as you need.

If you keep eating like this, you'll start looking less and less like your grandpa and more and more like something your grandpa would hunt. Which is why, if you want to shed that belly, it's a good idea to start paying some attention to calories, says Charles T. Kuntzleman, Ed.D., adjunct associate professor of kinesiology and director of the Blue Cross/Blue Shield Fitness for Youth program at the University of Michigan in Ann Arbor.

pounds, I know it's 100 calories a day. All you have to do is add a zero to the number of pounds."

This makes it easy, he says, to determine how much you need to reduce your calorie consumption or increase your calorie-burning activities.

Now, let's go back to that 500-calories-a-day deficit you're striving for. Does this mean you have to painstakingly count every calorie for the rest of your life? No. It may be as simple as eliminating your daily candy bar.

How to Get Fat Out of Your Diet

Or: You Wear What You Eat

We're about to tell you something that should make you very happy: You can go a long way toward banishing that belly without counting calories. (Not that you can ignore or forget about them entirely.) And you can do this by taking some fairly simple steps to avoid some of the fat bombs that we drop on our bellies every day.

Consider the 500-calorie Butterfinger candy bar. If you have been in the habit, say, of popping one of these out of the vending machine every day as a midafternoon pick-me-up, you could knock those 500 calories (and 20 grams of fat) out of your daily diet (and still get energized) just by taking a brisk walk around the building instead.

Do you automatically drop a dollop of butter on your baked potato? You could cut nearly 8 grams of fat and 68 calories out of your diet (and turn your potato into a towering inferno of taste) just by using a dash of Tabasco sauce instead.

What we're talking about here is changing your fat habits. That's right. Instead of focusing on the micro—counting calories or even fat grams—you can whittle that belly by focusing on the macro—which is to say, proteins, carbohydrates, and fats. You already know that your body handles them differently and is much more efficient at storing the calories you get from fat than those from protein or carbohydrates.

You also know that every gram of fat that you consume contains approximately 9 calories, as opposed to the 4 calories contained in each gram of protein or carbohydrate.

As Margery Lawrence, R.D., Ph.D., associate professor in the Department of Nutrition and Family Studies at St. Joseph College in West Hartford, Connecticut, points out, a substantial portion of the fat on your belly originally came from fat calories.

To put it bluntly, reducing the amount of fat you put in your belly can really reduce the amount of fat you put on it.

More Is Less

There's another good reason to focus on fat rather than calories, says Pat Harper, R.D., a nutrition consultant in the Pittsburgh area. Foods that are high in fat are usually high in calories. Which means that you can consume a heck of a lot of calories and still feel as though you have hardly eaten a thing. Not a good scenario for losing weight.

"I went out to lunch with a friend not too long ago, and she decided to skip the meal and just have the dessert," Harper says. "It was fried ice cream. I had the full meal, the chicken, the rice, the vegetable, the salad, the whole thing, and I actually ate fewer calories than she did."

Figure Out Your Fat Limit

There's nothing bad about fat, per se. You need fat to live; you just need a lot less of it than you're probably eating.

The U.S. Departments of Agriculture and Health and Human Services recommend that you get no more than 30 percent of your daily calories from fat. You may want to aim even a little lower. That way, given the way fat can creep across your lips, you can still get your daily intake down to the level they recommend.

Suppose that you're an average, 172-pound, totally sedentary guy whose daily calorie intake should be no more than 2,020. Since no more than 30 percent of those calories should come from fat, we'll just divide 2,020 by 30 to find out how many fat grams you can have every day. Answer: about 67.

Imagine, then, what happens when you order up a Double Whopper with cheese.

Twe-e-e-e BOOM! You bombard your belly with 63 grams (more than 12 teaspoonsful) of fat. Add to that a chocolate shake and an order of fries, and you're over your daily limit by nearly 23 grams. And this is just one meal.

Here's another point. That 67-gram fat limit is how much you want to take in just to maintain your weight. If you want to lose some, you have to reduce that number.

So, for example, if you want to get down to 165 pounds, your daily quota of calories and fat grams should be 1,950 and 65, respectively. In other words, if you can just shave a few grams of fat off your daily diet, you can shave them off your belly as well.

Pick Your Battles

Fat is in just about everything you eat. Even an apple, innocent as it looks, hides inside itself about half a gram of fat. So do you become paranoid? Obsessive? Start counting every gram you eat?

Not at all. Like we said before, you can lop off gobs of fat just by changing fat-intensive habits: the daily Butterfinger bar, the dollop of butter on your potato, the Double Whopper with cheese.

"Cut the things that don't count, that aren't important to you," Harper says. "There might be things that you really, really, really enjoy. Maybe you don't have to cut those if you cut everything else. Some people have to have butter on their corn or on their potato. Other people say, 'I don't really need the butter

Cracking the Code

Pat Harper, R.D., is a human encyclopedia on the subject of what's good for you. But for all her expertise, there is one phenomenon that baffles her: the legions of men who turn each aisle of the supermarket into an Aisle of Lost Souls.

"I see men picking up the packages, and they stand there and they look and read and look. I mean, they spend forever staring at that label," says Harper, a nutrition consultant in the Pittsburgh area. "And I wonder: What are they looking at? What are they reading for so long? Are they making decisions or are they just staring at this, trying to figure it all out?"

Harper guesses the latter. Food labels contain a lot of valuable information, but, if you don't know what you're looking for, they can be confusing. Which is why she has created a simple trick for cracking the code.

"If you're trying to watch your weight, look for the word 'fat' on the label and look for 3 grams or less," Harper says. "That's your cutoff. It doesn't matter what it is. It could be candy bars; it could be bread; it could be anything. But if it's 3 grams or less, it is by federal definition a low-fat product."

"This doesn't mean that you have to eat only low-fat products," she adds. "But the more products that you choose that are 3 grams or less, the more likely it is you are eating a lower-fat diet."

on that, I can just put pepper on my potato, but I just can't possibly live without butter on my such and such.' So where you have to have it, use a little, but if you don't have to have it, don't. Cut it there."

In other words, don't become a zealot, or you'll just end up hating your life (and soon be back to your fat old ways). Instead, look for daily opportunities to shun fat—and substitute healthier habits for your fat ones.

The best general guideline we can give you is to be alert to how much butter, margarine, oil, meat, milk, eggs, cheese, and sweets you're eating and then do whatever you can to cut back on them.

GO EASY ON THE BURGERS. "The number one source of saturated fat in the male diet is ground beef," says Melinda Hemmelgarn, R.D., associate state nutrition specialist for the Department of Food Science and Human Nutrition Extension at the University of Missouri in Columbia. Eating less ground beef can have a big impact on your weight.

Milk: It Can Do a Body Bad

When British explorers James Grant and John Hanning Speke were searching for the source of the Nile, writes Alan Moorehead in his book, The White Nile, they stayed for a time with Rumanika, the King of Karagwe.

Rumanika, Moorehead says, "kept an extraordinary harem of wives who were so fat they could not stand upright, and instead grovelled like seals about the floors of their huts." The usual diet, he writes, was "an uninterrupted flow of milk that was sucked from a gourd through a straw."

Is this what comes of drinking milk?

If you're still guzzling it the way you did when you were a teenager—which is to say, by the gallon a day—the answer can be yes.

An 8-ounce glass of whole milk contains nearly 9 grams (close to 2 teaspoons) of fat. So if you're putting away a couple glasses a day (maybe one on your cereal in the morning and another with those cookies you're having at night), you're taking in nearly 18 grams of fat a day. (We should add that this is a conservative estimate, given that an 8-ounce glass is just 1 cup—not the big tumbler that you may be in the habit of drinking.)

The solution? Switch to skim. You get just under half a gram of fat per 8-ounce glass, and you still get all that good calcium and other stuff your body really needs.

Better yet, when you eat a burger, choose lean ground beef, says Hemmelgarn.

Here's another way to reduce the amount of fat that you get from burgers. After cooking, press them between a couple layers of paper towels, says Harper. "Any way and every way that you can get the fat out or reduce it, that's smart," she says.

SKIN THAT CHICKEN. Since about half the fat that you'll find on poultry is either in or directly under the skin, one of the most effective ways to cut back on fat is simply to peel the skin off before eating the meat. While you're at it, forgo the drumsticks; they contain 8 grams of fat per serving—as much as top loin steak. A serving of skinless chicken breast, by contrast, has about 3 grams of fat.

DON'T FRY ANYTHING. Speaking of chicken, the absolutely worst way to prepare it (or anything else, for that matter) is to fry it. Frying adds tons of fat to whatever you fry. While a 3-ounce serving of chicken breast contains 3 grams of fat, that same serving, fried, has more than 15. So roast, bake, or microwave that chicken, but don't fry it.

TRADE IN THE BUTTER. If you're in the habit of cooking a lot of things in butter or oil, you're in the habit of injecting a lot of unnecessary fat into your veins. Whenever possible, replace butter and oil with a light misting of no-stick spray. Or at least use olive oil or canola oil, which are high in monounsaturated fats. These are better for your heart than the fats found in butter, margarine, or shortening, says Harper.

CUT BACK ON CHEESE. Cheese has a reputation for being a healthful food, but, in fact, it tends to be heavy on the fat. One ounce of Cheddar, which is to say a piece about the size of the top joint of your thumb, contains more than 9 grams of fat. And how many of those bite-size nuggets did you say you Hoovered off the snack tray last night?

SWITCH TO FROZEN YOGURT. If you're an ice cream eater, you should know that a mere 4 ounces of the stuff (about five good bites) contains anywhere from 8 to 17 grams of fat. By contrast, low-fat yogurts contain 3 grams or less; some contain virtually no fat at all. They may not be ice cream, but you'll be surprised at how close they can come.

UNDRESS YOUR SALAD. Nothing like a salad when you're watching your weight . . . unless you happen to like your greens swimming in dressing. Just 2 tablespoons of oil and vinegar contain more than 15 grams of fat. Go instead for the low-fat and nonfat dressings. Or try having your salad with fresh black pepper and a dash of balsamic vinegar or seasoned wine vinegar.

EAT MORE BEANS. The bean is perhaps the most underutilized source of protein in the United States. If you eat more beans and less meat, you'll get all the protein that you need and a lot less fat. Best of all, there are all different kinds of beans, from pintos to limas, so you don't have to get bored.

KEEP YOUR TUNA WET. Here's an easy way to cut back on fat: Buy your canned tuna packed in water instead of oil. You will save more than 6 grams of fat on every 3-ounce serving. In the war against fat, every gram counts.

WATCH YOUR PASTA. Pastas vary in more than just shape. For example, you can shave off 1.5 grams of fat by substituting a cup of macaroni or spaghetti for the same amount of rich egg noodles. Which is, perhaps, why Sophia Loren once said, "Everything you see I owe to spaghetti."

How to Keep Food Out of Your Mouth
Put Your Mind Where Your Mouth Is

"Honey, I'm starving. How 'bout you and me do the deed?"

Maybe this will fly in your house. Probably—unless you finesse it better than this—not. But it's still among our tips for keeping food out of your mouth.

Why? Because this approach to the problem is one of several in which our experts advise you to keep food out of your mouth by putting something else in it. Some of these tips will be more useful to you than others. True, if you ravish your mate on the kitchen table instead of ravishing that leftover pizza, you'll save yourself beaucoup calories. But how often can you do *that*? Certainly not every time you crave a cold slice of mushroom-and-pepperoni.

Which is why, rather than just giving you a list of things you might do instead of eating, we're going to give you an explanation of the principles underlying them. That way, you'll be able to come up with tips of your own. Because, after all, you need tips that are going to work for you, not for the sex-crazed newlyweds next door. (P.S. If you're the sex-crazed newlywed next door, see above.)

Pick a Personal Strategy

Okay, so you're suddenly struck by a craving. How do you deal with it?

"One approach would be to distract yourself," says Kelly Brownell, Ph.D., co-director of the Yale University Eating and Weight Disorders Clinic. "Another would be to engage in some activity incompatible with eating. Another would be to do something else rewarding. Another would be to resolve whatever's causing you stress."

There are many techniques that you can try, but they all boil down to essentially three approaches: diversion, confrontation, and moderation. Here's how they work.

Diversion

You can ride out your craving for food by turning your attention to something else, says Joanne Curran-Celentano, R.D., Ph.D., associate professor of nutritional sciences at the University of New Hampshire in Durham and nutrition research coordinator at the Center for Eating Disorders Management in Dover, New Hampshire. One of the best ways to do this is by doing something else that precludes eating. Have sex. Shoot some hoops in the driveway. Take a bath. Walk the dog. Go to a movie. Ride a bike. Paint a picture. Visit the driving range. Or, if you're at the office, get out and take a quick walk around the block. You get the idea.

Obviously, some of these things will take more time than you have to spend. So here are three quick—but effective—techniques for keeping your mind off the refrigerator.

DRINK A LOT OF WATER. We humans, imperfect as we are, often mistake thirst for hunger. Instead of drinking some nice, clear, calorie-free water when we're feeling thirsty, we stuff our mouths with calorie-packed snacks.

The next time you feel a hankering for something, try drinking a big glass of water first, says Judy E. Marshel, R.D., founder and director of Health Resources, a Long Island–based consulting and nutrition counseling company. You may find that's all you really needed.

"You know how people just grab?" asks Marshel. "They're so hungry that they just grab at anything that's available? If they satisfy their thirst a little, they settle down and don't grab as quickly or as much."

CHEW SOME GUM. Sometimes you can keep your mouth happy just by keeping it occupied, says Michele Trankina, Ph.D., professor of biological sciences at St. Mary's University and adjunct associate professor of physiology at the University of Texas Health Science Center, both in San Antonio.

In other words, just chew some gum. While you're at it, it's probably better to opt for the sugarless kind—not because of any calories you'll get from the sugar, but because it's better for your teeth.

BRUSH YOUR TEETH. A lot of people find that if they brush their teeth, that feeling of having a clean mouth stifles their desire to put something in it. Sort of like after you clean your house, you don't want the kids messing it up.

Confrontation

Another way to conquer food cravings is to look them in the eye and stand up to them, says Dr. Curran-Celentano. Imagine, for example, that there's a doughnut on the kitchen counter, and you can't stop thinking about it. Take control. Tell that doughnut, "Go away! I don't need you!"

If this is too confrontational for you, you can always succumb but in moderation (the third approach).

Moderation

"This is a pretty good approach," says Dr. Brownell, "because when people are watching what they eat, they tend to go into this restriction mode where they deny themselves food altogether, and that, of course, just sets up a great desire for the food. If you can eat what you're craving but just do so in small amounts, then you'll be better off."

Suppose you're in the habit of inhaling whole packages of cookies. Don't forbid yourself cookies. Instead, train yourself to eat just two and eat them very slowly. You will find that you enjoy them more that way, and you'll feel good about yourself at the same time.

Another trick to try when employing the less-is-more strategy is to use smaller utensils. If, for example, you go out and buy low-fat ice cream, and then come home and shovel about six servings into a big bowl and eat it, you're defeating the whole purpose of buying low-fat in the first place.

"One way to control that is to use a much smaller bowl," says Pat Harper, R.D., a nutrition consultant in the Pittsburgh area.

Preemptive Strikes

Of course, when it comes to keeping food out of your mouth, it doesn't hurt to plan ahead. Here are a couple of strategies for keeping it from getting in your face in the first place.

DON'T BUY IT. If you buy it, you will eat it. That is one of the great truths about human behavior. Which is why Harper suggests this rule: If you don't want to eat it all, don't buy it.

"If you do buy it and it's convenient, you're probably going to eat it," Harper says. "If you buy a dozen doughnuts, you're probably going to eat a dozen doughnuts. But you can control your destiny. If, instead, you buy one doughnut, you'll eat just one doughnut, because you're probably not going to go out at 10 o'clock at night in the pouring rain to buy more doughnuts. Certainly, you'd think twice."

Remember this principle when you do your shopping, Harper says. Instead of buying the 1-pound bag of chips, which you know full well you will sit down and eat, buy your chips in the small lunch-size bags, "even if it costs a couple cents extra," because you'll be less inclined to tear open several small bags of them.

EAT IT ONLY WHEN YOU GO OUT. Some people find it difficult to control themselves even when their food of choice is neatly contained in tiny bags. In that case, you may decide never to let it pass your door again.

"You can eat it when you go out but not at home," Harper says. "This way, you can control your environment so that you can achieve your goal."

THE 40 TOP FOODS
GRUB TO PUMP YOU UP

We asked experts on human nutrition to tell us the 40 best all-around foods you can eat, those "what gots the most juice" when it comes to things like vitamins and minerals.

But the experts balked. The first commandment of nutrition, they said, is "Thou shalt eat a wide variety of foods." In their view, it is a mistake to single out certain foods as being intrinsically better than others.

We tried putting the question another way: If you were stranded on a desert island, we inquired, and you could have only 40 foods, which ones would they be?

"You mean other than coffee and half-and-half?" responded Margery Lawrence, R.D., Ph.D., associate professor in the Department of Nutrition and Family Studies at St. Joseph College in West Hartford, Connecticut.

Still, it's clear that some foods—not counting "essentials" such as coffee—are a lot better than others. And at least one attempt has been made to quantify them. Nutritionists at the Center for Science in the Public Interest rated vegetables, fruits, beans, and grains by their vitamin, mineral, and fiber contents and came up with long lists of the best to the worst.

The nutritionists assigned each food a score based on what percentage of the Daily Value it supplied. They also gave points for fiber. So, for example, if a fruit supplies 100 percent of the Daily Value for vitamin A, it gets 100 points; if it also supplies 25 percent of the Daily Value for vitamin C, it gets another 25 points; and so on.

These are not only the most vitamin-, fiber-, and mineral-packed foods you can eat, by the way. They also happen to be great lean foods, says Bonnie Liebman, a licensed nutritionist and director of nutrition for the Center for Science in the Public Interest in Washington, D.C., where the study was conducted. Which is to say, if you eat more of these foods and fewer meat and dairy products, you will be eating a lot leaner.

"But not," Liebman adds, "if you were to cook those vegetables in butter. Or smother them with cheese. Or fry them."

But then, if you've read this far, you already know this.

The Top 10 Vegetables

There are no bad vegetables, but there are some that are pretty lame. Unfortunately, the lame ones tend to be the ones we Americans eat the most.

"Almost all of the top-selling vegetables in the country are garnishes for hamburgers," Liebman says.

Your average fast-food salad entombed in its plastic casket, for example, usually consists of a wad of iceberg lettuce, a couple slices of cucumber, a bloodless tomato, and maybe a dusting of carrot shavings. They aren't worthless, but you could do a lot better.

Fortunately, supermarkets stock plenty of options. Without further ado, here are the top 10 vegetables, in descending order from best to not-as-good.

- Collard greens (frozen)
- Spinach
- Kale
- Swiss chard
- Red peppers (½ pepper, fresh)
- Sweet potatoes (no skin)
- Pumpkin (canned)
- Carrots
- Broccoli
- Okra

Before we move on, let's just repeat that there are a whole heck of a lot of other vegetables out there, and if any one of them takes your fancy, by all means eat it. Don't worry about whether it is among the top 10. And don't worry if it's more nutritious raw than cooked. True, some nutrients are lost during cooking, but it's better to eat it cooked than not to eat it at all.

The Top 10 Fruits

Despite its reputation for having impressive medicinal powers, the apple, you may be surprised to learn, is nowhere near the top of the list. In fact, it doesn't even make the top 25. But again, this doesn't mean you should swear off apples. Even the modest McIntosh is a lot better for you than a candy bar.

At any rate, here are the 10 top fruits from Liebman's study.

- Papayas
- Cantaloupe
- Strawberries
- Oranges
- Tangerines
- Kiwifruit
- Mangoes
- Apricots
- Persimmons
- Watermelons

The Top 10 Beans

Full of fiber and protein and very low in fat, the bean, nonetheless, may be America's least-appreciated food. "It's a shame because they are so healthful," says Liebman. "I think the reasons people don't eat them are: Number one, they think of them as poor people's food; number two,

they're worried about gas; and number three, they don't know what to do with them." (They're not; don't worry about it; and check out a few ethnic cookbooks.) "You can eat them in very interesting ways," Liebman says.

Here are the top 10 beans.

- Soybeans
- Pinto beans
- Chick-peas
- Lentils
- Cranberry beans
- Black-eyed peas
- Pink beans
- Navy beans
- Black beans
- Small white beans

Incidentally, kidney beans, lima beans, and split peas are all really good for you, too.

The Top 10 Grains

Grains, you'll remember, are the base of the food pyramid we talked about in Nutrition Fundamentals on page 42. In other words, we are supposed to be eating more of them than anything else. Unfortunately, a lot of the grains we eat—such as in bland, billowy white bread—have had most of their nutrients processed right out of them. Anytime you can eat whole grains, you're better off.

Here are the 10 top grains.

- Quinoa
- Whole-wheat macaroni or spaghetti
- Amaranth
- Buckwheat groats
- Spinach spaghetti
- Bulgur wheat
- Pearled barley
- Wild rice
- Millet
- Brown rice

Quinoa and amaranth are grains that were originally consumed by pre-European Americans. Aztecs ate amaranth; Incas ate quinoa.

"I think of those as being similar to some exotic vegetables," Liebman says. "They're good for you, and you ought to try them, but don't think you have to go out of your way. I don't want to discourage people from eating plain old whole-wheat bread or oatmeal, the whole grains that are easy to obtain and that we know how to cook."

THE FACTS ABOUT FAST FOOD
IT'S WHAT YOU LEAVE OFF THAT COUNTS

Given that one out of three of us eats fast food on any given day, and since our number one, all-time favorite fast food is the almighty fatburger, it's really impossible to talk about weight loss without talking about food-on-the-run.

Approximately 22 percent of Americans, the truly hard-core, eat at convenience stores and fast-food restaurants an average of five or more times a week. Which explains why the signs in front of McDonald's restaurants have run out of room for zeros.

The problem, of course, is that fast food is usually fat food. When you make the decision to enter the drive-up lane, you know that you are not going to be pulling away with a lot of leafy green vegetables and wholesome grains. Can you eat fast food and still banish your belly? The answer is yes—but only if you take a few precautions.

A Question of Balance

"You can go to a fast-food restaurant nowadays and find something that will enable you to not go overboard on fat or calories," says Bonnie Liebman, a licensed nutritionist and director of nutrition for the Center for Science in the Public Interest in Washington, D.C. To do this, however, requires you to exercise considerable restraint.

Assume, for example, that your daily fat allowance is 67 grams, and that eating at McDonald's accounts for 36 of those grams, more than half your daily allowance. Obviously, you'll have to be extra vigilant the rest of the day to make sure that your additional fat intake adds up to no more than 31 grams.

"The problem is that the average person who eats at McDonald's isn't going to have his dietitian as his elbow saying, 'Oh, make sure you get the grilled chicken, and, oh yes, how about a salad with light vinaigrette?' " Liebman says. "The average person is going to have a Big Mac and fries."

One of the reasons diets don't work is that they usually require people to give up some (or all) of their favorite foods, which is no easy task. Clearly, a diet would be a lot easier to stick with if you were allowed to indulge your fast-food cravings from time to time.

On the other hand, if you blow your daily fat budget at one sitting, wolfing down some quadruple-bypass-bacon-and-cheese concoction, what on Earth are you going to eat for dinner? Clearly, there have to be some guidelines to help you navigate the perilous waters of this greasy sea. Fortunately for you, there are.

Fast-Food Tactics

Okay, so you're on the road, and you find yourself famished on fast-food row. On one side of the

Good Food on the Run

Not all fast food is fat food. Here are three ways to get a healthy, filling meal without giving up the speed.

Do yourself a mitzvah. When you're hungry and want something to eat that is both quick and portable, a bagel can be a great choice. "It has fiber, it's practically fat-free, and it's a complex carbohydrate that stays with you," says Pat Harper, R.D., a nutrition consultant in the Pittsburgh area. "When you eat a bagel, you know you've eaten, and you're not hungry in half an hour. And if you put some light cream cheese on it, that's a little bit of protein there. If you down it with a glass of juice, it's really a fine breakfast."

Give yogurt a try. A lot of men, if you suggest eating a cup of yogurt, will look at you as though you recommended eating a large spider. Which is too bad, because a cup of yogurt is the ultimate fast food. It's so loaded with nutrients that it's practically a meal in itself. And there are a lot of excellent brands on the market, many of which are 99 percent fat-free.

Take a hint from Bugs. Even if you're not a big fan of carrots, you may want to give the mini varieties a try. "There is a little bit of sweetness to them, and they are crunchy and real satisfying," Harper says. "They package them already peeled, and they are so handy. If you keep them in the refrigerator, maybe at eye level, chances are you'll grab them when you're hungry. They're an easy way to get vegetables, and they can take the place of a higher-salt, higher-fat food."

street is McDonald's, Burger King, Pizza Hut. On the other is Wendy's, Arby's, and Roy Rogers. Is there any way that you can eat lunch now without wearing it later?

SHUN THE FRIES. It's hard to think of another food that packs as much fat into so compact a package as the french fry. A large order of fries at McDonald's has roughly as much fat (and calories) as a Quarter Pounder. No sir, you're better off without them.

RECONSIDER THE CHEESE. Take one hamburger. Add one slice of Cheddar. Result: big increase in fat. Cheese essentially *is* fat. (With Cheddar, 74 percent of its calories come from fat.) The same goes for cheese on pizza. While whole-milk mozzarella is not as fatty as Cheddar, it still

has 6 grams of fat per ounce.

TAKE ON NO BACON. True, bacon adds a lot of flavor, but it also adds a lot of fat: 3 grams per slice, to be specific, which even shames the french fry.

PASS ON THE PEPPERONI. Skip the sausage, too. These are two toppings that take pizza into the fatosphere. Ten slices of pepperoni—about what you would get on two slices of pizza—gives you more than 24 grams of fat. One link of Italian sausage gives you more than 17. You are better off having peppers and onions instead.

FLEE THAT FILET-O-FAT. Fish—now there's a good alternative to a fatty beef burger, right? Nope. There are more than 20 grams of fat in that Fish Filet Deluxe, about as much as you would get from eating a Quarter Pounder.

UNDRESS YOUR SALAD. "Even with salad dressing, if you're not careful, the calories add up," Liebman says. "If you're going to get a salad and use a whole packet of ranch dressing, you'll get an extra 230 calories."

PUT TOGETHER A SMART MEAL. Mostly, we have been telling you what not to eat. Here are a few fast-food combos that you can enjoy and still stay in shape, says Liebman.

- A grilled chicken-breast sandwich (hold the mayo), a salad, and an orange juice.
- A small hamburger, a salad, and a cup of tea.
- A quarter-pound hamburger (with tomato, lettuce, and onion), an apple that you brought along, and ½ pint of 1 percent low-fat milk.
- A roast beef or turkey sub (with mustard, not mayo or oil), pretzels, and a juice.
- A slice of pizza, a garden salad (with light dressing), and bread sticks.

PLAY BEYOND THE BOARD. We have been talking about a few ways to enjoy fast food without overloading on unnecessary fat. But here is another point to consider: It's not all that difficult to get a fast meal without the drawbacks of the traditional burgers and fries.

Chances are, there are at least a few small grocery stores, convenience stores, or supermarkets somewhere along your route home. Rather than pulling up to a drive-up window, why not shop the salad or soup bars and zip through the express line? You will get your food just about as fast, but without all the fat.

ALL ABOUT ALCOHOL

HOW NOT TO GROW A "MILWAUKEE GOITER"

Better known as a beer gut, the legendary goiter of Milwaukee has long been linked in popular lore to over-indulgence in the brew for which that burg is famous.

Is there really a connection between your gut and the libations you pour into it?

The question is not that easy to answer. We know there are lots of calories in alcohol. Furthermore, your body burns alcohol before it burns fat, which means that when you drink, you are very likely to store (rather than burn) the fat from food. In addition, since the calories provided by alcohol can be used either as energy or converted to fat, it would stand to reason that at least some of the extra calories that you guzzle could end up on your gut.

Yet the connection between drinking habits and expanding waistlines isn't so clear. One study, which followed more than 7,000 men and women for 10 years, found that drinkers gained less weight than nondrinkers during that period.

Arthur L. Klatsky, M.D., who has done extensive research on the subject of alcohol and health and is senior consultant in cardiology at the Kaiser Permanente Medical Center and the Division of Research Group in Oakland, California, suggests that this is because alcohol is not an "extra" in drinkers' diets. That is, if they weren't drinking alcohol, they would be drinking something else with an equal or greater number of calories.

"Maybe you have a couple of beers a day instead of a couple of glasses of milk," says Dr. Klatsky. "People who drink regularly take the alcohol in place of something else, so it's not extra. It's their beverage; instead of Coca-Cola, they drink alcohol."

It would appear, then, that the drinkers have an advantage. While your average 12-ounce bottle of beer (the most caloric of alcoholic drinks) contains 146 calories, a 12-ounce can of cola contains 152, and a 12-ounce glass of 2 percent milk has 181.

A Beer a Day

This is not to say that, if you're worried about your weight, you shouldn't have a care about your drinking. Looking at it purely from a calories-in point of view, the effects of what you drink could be substantial. If you are an average American guy, somewhere between 5 and 7 percent of the calories you consume come from alcohol.

That means, if your daily calorie intake is the same as the national average (2,603) for men over 20, somewhere between 130 and 182 of those calories—about a beer a day—are booze-derived.

Given that there is virtually no nutritional

The big question is not how much you drink so much as how much that drink matters to you.

If you're a guy who likes a double bourbon every night with dinner, but you can take it or leave it, then you probably don't have anything to worry about. But if you gradually start drinking more, or you're a guy who spends the week staying sober but gets loaded every Saturday night, you probably have a problem, says Max Schneider, M.D., clinical associate professor of addiction medicine at the University of California, Irvine, School of Medicine and deputy chairman of the National Council on Alcoholism and Drug Dependence.

You know you most certainly do have a problem if your drinking is affecting your relationship with your wife, your work, or your health.

If your drinking is damaging you, you need to face the music and get help. Admit that you have a problem and then get to a chapter of Alcoholics Anonymous. Generally, men don't beat this thing alone; it's the kind of thing you need a support group to take on, says Dr. Schneider.

For the same reason, you should enlist your family in helping you to deal with it. They can be a great source of support and comfort.

Finally, lead yourself not into temptation. Steer clear of your old haunts, advises Dr. Schneider, if those haunts happen to be bars, and your old friends, if those friends only come with drinks attached.

---

value in alcohol, a guy could possibly lop a lot of lard off his abdomen simply by dropping his nightly bottle of belch. For example, if you're in the habit of swilling a brew every night when you get home from work, you could—at least theoretically—lose about 15 pounds in a year just by cutting it out.

You could do that. But let's face it, you would be depriving yourself of one of life's little pleasures. And since life is a fairly barren furrow without those little pleasures, what's the point in that?

Moreover, there is some very strong evidence that by depriving yourself of your nightly libation, you are not just cheating yourself out of a small pleasure, you may also be denying yourself a longer life.

Healthy Drinking

It's true. The guy who quaffs an ale, sips a flute of wine, or even throws back a shot of scotch at the end of the day is likely to stay healthier and live longer than his teetotaling twin.

This is because studies have consistently shown that men who consume a moderate (note that word *moderate*) amount of alcohol on a regular basis are less likely to suffer heart attacks and ischemic strokes (that is, strokes caused by the blockage of a blood vessel) than men who don't drink.

Researchers still don't understand the whole mechanism of this effect, but they do know that alcohol increases the level of high-density lipoprotein (HDL) cholesterol (the good kind) in your bloodstream. There is also, says Dr. Klatsky, the possibility that some alcoholic beverages have a mild antioxidant effect, which may prevent low-density lipoprotein (LDL) cholesterol (the bad kind) from clogging up your arteries.

How much does moderate drinking reduce your risk? That depends on which study you look at. The figures range from 25 to 40 percent.

With alcohol, though, it is easy to have too much of a good thing. You don't need us to tell you this if you have ever spent a night, as the Australians put it, "laughing at the ground." But the ill effects of heavy drinking go way beyond the next day's hangover. Too much sauce can lead to some really serious life-threatening stuff.

We are not saying that the odd night on your knees will kill you, but if your only exercise routine is bending your elbow at your local pub; if your friends often have occasion to describe you as swacked, plastered, shellacked, lit, or loaded; if, we say, your ship often lists to starboard, decks awash, with three sheets to the wind, then you're a prime candidate for a grim variety of serious health problems, from heart irregularities, various cancers, and gut trouble to cirrhosis of the liver.

In short, you could end up like Nicolas Cage in the movie *Leaving Las Vegas*.

The French Paradox

There is a prevailing notion that red wine is supposed to be better for you than other alcoholic drinks. This belief has its origins in a concept known as the French paradox, which, as it happens, is a good example of how a little science can go a wrong way.

Attempting to understand how Frenchmen could eat so much rich food and still have much lower rates of heart disease than Americans, researchers hit upon the notion that it must be something in all that red wine those Frenchmen drink.

Specifically, they focused on phenolic compounds, antioxidants found in red wine that seem to prevent the oxidation of LDL cholesterol. Less oxidation of LDL means a decreased chance of getting clogged arteries.

When news of this research made its way to television's 60 Minutes, herds of Americans stampeded to their local liquor stores and guzzled the grape like Lourdes' water.

This was wonderful news for the wine industry, of course, but subsequent research has raised serious questions about whether there is really any big benefit in wine over beer, bourbon, or other spirits.

Indeed, in a review of 25 studies, Dr. Klatsky and other researchers found that it really doesn't matter what you drink because it is the alcohol that provides the main benefit in drinking.

"Alcohol is overwhelmingly the major thing," says Dr. Klatsky, "and if there is some other factor, it's a minor factor. There are data that show that small amounts of alcohol, independent of the vehicle, are likely to protect the heart."

Dr. Klatsky suggests that many of the studies seeming to show the benefits of moderate wine drinking may be misinterpreted because they may not consider other lifestyle factors that may come into play. American wine-drinkers, for example, tend to be more educated and richer, and therefore may eat better and get better health care than liquor or beer drinkers.

Belly Up to the Bar

Let's return to the issue of drinking and weight. One study did show a correlation between beer swilling and gut building, suggesting that, given the choice between a glass of wine or a bottle of brew, you who choose the brew will put more rubber on your spare. The study, which looked at more than 12,000 men and women, found that those who drank more than six beers or other non-wine alcoholic drinks a week were 1.4 times more likely to have a big belly than those who drank less than one. Meanwhile, those who drank

What Is a Drink?

When it comes to drinking, most experts define <u>moderation</u> as no more than one drink a day for women and no more than two drinks a day for men.

This is an okay rule of thumb, but not something you should adhere to slavishly. For example, if you are a small man, two drinks a day might be more than is good for you. If you are a big woman, two might be just fine. Body size aside, some of us just don't handle booze as well as others. So if you are going to err, it's better to err on the side of caution. With drinking, less is more.

So what, officially speaking, counts as a drink? According to the government's dietary guidelines, a drink is defined as the following:

- **One bottle (12 ounces) of beer**
- **One glass (5 ounces) of wine**
- **One shot (1.5 ounces) of 80-proof liquor**

more than six glasses of wine a week actually had littler middles than those who didn't drink at all.

The researchers who did this study, however, admitted that the difference in adiposity between wine and beer drinkers could, in fact, be due to factors other than the booze, such as different eating habits between wine and beer drinkers.

So What'll You Have?

The bottom line is that a little light drinking probably won't hurt, and may even help you. Here are a few guidelines.

DRINK LESS. If you're drinking three or more drinks a day, you're a heavy drinker, and you're not doing yourself any favors. You should have no more than one or two drinks a day; more than that is not good for either your health or your belly, says Max Schneider, M.D., clinical associate professor of addiction medicine at the University of California, Irvine, School of Medicine and deputy chairman of the National Council on Alcoholism and Drug Dependence. If you sit down and swozzle a six-pack, you're not only doing damage to your brain but you're also taking in almost a thousand calories.

DRINK MORE. On the other hand, "if I meet a person who is at a high risk for a heart attack and has the occasional drink, but who really doesn't drink very often, I sometimes encourage that person to have one drink more often," Dr. Klatsky says. "If you have heart trouble, I think you should do every reasonable thing you can to reduce the risk of an attack." And moderate amounts of alcohol, as we have seen, may help.

ABOVE ALL, KEEP TRACK. Pay attention to how much you are drinking. A drink is not a big old tumblerful of scotch; that's two or three drinks in one. If you're in the habit of tipping a bottle of scotch or bourbon over the rocks every night, you should try using a shot glass to measure it, just so you know how much you are really drinking.

WATCH THE CALORIES. There is no question that alcohol will add calories to your diet. If you are counting calories, factor it in. A glass of wine is roughly equivalent to a slice of bread; a beer, to two slices.

TRY WINE. Which, come to think of it, is why it isn't such a bad idea to switch to wine. "As far as weight loss is concerned, wine is probably the lowest-calorie beverage per standard drink," says Dr. Klatsky. "So you could make more of a case for wine in that regard."

DRINK BETTER. If you're not offing a six every night, you can afford to buy something better. Savor one richly flavored microbrew instead of swilling several cans of cheap mass-market, assembly-line horsewater. Same goes for wine or scotch. Go for the fine bordeaux; go for the single malt. Enjoy. Life is short.

DON'T DRINK IF YOU CAN'T. Obviously, there are some of us who cannot drink. If you have had problems with alcohol in the past, stay away from it. "Most men who are nondrinkers have a solid reason to be a nondrinker," Dr. Klatsky says. "For example, they may have had a problem with alcohol or a father who was an alcoholic, or they might have religious reasons. Something. There are exceptions, but generally these people are best left alone. In any case, drinking is not the most important thing that you can do to protect your heart."

SCENARIO **1**:The Late Show

AGE: 44

WEIGHT: 215

LIFESTYLE: A dispatcher for a large trucking firm, he has never had to worry about his weight too much. In recent years, however, his increasingly sedentary lifestyle—too much time at work, not enough time doing things outside like riding his bike—has taken a toll. He is not fanatical about losing weight but would like to drop a trouser size or two.

WEIGHT GOALS: Wants to lose about 15 pounds.

PROBLEM: This is a guy who eats pretty healthfully during the day—his diet is generally low in fat and sweets and high in grains and vegetables—but every night, a couple hours after dinner, something snaps. There's that carton of ice cream beckoning from the freezer, or that bag of potato chips serenading from the pantry, or those cookies calling out from the jar. Whereas during the day he finds such come-ons easy to resist, in the still of the night, he finds them irresistible. It's as if he has used up his daily ration of willpower and, as bedtime approaches, must succumb or run screaming into the night.

Like Ulysses, this man could have himself bound to his galley's mast to resist the siren's call, but then, how many of us these days have masts or galleys or crews to bind us? No, better to avoid those siren songs entirely.

According to Pat Harper, R.D., a nutrition consultant in the Pittsburgh area, this man simply shouldn't keep things like ice cream, potato chips, and cookies around the house. If they are not there to tempt him, Harper says, he is not likely to eat something less tempting. Nor is he likely to get in his car at 10:00 at night and go out in search of them. But if they are there, not only will they tempt him, but more than likely he will succumb to the temptation.

Instead, he should make it a rule that ice cream or chips or cookies—or whatever his particular nemesis

might be—are not something that will be a part of his home environment but will be something he is allowed to eat when he goes out. Indeed, reserving his daily snacks for special times will make them more special, too, and he is likely to enjoy them more than when he simply devours them at home.

If this seems too drastic—if, for instance, he occasionally has his nephews over and doesn't want to deprive them—he could try taking a middle path by buying chips or cookies or whatnot in small packages. He will be much less likely to open several small packages than to clean out one large one, Harper says.

"If he buys his chips in those little lunch-size bags, he might just open up one of those and go through it. It's a way of controlling portions so he doesn't have to give them up," Harper says. "The problem is not the food, it's the amount that he eats. If he eats a pound of them, he has a problem."

Another part of the solution to this man's dilemma is to make healthy substitutions by choosing nonfat or low-fat versions. We are not saying that he can't snack, after all. He may, in fact, need a light snack. So someone, buy him an air popper. Let him eat popcorn—it's healthy, good for digestion, and low in calories, particularly when it's made without oil or butter. Sprinkle on some Cajun spices for a funky variation.

A terrific snack is fresh fruit, of course. A late-night apple or slice of watermelon is satisfying, filling, and far less apt to put a ring around the belly.

Finally, while we don't know enough about this guy to get into his head, we have to wonder: Why the late-night gorging? Is he actually hungry? Then maybe he needs to look at how he is eating during the day—a well-balanced diet shouldn't leave him in need of food at 11:00 P.M. And if he's not hungry, but gobbling food anyhow, well, why? Boredom? Just a bad habit? Deep-seated demons gnawing at his soul? There may be some lifestyle issues to work out rather than just worrying about the food itself. Or maybe the guy just needs a hobby (say, exercise?) to divert his attention from food.

SCENARIO **2**:Comfort Food

AGE: 34

WEIGHT: 285

LIFESTYLE: An account executive at a large advertising firm, he spends 10 or more hours a day at the office. The long hours aren't due only to job demands; rather, he spends so much time on break—in the cafeteria, the snack room, or away at lunch—that he needs the extra time to get things done.

WEIGHT GOALS: His doctor has told him to lose at least 70 pounds if he wants to see the other side of 50.

PROBLEM: This man is truly addicted to food. Eating is what he does—in the car on the way to work, at his desk, in the living room at home, and in the bedroom at night. He has tried for years to successfully cut back on the amount of calories that he takes in, but he finds it extremely difficult—more difficult, in fact, than giving up smoking (which he finally did last year). Hunger isn't the issue; even after a large meal, he is back in the kitchen an hour later.

It's pretty obvious that this man is eating for all sorts of reasons that have nothing to do with hunger, says Joanne Curran-Celentano, R.D., Ph.D., associate professor of nutritional sciences at the University of New Hampshire in Durham and nutrition research coordinator at the Center for Eating Disorders Management in Dover, New Hampshire. He may be eating because he's nervous, angry, lonely, tired, or bored. Or maybe he's eating simply because it has become a habit. And food, and the habit of eating, can become a real comfort.

This is not to say that this man may not have a physical problem with hunger itself; some people lack the appropriate "switch" that tells them they have had enough. But in this man's case, the issue appears to be more psychological than physical. What he needs to try to figure out is why he is eating all the time. Dr. Curran-Celentano recommends that he keep a record of what he eats, when

he eats it, and where he eats it.

"Once he sees patterns emerging, then that can tip him off about appetite," Dr. Curran-Celentano says. He may discover, for example, that his omnivorousness is the product of stress or loneliness. If so, he can work at developing new responses to these feelings.

He can distract himself by doing something that's "incompatible with eating," like keeping his hands busy while working in the yard, says Dr. Curran-Celentano. Or he can keep himself occupied—and his mind off food—simply by doing something else that he enjoys, be it shopping, working on his truck, or cleaning the garage.

One of the best things that he can do is confront his cravings head-on. The next time he finds himself reaching into the cookie jar, he should pause and ask himself, one, if he's really hungry, and two, what's happening at that moment to lead him to eat—and what he can do to resolve it.

He also needs to try to get in touch with his body enough to distinguish real hunger pangs from mere appetite, says Nancy Clark, R.D., director of Nutrition Services at SportsMedicine Brookline near Boston and author of *Nancy Clark's Sports Nutrition Guidebook*.

"Appetite is just a desire to eat," Clark says. "And that doesn't always mean that your body needs calories."

But for this guy in particular, distinguishing between hunger and appetite won't necessarily be all that easy. This is because he has eaten in so many different places, so many different times, that the very places themselves may be hunger triggers, says Dr. Curran-Celentano. Most of us, when we walk into a kitchen, think about food. For this guy, every room in the house is a kitchen.

And that is why, finally, he needs to deprogram himself by restricting his eating to specific venues. The kitchen should be the place for eating—not the car, not the desk in the office, not the couch in front of the television set, not the easy chair in the living room, and not the bed in front of *Letterman*.

SCENARIO 3: On the Road

AGE: 28

WEIGHT: 180 and gaining

LIFESTYLE: A salesman for a large telecommunications company, he spends his days on the road trying to sell long-distance services to corporate clients. Since he drives more than 200 miles a day, he leaves the house early and gets home late, with little downtime in between.

WEIGHT GOALS: Only needs to lose a few pounds to get down to 172—his best weight.

PROBLEM: An inordinately large proportion of this man's diet is fast food: eggs, sausages, butter, burgers, fries, pizza, subs, and more. He knows his heart is under siege, but given his hours and the amount of time he spends on the road, he doesn't see an easy alternative.

Clearly, this man needs to get out of the fast lane to the cemetery by getting off fatty fast food. True, his job requires that he spend a lot of time on the road, and the nation's highways aren't known as a haven for healthful cuisine. But there are many ways in which he could avail himself of healthier food without overhauling his entire diet.

A key question is whether he is actually eating while driving or sitting down in a restaurant to eat. Let's assume that he is doing both over the course of a week.

Let's look at eating while driving first. (We won't comment on the safety or appeal of this; wrong or right, it's what guys do.) Our man could vastly improve his diet if he would occasionally pack his own lunch and keep it in a cooler in the car, says Margery Lawrence, R.D., Ph.D., associate professor in the Department of Nutrition and Family Studies at St. Joseph College in West Hartford, Connecticut.

The goal is to come up with a well-balanced assortment of food that can be eaten with one hand, without dripping or making lots of waste and without having to divert one's eyes from the road. The answers? Pretzels. Apples, pears, peaches. Sliced carrots, celery, cucumber. Turkey sandwiches. Roast beef sandwiches. Peanut butter and jelly sandwiches. Juices. Cherry tomatoes. Trail mix. Hunks of cheese. The list is as long as your imagination. Any of these would be a vast improvement over his usual diet. If he does this even occasionally, it will do his belly—and his wallet—a world of good.

Now let's assume that this guy wants to be in and out of a restaurant in 20 to 30 minutes. Why limit it to fast-food restaurants? He could go to a diner and get just soup and salad. Go to any Asian restaurant and get a large bowl of noodle soup. Go to a sandwich shop and get a turkey sub and some pretzels. Go to a pizza shop and get two slices and the house salad. Again, the options are endless—once you think about it.

If he still wants the convenience of the national fast-food joints, then he should choose his fast food wisely. If he is careful, he can go into a fast-food restaurant and put together a meal that's not too bad for him, says Bonnie Liebman, a licensed nutritionist and director of nutrition for the Center for Science in the Public Interest in Washington, D.C. But he has to watch himself.

One other excellent option is to skip the restaurants and pull up to a supermarket. There, our man can pick up a quick cup of low-fat yogurt, hit a salad bar, grab a piece of fruit, and, just so he doesn't feel deprived, a little package of low-fat cookies, says Pat Harper, R.D., a nutrition consultant in the Pittsburgh area.

Of course, he should be careful that he's not starving when he hits that grocery store, or he may tote out a lot more stuff than he meant to. But really, almost anything he buys will probably be better for him than the hamburgers on fast-food row.

It isn't likely that this man will forsake fast food entirely (nor, given his preferences, is it desirable). He likes it, and if he tries to give it up entirely, he will soon get bored and frustrated with his new diet and may decide to forget the whole thing. But if he makes it a point to eat healthier food several days a week, then he can still enjoy some of his fast-food favorites while managing to drop a few pounds.

SCENARIO 4: The Follies of Fat-Free

AGE: 60

WEIGHT: 180

LIFESTYLE: He manages a small bookstore in a suburban shopping mall and is just a few years away from retirement. Although he has never had serious weight or health problems, he is honest enough with himself to know that he is at an age where little things can make a big difference. He wants to stay as healthy as possible for as long as possible and is motivated to make the necessary changes.

WEIGHT GOALS: He wants to lose 10 to 15 pounds.

PROBLEM: He has recently become very conscientious about eating a low-fat diet. He reads labels religiously and cooks using low-fat ingredients. But despite his efforts, he keeps gaining weight.

This man is in many ways representative of the state of the American stomach today. While he knows that he should lower the amount of fat in his diet and has made serious efforts to do so, he has made one fatal assumption: that he can eat pretty much as much as he wants because he is eating low-fat or nonfat foods. So when he polishes off a bag of baked tortilla chips, he thinks to himself, "That's okay. They're fat-free."

The problem, of course, is that he is still taking in more calories than he is burning, and those calories have nowhere to go but into storage, says John B. Allred, Ph.D., professor of nutrition in the Department of Food Science and Technology at Ohio State University in Columbus and co-author of *Taking the Fear Out of Eating: A Nutritionists' Guide to Sensible Food Choices.* In other words, he can cut out all the fat he wants, but calories still count.

Since he has already gotten into the habit of reading labels, he just needs to read them a little more closely. It's not enough just to look at how many grams of fat there are per serving. "The most important number on a food label is serving size," Dr. Allred says.

With snack foods, in particular, the official serving size—say, two cookies, or one snack cake—is often unrealistically small. Which means that people often eat a lot more than the amount recommended on the label. If this man is eating several servings of his low-fat whatever, he is not benefiting by eating low-fat because he is still taking in too many calories.

That's why the second most important number on that label is calories. A food may be low-fat and still be just as high in calories as its fattier cousins because a lot of food manufacturers pump their low-fat offerings up with extra sugars to make them taste good.

The problem is, though, that they still don't satisfy the appetite like the fatty stuff.

"Talk to someone who just eats one or two SnackWell's," says Melinda Hemmelgarn, R.D., associate state nutrition specialist for the Department of Food Science and Human Nutrition Extension at the University of Missouri in Columbia. "Chances are, you'll eat four or five of those things or even half a box. If you're just eating one or two, it's a great way to save a few grams of fat, but most people don't look at them that way. The connotation for most people is 'They're fat-free, I can eat all I want.'"

Obviously, if this man is serious about staying trim and healthy, he has to do more than monitor his intake of snack foods. He also needs to eat more fruits and vegetables and fewer Snack-Well's.

"One very easy way to trim calories," Hemmelgarn says, "is to substitute other foods—primarily fruits and vegetables—for the nutrient-poor, calorie-rich foods." Eating more good foods will provide an abundance of vitamins, minerals, and other healthy compounds. And at the same time they will help keep him full so that he will naturally find himself eating fewer snacks.

SCENARIO 5: The Taste Challenge

AGE: 42

WEIGHT: 165 and rising

LIFESTYLE: An auto mechanic and recently divorced father of two, this man has always been a tightly wound sort who is only comfortable when doing things in their proper order, at the proper time, and most important, "as they've always been done." This attitude has helped make him an excellent mechanic, but he also has a tendency to be a little rigid in his thinking.

WEIGHT GOALS: A small man, he needs to lose about 10 pounds.

PROBLEM: Not surprisingly, this man is fairly rigid about what he will and will not eat. His response to the offer of new foods and cuisines—"I know what I like, and I don't like that"—is so automatic that it ought to be his motto. Unfortunately, he eats pretty much the same way that he did when he was a kid. His preferred diet is heavy on the meat and potatoes and light on everything else. In addition, he has a sweet tooth. He rarely gets through a day without ingesting something from the cookie–cupcake–ice-cream–candy-bar food group.

This man needs to open his mind and his mouth to the wonderful world of food that's passing him by. Not only is he doing his belly and his health no favors by living on this meat–and–potatoes–and–pecan-pie diet, he is also opting his taste buds out of life's rich pageant, says Pat Harper, R.D., a nutrition consultant in the Pittsburgh area.

He should try all over again everything that he has ever tried and hated, Harper recommends. After all, the last time this guy tasted—and rejected—a brussels sprout was when he was five. So he is well overdue to try one again. He may well discover that—once he gets over the shock of something green on his plate—he really likes it.

It is not at all uncommon for adults to enjoy foods they despised when they were kids. One theory is that adults have far fewer taste buds than children do. He may find that the stronger tastes he hated then are more appealing than appalling now.

He should also, Harper adds, be adventurous and try some things that he has never tried before. He may discover several foods to which he will say, "Where have you been all my life?"

Most of all, though, the foods this guy needs to try to befriend are citizens of the Plant Kingdom. The connections between belly fat and meat consumption or vegetable consumption are fairly easy to state, says Henry Kahn, M.D., an internist and associate professor of family and preventive medicine at Emory University School of Medicine in Atlanta. The more meat you eat, the more likely you are to gain a belly. But the more vegetables you eat, the more likely you are to lose one.

"I would tell him to move away from saturated fats, meaning animal fats in particular, and toward a wide variety of vegetables prepared without the addition of saturated fat. Simple advice such as 'More vegetables, less meat' will probably do it."

The other thing that this man has to do is rein in his sweet tooth. Not give up sweets entirely but simply eat less of them, says Margery Lawrence, R.D., Ph.D., associate professor in the Department of Nutrition and Family Studies at St. Joseph College in West Hartford, Connecticut.

He should decide, for example, what's most important to him—that afternoon candy bar or that after-dinner dish of ice cream—and choose to have one or the other, but not both, on any given day. He might also, Dr. Lawrence says, try substituting a piece of fruit for one or the other of those things. Or he might try having a little smaller bowl of ice cream and add a piece of fruit.

SCENARIO 6: Going to Extremes

AGE: 39

WEIGHT: 222

LIFESTYLE: A bricklayer and part-time surveyor, this man deals in incredible precision, measuring slopes and angles to fractions of an inch. The focus that he brings to his job extends to his life as well. He doesn't like guesswork and always wants to know exactly where he is going.

WEIGHT GOALS: Needs to lose about 25 pounds.

PROBLEM: This is a man at war with himself. For many of the last 15 years, he has been trying to lose weight. And because he never does anything by half, his diets haven't always been undertaken wisely. He once tried to lose weight by putting himself on a severe regimen of cabbage soup, lettuce leaves, and ice water. Another time he decided to cut out excess calories by eating only one meal—dinner—a day. Needless to say, his diets haven't lasted long. After a week or so of self-abuse, he usually has lost 10 pounds, but also his patience. It doesn't take long before he has given up in frustration and is back to his old weight or—worse—even heavier.

This guy's approach to weight loss is guaranteed to fail, says Colleen Pierre, R.D., a nutrition consultant in Baltimore. Nobody is going to stay on a regimen that they hate, and he's not doing his body any favors by jerking it around this way.

The bottom line is that diets—even fairly sensible diets—frequently don't work.

When a guy's a dieter, Pierre says, "I ask him, 'Have you ever been on a diet before?' And he'll tell me, 'Oh, I went on this one diet, and it really worked.' Obviously, though, it didn't work, or he would have lost the weight and kept it off."

The problem with diets is that, by definition, they're short-term plans. You diet, you lose weight, and then you don't diet anymore. And what happens? You gain back all the weight that you lost.

So you diet again. And again.

The only way this man will lose weight and keep it off, Pierre says, is to develop a truly livable plan—one that he can live with, day after day, without feeling as though he is being deprived.

It doesn't have to be complicated. The most efficient plan is also the simplest: He should eat a wide variety of foods based on the government's Food Guide Pyramid—that is, a lot of grains, legumes, fruits, and vegetables and a lot less meat and full-fat milk, cheese, and other dairy products. (For more information, see Nutrition Fundamentals on page 42.)

Since most men don't want to count calories, he would be well-advised to at least keep a food record, writing down everything that he eats or drinks for a few days, says Pierre.

"I might look at his food record and see that every afternoon he drinks a Coke and has a candy bar. I might say, 'Suppose you could go the rest of your life and have a Coke and candy bar every afternoon. Do you think you could live with that?' " Once this man agrees that having a daily Coke and candy bar would be perfectly okay by him, then he should start seeing what other changes he will need to make in his diet to accommodate them.

For example, Pierre says that she would allow him about 200 free calories a day. He could spend those calories on anything he wants: Cokes, pretzels, candy bars, whatever. Of course, 200 calories doesn't go very far, so he might have to save them for a few days to get something really good—a big piece of pie, for example. "The idea is that he doesn't have to cheat," she says. "Normal eating includes having some of these things—but they're treats, not diet staples. He needs to see that the real staples are fruits and vegetables, breads and cereals, a little bit of meat, and a little bit of dairy."

Allowing himself occasional treats will work much better than dieting, says Pierre, because it moves foods out of the forbidden category—which is always where he will encounter the most temptations—and makes them a normal part of the week.

SCENARIO 7: Changing Habits

AGE: 55

WEIGHT: 209

LIFESTYLE: A high school teacher for nearly 30 years, he is a firm believer in using systems—from seating charts to detailed lesson plans—to keep things running smoothly. In the rest of his life, as well, he is more than a little set in his ways. He has found that uncertainty breeds chaos, which, as a career teacher, he has learned to avoid at all costs.

WEIGHT GOALS: Has to get down to 180.

PROBLEM: This man has been warned by his doctor that he is seriously overweight and his cholesterol levels are way too high. He knows that he needs to reduce the amount of fat in his diet, but he is a walking lifetime of bad habits that need changing. Needless to say, these habits have resulted in a fine heap of a belly.

Obviously, this man needs to make radical changes in his diet, but it's going to be very difficult for him to begin. He is going to have to change many of the things that he has taken for granted all his life—like the privilege of grabbing a double burger with fries whenever the urge strikes. And nothing's harder to change than ingrained habits.

Still, he has to take that first step. "First of all, he has to examine what foods he currently eats," says Keith-Thomas Ayoob, R.D., Ed.D., assistant professor of pediatrics at Albert Einstein College of Medicine of Yeshiva University in New York City. "And one of the ways he can do that is to keep track of everything he eats for three days and be as detailed as he can. He can't just say that he had chicken. Is it fried? Is it a breast? Is it a leg? He will find that doing this provides a lot of information like 'Oh yeah, I forgot that brownie I had at 11 o'clock and that extra soda at the end of the day.' "

Once he knows exactly what's going into his mouth each day, he has to consider which of these foods he may want to do without. "I wouldn't want him to forgo all the foods that he likes," says Dr. Ayoob. "I would work with him to fit them in, but to fit them a little less often or in smaller portions. I wouldn't want to send him home thinking, 'Oh, I have to live on a diet of seaweed and water.' "

The third thing he has to do, says Dr. Ayoob, is take a hard look at his activity level. "We often leave that out of the diet equation, but it is almost impossible to lose weight and keep it off without taking into account activity levels. I don't think a person has to run marathons, but he should look at what activities he is doing and think of where he can begin to change."

"I'll give you one example of what actually happened with a patient of mine. I said, 'Look, between now and next week, walk around the block once.' The person really resisted, and I said, 'You walked in here, I know you can do that.' And the next week, I said, 'Walk around the block twice.' Well, within six weeks this patient was walking half a mile a day and eventually got up to a mile a day."

The point is that by starting slowly and being very consistent, this man can make a lot of progress in a short period of time. "If somebody's doing one push-up a day, and then every week, he ups it one, well, in six months he's doing 26 push-ups a day. I think we need to be a little more patient about how quickly we go with things."

Exercise will do a lot to help this man shed some pounds, but because of his high cholesterol, he really has to make substantial changes in his diet. "Most fruits and vegetables are loaded with vitamins and minerals and phytochemicals, and researchers are finding very strong links between phytochemicals and protection from cancer, heart disease, and diabetes."

"If he eats as many as five fruits and vegetables a day, not only would that go a long way toward lowering his total calorie intake, but it would also go a long way toward improving his health," says Dr. Ayoob.

Again, the idea is to make the changes gradually. He should begin by laying in a small supply of fruit—just apples, say. Every day he should have one or two of them—maybe grabbing them on his way out the door, for instance, or eating them for dessert after supper.

"It's going to take him several weeks to adapt," says Dr. Ayoob. "We are really talking about a long-term approach. The weight didn't come on quickly; it's not going to come off quickly. This is fine, though, because we find that gradual changes are more likely to become permanent changes."

PART III

THE LEAN LIFESTYLE

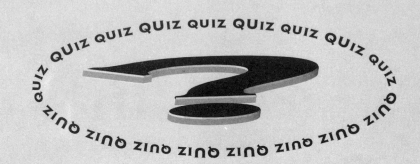

DOES MY LIFESTYLE SUPPORT LEANNESS?

Losing weight, as you know by now, has less to do with any particular diet or exercise plan, and a great deal to do with how we live our lives every day. It's the little decisions—buying one doughnut instead of a dozen, say, or occasionally walking instead of driving to get the paper—that determine whether we'll be lean or larded.

1. When I go to the mall to do some shopping:
   a. I park wherever I can find a spot and walk in.
   b. I drive around the parking lot for as long as it takes to find the perfect parking space—that is, the one closest to the door.
   c. I park—illegally—in a space reserved for the handicapped.
   d. I don't go to the mall; I do all my shopping on-line so that I never even have to get out of my chair.

2. During coffee breaks I always:
   a. Grab a cheese Danish.
   b. Grab an apple.
   c. Grab a quick walk around the building.
   d. Grab an apple and a quick walk around the building.

3. For lunch I usually:
   a. Dash out for fast food.
   b. Construct an elaborate salad at the cafeteria salad bar, then eat it, elaborately.
   c. Go for a run or work out at the gym.
   d. Eat at my desk so I can do more work.

4. I usually spend my evenings:
   a. Watching TV until I fall asleep.
   b. Watching TV for just an hour or 2. Well, maybe sometimes 3.
   c. Watch the news, then turn it off and do some chores.
   d. Watch the sun set as I take the dog for a nice, long walk.

5. I get some kind of exercise:
   a. At least half an hour a day.
   b. At least three times a week.
   c. Once in a while.
   d. I don't have time to exercise.

6. Exercise:
   a. Is something I do when I can fit it in to my schedule.
   b. Often gets pushed out of my day by other things that demand my time.
   c. Is something I schedule into my day, and I religiously stick to my schedule.
   d. Sometimes gets bumped by something else, but when it does, I still make time to do it.

7. When I go to the gym:
   a. I feel like a dweeb next to all those behemoths pumping free weights.
   b. I feel all right, I guess, but there are about a thousand other places that I'd rather be.
   c. I feel good that I'm there but even better when I'm done.
   d. I feel good because each time I go, I push myself a little harder and a little further.

8. On the days when I just can't seem to get myself motivated to work out:

   a. I just blow it off.

   b. I focus my thoughts on how good it's going to feel when I'm done. Then I do it.

   c. I do some other exercise, like taking a walk.

   d. I treat myself to an ice cream sundae.

9. My goal is to:

   a. Banish my belly.

   b. Live longer.

   c. Be healthier.

   d. Exercise several times a week.

10. It's a lazy Saturday afternoon. The kids are at friends', the wife's out shopping, and I:

   a. Am sprawled in my La-Z-Boy recliner, sucking down brewdogs and barbecued potato chips, while watching the game.

   b. Am out rototilling the garden.

   c. Am playing a game of pickup basketball at the park.

   d. Am driving around the mall parking lot searching for the perfect parking space.

ANSWERS

It doesn't take genius to know which answers you were supposed to give. But it's worth taking a minute to see how all of these issues—which are just a sampling of everyday lifestyle changes that can help you lose weight—can add up to substantial gains in fitness.

1. (a) Obviously, you're going to burn off more calories walking across the parking lot than you will sitting in your car (or sitting anywhere else, for that matter).

2. (d) If you're a guy who passes on the Danish in favor of an apple and burns off a few extra calories while you're at it, you're doing nice work on both sides of the calories-in/calories-out equation.

3. (c) In the best of all possible worlds, you would have time to eat and exercise at lunch. Maybe you don't have time for a full workout, but you'll be healthier if you squeeze in a walk as well as a salad.

4. (d) The key to losing weight is very simple: The more movement the better. Walking the dog is better for you and your dog than any number of Benji film festivals.

5. (a) Fitness pros agree that everyone should get at least half an hour of moderate exercise every day. Can't get much simpler than that.

6. (d) It would be nice if we could set a workout schedule and stick to it, no exceptions. But life isn't like that, which is why you have to be flexible.

7. If you answered (c), that exercise is something you do knowing you will feel good later, you're more than halfway there. Anything that keeps you coming back is good. But the place you really want to get to is (d). Once exercise has become its own reward—you do it because you look forward to it, and it feels good while you're doing it—it's a solid part of your life, and chances are that you'll stick with it.

8. (b) No matter how much you make exercise a habit, there are going to be days when you don't feel like doing it. The best way to get past this hurdle is to remember what it's going to feel like when you get to the other side.

9. This is a trick question because all of the answers are worthy goals. But the best answer is (d), because it's specific. You're not promising yourself pie-in-the-sky success and then getting discouraged when you don't measure up.

10. Sorry, another trick question. Yes, pickup basketball is good. But the answer is (b). Why? Because working in the yard—or organizing the garage or walking the dog—is a daily activity that doesn't require a lot of commitment or advance planning. The important thing is to do something physically challenging that you also happen to like doing.

How to Shed Your Past

It's You against You

Take off your shirt and take a look in the mirror. See that thing around your middle there? That's your past. That's all the days you guzzled grease-burgers with gargantuan fries and all the nights you lounged on the couch like a walrus on a sandbar. In short, a man's belly is the product of his lifestyle, which, for many of us, is all the years we lived large and lazy.

It goes without saying that to shed your past, you have to shed some of your bad habits. Essentially, this means redefining yourself, replacing old habits with some new, good habits in order to create a new, lean, lively you.

It sounds like a tall order, and it would be if you tried to transform yourself overnight. But if you make gradual changes in your eating habits and ease into getting more active, you will transform yourself—not instantly but surely. What you're doing, after all, is not changing just a few habits but changing your life.

The tricky part, really, is sticking with your new "habits" long enough for them to become habits. And how to do that is the focus of this chapter. According to Rod K. Dishman, Ph.D., professor and director of the Exercise Psychology Laboratory in the Department of Exercise Science

at the University of Georgia in Athens, "Good habits, once formed, are no more difficult to maintain than bad habits." (Hey, that's why they call them habits, right?)

Obviously, there are obstacles on the way to forming those good habits. If, for example, you're like most of us, once you start eating leaner and working some exercise into your life, you may see some fairly quick results . . . initially. You are, however, going to reach a point where those results flatten out and you don't seem to be making much progress.

"Later gains occur more slowly than initial ones," says Dr. Dishman. "This is very frustrating when constant improvements are expected."

This is the critical juncture where a lot of guys get discouraged, give up, and drop out. In fact, about 50 percent of all new exercisers quit somewhere between six months and a year into their new programs.

In the following pages are some excellent strategies for keeping with the program. Shedding the past isn't hard, but you have to take it one step at a time.

Rule 1: Don't Compete against Others

Picture yourself walking into the gym, determined to work through a few sets of repetitions on the free weights. Chances are, there's a bunch of bulked-up guys in there tossing the weights around like Frisbees. This can make you feel, well, kind of small.

There is nothing at all wrong with being competitive, but you don't want to be measuring your performance against others, for the simple reason that you're more likely to give up when you don't feel that you measure up.

"There's always going to be somebody better than you," says Charles T. Kuntzleman, Ed.D., adjunct associate professor of kinesiology and director of the Blue Cross/Blue Shield Fitness for Youth program at the University of Michigan in Ann Arbor. "They're either going to be younger or they're going to be more skilled or they'll have more talent, training, a better day, whatever."

Obviously, then, if you focus too much on the superior skills of the competition, you may end up saying, "What's the point?"

Rule 2: Do Compete against Yourself

Even though you can't control what others do, what you do is very much in your control, says Lavon Williams, Ph.D., assistant professor of sport and exercise psychology in the Department of Physical Education at Northern Illinois University in DeKalb.

Researchers have found that athletes who measure themselves against themselves, who focus on their increasing competence in performing a task, are the ones who are most likely to achieve greater mastery of the task, to maintain greater interest in it, and to expend more effort in improving their performance.

"Individuals who define success relative to past performances or to themselves are more apt to be intrinsically motivated, which can lead to greater effort," says Dr. Williams. "That's kind of the bottom line."

In fact, exercise and that sense of competence tend to reinforce one another. The more competent you feel in your chosen form of exercise, the more likely you're going to do it, and the more you do it, the more competent you're going to feel.

If, for example, when you walk into that gym, you focus not on all those bulked-up guys but on how much more weight you can press this week than you could a month ago, you're going to find your own

Find Yourself a Faster Class of Friends

When you talk about what makes one guy stick to his exercise program and another guy fall off, you have to talk about those things that your Mama used to call your inner resources.

(As in: "Mama, I'm bored. There's nothin' to do around here." To which she would reply, "Boy, don't tell me that. It means you have no inner resources.")

There's no question that some of us have more inner resources than others, but that doesn't mean that you can't use a few outer resources to charge yourself up.

One of the best and most time-honored of these is peer pressure. Nothing so motivates a man as the fear of his peers.

"I think of one guy in particular," says Brian Wallace, Ph.D., chairman of sport fitness at the U.S. Sports Academy in Daphne, Alabama. "He was highly motivated, and he talked his friends into working out, too. He was a good salesman, and they all wound up doing it together, and that made them stick with it."

In fact, when you're trying to get active, it's a good idea to find people to be active with, says Dr. Wallace. "If you go home and your friends and family are not doing anything, you're not going to do anything either. Whereas if they are, you'll cross that threshold. Instead of saying, 'Nah,' you'll say, 'Okay, I'll do it.' And after a while, you'll feel guilty if you do miss."

progress a powerful motivator to keep on going.

Researchers define a person who measures his success by outperforming others as "ego-oriented" and a person who measures his success in his own performance as "task-oriented." Clearly, nobody is all one or the other, but if you focus on improvement in your own performance or are task-oriented, you are more likely to view yourself as successful.

"For example, we could be playing a game of basketball," Dr. Williams says. "You may win. If I were highly ego- and low task-oriented, I might not feel successful. But a high task-orientation can allow me to lose the game and yet feel successful because maybe I lost the game, but I played better than I ever played before. Relative to my own standards, I played well even though I lost to you."

Top Machines

Although gyms provide a lot of benefits—like good equipment, competent instruction, and free hot water—not every man feels comfortable baring his out-of-shape physique in front of a bunch of strangers. Which is why many men prefer working out at home.

But before you invest big bucks in expensive gear, it's worth considering which of the home-gym machines provide the most benefits. Researchers at the Medical College of Wisconsin and Veterans Affairs Medical Center, both in Milwaukee, looked at six indoor exercise machines and compared the number of calories each burned at similar levels of exertion.

The treadmill was clearly number one. Exercisers working out "somewhat hard" on the treadmill burned more than 200 more calories per hour than they did when working out at the same level of exertion on the stationary bike, which was the lowest ranked of the six machines.

Here's the complete ranking, from the best to the worst.

- **Treadmill**
- **Stair-climber**
- **Rowing machine**
- **Airdyne machine**
- **Cross-country ski machine**
- **Stationary bike**

Of course, if calories burned per hour were your only consideration, the choice would be clear. But you have to consider your personal preferences as well. If you hate treadmills but love cycling, you may be better off buying the stationary bike. Because even a great treadmill won't help you burn calories when it's catching cobwebs in a corner.

Rule 3: Do Keep Records

Since tracking your own progress can be a powerful motivating force, many experts suggest that you keep a log of how far you run or how much you lift each day. It's something to buck you up when you're in a slump. You can go back a few pages to see how you were doing a few weeks or months ago, and you'll get a sharp reminder of what a distance you really have come.

"The challenge of finding out what you're capable of doing is a far greater motivator than comparing yourself to somebody else," says Dr. Kuntzleman. "It's that inner self that really is crucial."

Beware, however, of using your log as a stick to beat yourself with. If you're a hypercritical sort, you may be tempted to view the record of your performance as less than stellar. If you do, you're going to undercut yourself completely.

"It depends a lot on your perception," says Dr. Williams. "I could be on the verge of burning out, and I could look back on that and see that as pressure. Like I used to run 5 miles a day, and now I don't want to, so what's wrong with me? If you're going to punish yourself with the information, it wouldn't be good. But if you can use it as a motivator, then it would be."

Rule 4: Do What You Like

It is amazing how many men choose an exercise—running, say—that they really don't enjoy very much. They do it because it's good for them. That's admirable as far as it goes, but it raises the question of how long they will likely stick with it.

Experts are unanimous on one point: Don't choose an exercise only because it's good for you; choose one that you enjoy. "It doesn't necessarily have to be, quote, 'exercise,' like doing a certain number of sit-ups," says Dr. Williams. "Instead, you could go out and do something that you enjoy. Pickup basketball, for example, can be a good workout. And if you're more apt to do it, I would encourage you to do that rather than something that you don't enjoy as much."

Rule 5: Don't Overdo It

It's a common trap. You discover a wonderful new sport or exercise—playing golf, say, or lifting weights. Naturally, you're enthusiastic, and you can't wait to get very, very good at it—immediately. So you blast into a 5-mile run on your second day out. Or try to lift 75 pounds when 50 is your limit. Or play 18 holes of golf even though you're exhausted after 9.

You wanted to get fit. Instead, you got hurt. Which means that whatever it was that struck your fancy all of the sudden doesn't seem like fun anymore.

The only way to stick with the program is to "choose an intensity that allows you to feel at least as good when you finish as when you started," says Dr. Dishman. Put another way, you want to choose a level of intensity that allows you to enjoy the workout rather than merely being relieved when it is over.

How much is too much? Ideally, you should exercise at a pace that feels somewhat hard but that doesn't make you gasp for breath, says Dr. Dishman. "The pulse rate will likely be in a range of 120 to 150 beats per minute. At this level, most healthy people can safely increase fitness and health while avoiding discomfort."

Rule 6: Don't Set Unreasonable Goals

Goals can be great motivators, but only when you achieve them. Setting expectations too high guarantees that you won't succeed, and nothing takes the wind out of an exercise program like falling on your face—figuratively and literally.

Suppose, for example, you promise yourself that you'll lose 20 pounds in two weeks: You're sabotaged from the outset because there is virtually no way you're going to succeed.

This isn't to say that you don't want to be ambitious. For example, promising yourself that you're going to lose 20 pounds (but without the time limit) gives you something to shoot for. But you should also plan a series of short-term, step-by-step goals that *are* attainable and that will bring you closer to your ultimate objective.

Rule 7: Do Set Reasonable Goals

Although long-term goals like "I want to live longer, be healthier, and banish my belly" are all very well and good, they're not going to keep you motivated in the day-to-day. For that you need short-term goals—as long as they are specific, realistic, achievable, and measurable.

Telling yourself, for example, "I will lose 3 pounds this week," is risky. After all, you may not lose the weight, and then you'll feel that you failed. A better goal would be "I will work out three times this week." The latter is better because it is totally achievable, and achieving that goal is a kind of reward in itself. In short, it is better to focus on what you can do than on what your bath-

---

Engineer Your Environment

There are lots of reasons for not exercising, from "I'm too tired" to "You don't really expect me to exercise in this weather, do you?"

Obviously, if you really don't feel like working out, there is no talking you into it. On the other hand, if you sort of feel like exercising but could just as easily talk yourself out of it, there are ways to push yourself in the right direction.

"Engineer your environment so that it is difficult, not easy, to talk yourself out of exercising," says Rod K. Dishman, Ph.D., professor and director of the Exercise Psychology Laboratory in the Department of Exercise Science at the University of Georgia in Athens.

For example:

- **Put exercise equipment near your bed at night so that it's the first thing you see in the morning.**
- **Keep workout clothes in your car or office so that you can't say, "I don't have them with me" when a workout opportunity arises.**
- **After work, take routes home past exercise facilities, not your favorite lounge.**
- **Put exercise signs or cartoons on the doors of your house, office, car, and refrigerator.**
- **Shame yourself into starting and reward yourself for finishing.**

---

room scales might tell you.

Set a lot of short-term goals and then reward yourself well when you meet them, recommends Kelly Brownell, Ph.D., co-director of the Yale University Eating and Weight Disorders Clinic. Indeed, he suggests shooting for a number of different goals at the same time. This not only provides variety but also guarantees that you'll meet at least some of them.

"So somebody might say, 'Okay, my goal for this week is to exercise three times, and I want to lose a pound, and I want to eat a healthy diet.' At the end of the week, let's say that they're unlucky and the scale doesn't show any change. They can still feel good when they succeed in those other areas."

Indeed, it doesn't always hurt to set up specific rewards for meeting your goals. You might, for example, say to yourself, "If I exercise three times this week, I'll buy that new Neil Young CD that just came out."

Rule 8: Don't Get Off the Track

Be careful, though, about letting rewards loom too large in your motivation. These are what researchers call extrinsic motivators, which is a fancy way of saying that they are reasons you give yourself to exercise (or do anything else) that have nothing to do with the real reasons why you should be doing it.

"An extrinsic motivator might be 'I'm going to run this race because I want to get this really cool T-shirt,'" says Dr. Williams. "So I might be training and running not for the purpose of being a more healthy individual but because I want something. The thing about extrinsic rewards is that once they're gone, whatever it took to get the reward is gone as well."

In other words, if you're trying to lose weight only because you have a class reunion coming up, your motivation is going to be all used up once that particular occasion is history.

On the other hand, sometimes extrinsic rewards can help give you the boost you need, particularly when they're contingent on your behavior. For example, no cappuccino on the patio until you have done your run, ride, or stroll.

"A friend of mine who wanted to start exercising just couldn't do it, so she started this thing where every time she exercised, she would put 50 cents or a dollar into a pot," says Dr. Williams. "It wasn't a great reward, but it kept her going because when she accumulated enough money, she could buy something she wanted. At first I thought, 'Ooh, that doesn't sound too good,' but what it did was keep her exercising long enough to where she started to reap the benefits of exercise and could exercise without those rewards."

Rule 9: Do Make Exercise an End in Itself

The ultimate goal of any sport or exercise plan is getting to the point that you're doing it for no other reason than that you enjoy it. Although you can have many good motives for starting an exercise program—to look good, live longer, and so forth—none of these has the kind of staying power as doing something because you like it.

Indeed, researchers (and long-term exercisers) agree: Once you have been exercising long enough, once your daily routine has become a habit, it will start feeling bad not to do it. It's at this point that you'll be intrinsically motivated, and that's a very powerful place to be.

Obviously, to achieve this level of "exercise nirvana," you have to find your own way. "Ignore fitness experts who know that they have the better plan for everyone," Dr. Dishman says. "Find the activities, the goals, the motivators, even the times of day that are right for you."

The rewards of exercise don't have to be deferred to some point in the distant future. The rewards are in the way exercise makes you feel every day, right now. "Your exercise program should make you feel better," says Dr. Dishman. "If it doesn't, change it until it does."

LIVING LEAN

27 EFFORTLESS (REALLY) WAYS TO PARE DOWN YOUR BELLY

This book is filled with exercises to make you sweat.

And we won't kid you: If you really want your gut to be its flattest, there's no getting around the fact that you have to put out some effort.

On the other hand, there are a multitude of ways to whittle your middle that are virtually painless. These "effortless efforts" require making only minor tweaks to your lifestyle. We have already showed you how, for example, you can burn off more than 5 pounds of fat in a year just by taking the stairs instead of the elevator at your office every day. That's the kind of thing we're talking about: Doing things that you have to do anyway but doing them the "hard" way. That and weaving a little more activity into the fabric of your day.

In the following pages the figures are for the average-size, 172-pound guy. If you weigh more, you'll burn a little more; if you weigh less, you'll burn a little less. The calculations are based on the calorie-burning computations of Charles T. Kuntzleman, Ed.D., adjunct associate professor of kinesiology and director of the Blue Cross/Blue Shield Fitness for Youth program at the University of Michigan in Ann Arbor, and on the fact that you have to burn off 3,500 calories to lose 1 pound.

Here, then, is the lazy man's guide to banishing your belly—more than 25 easy, virtually sweat-free methods to make your middle thinner.

1. Deliver your own paper. Good morning. It is, as Mr. Rogers says, a beautiful day in the neighbor-hood. So why not, instead of having your newspaper delivered to your doorstep, walk down the street a couple blocks to the nearest honor box? During this 10-minute excursion you can listen to birds tweeting, view the dew on the grass, and burn, depending on how fast you walk, anywhere from 34 (a leisurely stroll) to 121 (a wind-whistling-through-your-ears power walk) calories.

Either way, not a bad way to start the day. Even at the slowest pace, you can burn off 3½ pounds in a year. And at the fastest, 12½ big ones.

2. Work for your breakfast. Having scrambled eggs for breakfast? Or whipping up a batch of flapjacks? Don't use the electric mixer—beat your breakfast by hand. You'll burn 1 extra calorie for every minute you do it. Maybe not a huge thing, but every little bit counts. (Of course, you would be better off not beating anything but having a high-fiber cereal and some fresh fruit instead.)

3. Bike to work. If you're not that far away from your workplace, you can burn big by riding a bike instead of driving that boat to the office every day. At a moderate pace of 10 miles an hour, you can burn 175 more calories in a half-hour than you would driving—and that's just going one way. Round trip: 350. Do this every workday for a year, and you'll burn off 24 pounds.

4. Drive a stick. If it's not practical (or sane, due to traffic) to bike to work, you can burn a few extra calories in traffic by driving a stickshift. In a half-hour commute, you'll burn 20 more calories than that guy in the Continental, and 20 more on the way back home. We're talking, with holidays and two weeks off for vacation, more than 2 pounds a year.

5. Stand, don't sit. Even if you work at a desk all day, you can still work in a little more moving around. For starters, try standing up instead of sitting down whenever you're on the phone. Even if you're on the phone for just an hour a day, you can burn an extra 25 calories in that hour just by standing. That's more than 1½ pounds in a year.

6. Dump the Danish. Break time—and here comes the coffee cart. But instead of spending 10 minutes schmoozing while you inhale a Danish, take a brisk walk around the building. Doesn't matter whether it's inside or out. You can—even at a moderate pace—burn 58 calories in that 10 minutes. And if while you're walking you eat, say, an apple instead of that cheese Danish, you can subtract another 272 calories. Take that walk every workday, and you'll burn off nearly 4 pounds in a year. Substitute an apple habit for a cheese Danish habit, and you'll subtract another 18 pounds.

7. Schmooze to lose. Don't tell your boss we told you this, but you actually burn more calories schmoozing in the breakroom than you do reading, writing, or talking on the phone while sitting at your desk. Not a lot more, mind you. Only .09 calorie more a minute, in fact. But, hey, if you're one of those guys who spends a couple hours a day gossiping instead of working, you're almost 11 calories ahead of the deskbound and diligent. Sure, your co-workers may hate your guts, but, at the end of a year, your guts will be about ¾ pound lighter than theirs.

8. Stroll at lunch. Now is a great time to get to the gym or go for a run or do some other strenuous exercise-type thing. Obviously, if you do this regularly, you're going to burn beaucoup flab. But since this is a chapter about "effortless" ways to burn it, we won't go into that here. Instead, let's just say that you shouldn't let eating (and socializing) monopolize your lunch hour. Squeeze in another 10-minute stroll around the grounds, and in a year you're down another 4 pounds.

9. Shake yourself up. Slipping into that midafternoon drowse? You can break up your day by shaking yourself awake. Get up, stand up, and run in place for a couple of minutes. Even at just a moderate pace, you'll burn more than 15 extra calories. Do this a couple of times a day, and in a year you will have burned more than 2 pounds. Of course, when your co-workers see you running next to your desk like a hamster in a treadmill, they may look at you funny. But who cares? They're fat and you're not.

10. Do some yoga. Another way to wake yourself up while burning a few calories is to do a few minutes of yoga. Five minutes of stretches twice a day will burn 26 more calories than you would just sitting there. Loss in a year? About 1½ pounds.

11. Park far away. Finally! The whistle blows, and you're out of there. But you have to stop off at the supermarket on the way home. When you get there, park your car at the far end of the lot and hoof it. Even in the biggest parking lots, the walk probably won't amount to more than 5 minutes, but you'll still be burning an extra 25 to 30 calories (or more, depending on how much stuff you tote out of the store). Which means that if you go to the market or the shopping mall three times a week, you'll easily burn another pound in a year. Not only that, but you'll never again have trouble finding a parking space.

12. Don't do the drive-up window. By the same token, if you're having fast food for dinner tonight, you should slow it down. You're better off not having it in the first place, of course, but if you are, you should park your car and get up off your duff to walk in and place your order at the counter. Maybe you'll only burn 10 to 15 extra calories doing this, but if you do it a couple of times a week all year, you'll burn off at least one of those Double Whoppers with cheese and perhaps an order of fries.

13. Pump yourself up. When you have a choice between full service and self-service, always choose the latter. Pump your own, and while you're at it, wash the bugs off the windshield. You'll burn 2.42 more calories per minute than you would just sitting in the car. Not a lot in one sitting, but if you spend 10 minutes filling up every week of the year, that's one-third of a pound.

14. Ride into your television. Home at last, you flip on the tube. If, instead of just sitting there while you watch TV, you pedal away on a stationary bike—nothing frantic, just a nice steady pace—you'll burn an extra 3 calories every minute. An hour of pedaling nets you 180 calories. Do it every day, and you are down nearly 19 pounds at the end of a year.

15. Shoot some hoops. Trade in a half-hour of that tube time for a half-hour of shooting baskets in your driveway. We're not talking savage one-on-one here; we're just talking dribbling around and working on your hook shot. You'll burn 265 more calories than you would watching *Gilligan's Island*. Do this just a couple times a week for a year, and you lose more than 7 pounds.

16. Walk the dog. Is Bowser looking more like a hassock than a basset hound? Take him for a walk. A relaxing 20-minute stroll with your barker on a leash can burn 68 calories. Do this every day like a good dog owner should, and you can drop 7 pounds in a year, not to mention that Bowser will begin to resemble a dog again.

17. Roll out the barrel. It's Friday night, and the love of your life wants you to take her dancing. Ugh. But sometimes you have to make sacrifices for love. As long as you are doing that, do it right. Forget the fox-trot, forget the waltz, and forget that worthless wiggling everybody does to rock 'n' roll. What you want to do is the polka. It's the ultimate calorie-burning dance. You'll burn 10 big ones a minute, more than twice as many as those other dances. If your sweetheart drags you on the dance floor to polka for a couple of hours every couple of weeks, you'll be almost a pound lighter at year's end. (Next best type after the polka? Square dancing.)

18. Stay on top. Speaking of love, it's worth mentioning that as calorie-burning activities go, it's overrated. Still, you do have one big advantage over your mate—if, that is, you stay on top of the situation. You'll burn more than twice the calories per minute (5.58) when you're on top than she will on the bottom (2.5). In fact, she would burn more calories per minute if she went shopping. Spend 10 minutes every time you do it and do it twice a week, and love's labors will lose you about 1½ pounds a year.

19. Groom thyself. It's Saturday morning, and you don't have to go to the office, so why bother with the razor? Two reasons: You'll be a lot easier to look at, and that time spent grooming means calories burned. You'll burn 3.75 calories a minute showering, shaving, brushing your teeth, combing your hair, and getting dressed. All those weekends when you let yourself go to seed are opportunities to lose lard. If it takes you a half-hour to groom yourself, and you do it every weekend, you'll burn off more than 3 extra pounds a year.

20. Push, don't ride. First on your list of Saturday morning chores is mowing the lawn. Your neighbor, who didn't waste time grooming himself, is already out there jiggling around on his lawn tractor. Do you (a) get on your tractor and jiggle around, too; (b) crank up your old power mower and push it around; or (c) get out your old-fashioned push mower and make a day of it?

Obviously, you'll burn the most calories with the push mower, but let's be realistic. When you have a lawn of any size, you don't want to be dedicating your life to it. Fortunately, though, if you push a power mower instead of riding, you'll still burn 2.34 more calories a minute than your neighbor will and be almost a pound lighter come the end of summer.

21. Don't blow it. Of course, no sooner do you get past the mowing season than you find yourself deep into the leaf-raking season. Your neighbor is out in his front yard piloting a high-speed leaf blower (the high-decibel equivalent of banshees in a sack), burning off about as many calories as he would standing still. You, on the other hand, get out your trusty rake and burn more than 4 calories a minute. If you happen to live in big-tree country, you could easily have half a dozen weekends each fall where you spend 3 to 4 hours at it. If so, you can drop more than a pound when the trees drop their leaves.

22. Catch the drift. Suddenly, you find yourself under a foot of snow. Your neighbor, of course, is out there with his blower. You, however, go at it with a shovel. This is big-time calorie burning. If it's just a light snowfall, you'll burn more than 11 calories a minute; if it's heavy, you'll burn almost 20. You can burn more than a thousand calories in the hour it takes you to clear your walk and driveway. Three good snowstorms, and you're a pound lighter.

Of course, shoveling snow hardly qualifies as an "effortless" way to lose weight. But you have to do it anyway, so why not do it in such a way that you gain more than a clean driveway?

Just don't hurt yourself out there. Take small amounts of snow—no more than 3 inches at a time—and shovel slowly, says Dr. Kuntzleman. If the snowfall is wet and deep, pay the neighbor's kid to do the job for you.

23. Start chopping. When you get done shoveling all that snow, you can come inside and stretch out in front of the fire. Right? Only if you chop some wood. With ax in hand, you burn more than twice as many calories a minute (8.33) as your neighbor with his power saw. Let's say that you just have fires on weekend days and that you spend 20 minutes each weekend day chopping the wood you need for those fires. In the winter months of December, January, and February, you can burn off more than a pound of fat just by chopping wood.

24. Cast off that flab. Spring brings an end to the snow shoveling and wood chopping. Better yet, it brings the beginning of the fishing season. You can catch more than crappie depending on how you fish. The guy who wades upstream in pursuit of trout burns more than twice as many calories a minute as the guy who just sits in a boat and watches his bobber drift. If you're a wader, 3 hours of fishing will net you more than a thousand calories burned. Three Saturday mornings spent in pursuit of the rainbow will net you almost a pound.

25. Golf religiously. What, after all, are Sunday mornings for? Not that we're advising you to favor your mortal belly over your immortal soul, but the fact is that you'll burn a heck of a lot more calories playing the back nine than you will sitting or kneeling in church—6.59 more a minute, to be exact. Of course, if you ride in a cart, you'll burn a lot less. You have to carry your own clubs. If you do, you'll burn 70 calories for every hole you play.

Of course, you may also burn in hell. But then, that's your lookout.

26. Don't just sit there. Go to bed. Okay, here we go with the most effortless way to lose weight: Sleep. Granted, you don't burn a lot of calories sleeping, but you actually do burn more calories when you snooze than you do just sitting still—three times as many, in fact. Maybe this is because, like old Bowser barking and running in his sleep, you "do" more stuff in your dreams than you do just sitting. How many calories do you burn sitting?—.41 a minute. Sleeping?—1.25 a minute.

27. Read yourself thin. Of course, just about any other activity that you can name beats sleeping. Even watching TV beats it, though not by much (.16 calorie a minute more, if you really want to know). But if it's late and you can't sleep, and you have your choice between watching TV and reading a book, you'll burn a quarter calorie more a minute if you read. Which, if you think about it, could really add up, given that the average American guy watches more than 3½ hours of the tube a day. If you're that average American guy, and you started reading instead, you would be—yes, we're really going to tell you this— more than 5 pounds lighter in a year. Now, that's a good argument for literacy.

Coping with the Ups and Downs
Especially the Downs

You are right. It is a dumb title. Who needs help coping with the ups?

The downs, though—now there's something to cope with.

There will be times when you just can't seem to find the wherewithal to strap on those running shoes, and the mere thought of going to the gym exhausts you. And there will be times when you succumb to old habits and toss a couple pounds back on your gut just by spending the weekend eating junk.

So how do you find the strength, stamina, stubbornness—whatever you want to call it—to deal with that?

The answer is as old as Epictetus, the philosopher who, nearly 2,000 years ago, propounded the principles of Stoicism.

"Everything," he said, "has two handles—by one of which it ought to be carried and by the other not."

Say, for example, you skipped the gym for a few, dined at the D.Q. and Fat Boy's Bar-B-Q, and put a couple more pounds to the round on you. How will this affect your overall progress? It all depends on which handle you try to carry it by.

If you try to carry it by the handle of "This means I'm a failure," you'll be dragged down by the weight of it. But if you choose the handle of "Okay, so I took a little vacation," you can not only carry it but you can also shake it off and move on.

Get Real

Fast-forwarding to the soon-to-be twenty-first century, we have gotten no wiser than Epictetus.

Daniel Kosich, Ph.D., a senior consultant for the International Association of Fitness Professionals and author of *Get Real: A Personal Guide to Real-Life Weight Management*, stresses the same principles as those stressed by the great Stoic.

If you fall down, he says, get up, dust yourself off, and get on with it (handle number 2). As for keeping up when you just don't feel like it, Dr. Kosich suggests that you start being realistic and honest with yourself.

First of all, "getting the physique of an elite athlete only happens when you train like an elite athlete," he says. "Regardless of the number of commercials we see that say that there's some easy, simple way to get to look like people who work out 2 hours a day, it doesn't happen unless you work out 2 hours a day."

Second, he says, "Let's be honest: You aren't always going to look forward to exercise. I don't know about you, but there are lots of mornings that I wake up and I don't want to go on my bike ride. But I know that if I do the bike ride, I'm going to feel good afterward. It's not always going to be fun. You can't expect it to be fun. If you think it is, you're going to drop out."

Third, "try focusing on the afterward part instead of trying to trick yourself into thinking that interesting. Certainly, the more fun you make them, the more likely it is you'll stick to them.

And how do you do that? By adding variety to your exercise diet.

"I think that people who do the same things all the time for a long time either are involved in some form of competition or else they are going to drop out or get injured at some point," says S. Boyd Eaton, M.D., associate clinical professor of radiology and adjunct associate professor of anthropology at Emory University in Atlanta.

"It's much better," says Dr. Eaton, "to have a situation where you vary your exercise activities. If you can jog and bicycle and swim and do things like that for aerobic exercise, that's great. And if you do resistance training, you need to vary your program at intervals so that you can be working on different muscles or working on the same ones from a different approach."

This type of varied approach—weight lifting plus aerobic exercise or jogging plus swimming—is called cross-training. We talk about it further in Cross-Training on page 123. For now, let's just say that mixing up your workouts is a great motivator. It's hard to get bored when you're doing three or four (or more) activities a week. In addition, cross-training hits your muscles and joints from different angles, so you get a better overall workout.

Here's the kicker. You'll burn more fat cross-training than you will sticking with just one exercise. For example, a study found that men and women who split their half-hour workouts into equal parts of strength training and aerobic conditioning lost twice as much weight as those who did only aerobic exercise.

Keep the Big Picture

Finally, don't look at any of this as a thing apart from the rest of your life. Recognize instead that it's an integral and necessary part of your life, and "you do it the same way that you brush your teeth and take a shower," Dr. Kosich says.

"It's just an important thing to do because it's part of taking care of yourself. If you can adapt that kind of a positive outlook at the way you're taking care of yourself, the whole weight-management thing just fits into your lifestyle. It's just all part of the mix," he says. "And doing the kinds of things that we know we need to do sets the stage for a much healthier outcome."

you ought to be really looking forward to the beginning part of it," Dr. Kosich says. "There are a lot of parts of physical activity that aren't fun at all, but I've never known an occasion when it didn't feel better afterward."

Find Fun

Boredom will sabotage any workout plan, so you should make an effort to keep your workouts

MAKING TIME FOR EXERCISE
TIME WAITS FOR NO ONE

Imagine for a moment that you've just gone to the doctor and he's given you the bad news: You have kidney disease. The good news, though, is that you can live a lot longer if you'll do dialysis three times a week.

What's the likelihood that you're going to say, "Sorry, Doc, I just don't have time for that"?

"As you well know, one of the major detractors from staying with exercise programs is saying, 'I just don't have enough time,'" says Daniel Kosich, Ph.D., a senior consultant for the International Association of Fitness Professionals and author of *Get Real: A Personal Guide to Real-Life Weight Management*.

But, he adds, if a doctor says that you need dialysis, "all of a sudden that goes right to the top of your priority list. And it's not a question of 'Well, I don't have time because I have this appointment or I have some other commitment.' You go do it because it's important to your health."

So why don't most of us find time to exercise? Mainly, Dr. Kosich says, because we don't recognize that it's just as important to us as dialysis is to the kidney patient.

"It's not such an acute situation that people will put it in the perspective of saying, 'This needs to be a priority for me, this needs to be something that I recognize is so important for me and my health

and the long-term quality of my life that I have to prioritize it,'" Dr. Kosich says.

Once you recognize how important exercise is to living a long and healthy life, you'll make time to incorporate it into your daily routine.

"And maybe it means that I don't go to the meeting, or maybe it means that I don't have this commitment or I don't make the engagement because my active lifestyle becomes a higher priority," he says. "It's kind of a readjustment of what people think are the most important things."

Unfortunately, a lot of us don't make that readjustment until we have a heart attack. Then, if we survive it, we suddenly get religion. We finally realize that if we can't find time to exercise, we may be—game over—out of time.

Incredible Time-Savers

So much for the sermon. That still leaves you with the very practical problem of finding time in your busy schedule for exercise.

Fortunately, there are some very practical solutions.

To begin with, you have to recognize that you really do have the time, if you want to.

"It's all about how you choose to spend your time," says Harriet Schechter, co-author of *More Time for Sex: The Organizing Guide for Busy Couples* and founder of The Miracle Worker Organizing Service in San Diego, which, since 1986, has helped thousands of people (and businesses) organize their lives. "You have to realize that you have a choice. Stop giving away your choice by saying, 'I don't have time to do this.' You know that's just an excuse."

Here are some of her suggestions for getting your time (and your life) under control.

Make a Time Budget

For starters, Schechter says, you need to figure out where all your time is going now.

There are only 168 hours in a week. How are you spending them? Estimate—in writing—how much time you spend each day sleeping, eating, working, grooming, exercising, commuting, doing chores, running errands, hanging out with friends and family, making whoopee with your mate, and just generally amusing yourself (going to the movies, watching TV, and reading books, magazines, and newspapers). Also, how much time are you wasting each day looking for your car keys, wallet, or glasses or sorting through the same piles of papers on your desk?

Now, take a hard look at your record. You may be in for some rude revelations, but they can suggest some immediate solutions.

Unplug Yourself

If you're an average American male, you're watching more than 3½ hours of television per day. Indeed, says Schechter, this is where many people's "missing" time goes.

Hey, dude, that's more than 24 hours a week! You're spending one day out of every seven watching TV!

And that means you're spending 53 days a year in a daze. Think about it. If you live to be 70, you'll have spent 10 years of your life on Planet Television.

Obviously, this suggests at least one area where you may find some time to exercise. Cut just 1 hour of television out of every day, and you have 7 hours a week in which to get fit.

Don't Answer That!

Another appliance that takes great bites out of our day is the telephone. Invented to serve us, it has become our master. Its random intrusions and interruptions play havoc with any kind of schedule, and yet we cannot let it just ring.

Indeed, so complete is our enslavement that what was once a sanctuary—the automobile—is now just a rolling telephone booth. Some of us even go so far as to carry a cellular phone with us when we go for a walk in the woods.

This kind of "addiction" leads to situations where you lose control of your day. If you duck out for a midday workout, for example, and then on the way to the gym take a call in your car, that call can tie you up long enough to rob you of your workout.

So if you truly want to take control of your life and have the time you need to do what you want to do, you should screen your calls with voice mail or an answering machine, Schechter says. "You don't have to answer every time it rings."

Instead, ask yourself, who's in charge here: me or my telephone? "It's really about stepping back and saying, 'I don't have to do that,'" Schechter says. "It's about changing your perspective on it."

Schechter has a few other phone tips. If it's a business call, make a quick list of items to be discussed and stick to it. If the person you're calling is a talker, let him know up front how much time you have to chat.

She has an interesting way of doing that: "I will use a ticking timer. If I have somebody who talks more than I do, then I'll make sure they hear the ticking. When the timer buzzes, it gives me a way to get off the hook."

Another approach that she recommends is to use your fax machine instead of your telephone to send quick notes to someone. Faxes don't require you to squander time on gossip and pleasantries.

Organize Your Paperwork

Another great sinkhole of time, Schechter says, is the time we spend trying to find things: bills, letters, business cards, notes, receipts, and records.

Most of us don't have any systematic method for keeping our paperwork in order; instead we subscribe to the big-pile-on-the-kitchen-counter method or the big-pile-that-was-on-the-kitchen-counter-but-now-is-stuffed-in-a-drawer-because-company's-coming method.

And every time we need something, we waste time ransacking that same pile (or, even worse, multiple piles) of paper.

To get an idea of just how much this is costing you, Schechter provides this formula: Estimate how much time you spend looking for things each day and multiply that number by your hourly wage (or whatever you think your time is worth). Then multiply that figure by the days in a year. If your hourly wage is $20, say, and you spend 10 minutes a day looking for stuff, you're wasting more than $1,000 a year.

The solution? Set up a "paper-flow" or "action-file" system of several clearly labeled files or stacking trays. Categories can be anything you like, but Schechter suggests that they might include Bills to Pay, Catalogs, Coupons, Letters, Invitations, To Do, To File, and To Read.

Then, when paper comes into your house, categorize whatever you can and deal with it immediately. If it's a bill you have to pay, pay it; if you can't pay it just then, file it in the Bills to Pay tray. Also, don't forget to make good use of your "circular file" for any junk mail that comes in. Indeed, the quickest way to process mail is to stand next to a wastebasket while you go through it.

Toss It

Speaking of which, one of your goals should be to toss as much stuff as quickly as you can. After you have paid those bills, answered those letters and whatnot, you should decide what to do with

Exer-snacks

The Centers for Disease Control and Prevention in Atlanta and the American College of Sports Medicine, which is headquartered in Indianapolis, have recommended that "every U.S. adult should accumulate 30 minutes or more of moderate-intensity physical activity on most, preferably all, days of the week."

This doesn't mean that you have to carve out 30-minute blocks of time. You can gain tremendous health benefits just by grabbing little bits of exercise—5 minutes here, 10 minutes there—the same way you might grab a snack.

"There's good data showing that minimum amount has a clear effect even if it's broken up into smaller amounts of time," says David Levitsky, Ph.D., professor of nutritional sciences and psychology at Cornell University in Ithaca, New York.

So, for example, if you take the stairs instead of riding the elevator, walk instead of driving, do a quick 10-minute walk around the office instead of taking a coffee break, pedal a stationary bike instead of sitting while watching TV, garden, do housework, rake leaves, or throw the old pigskin up and down the backyard with your kids, you're accumulating time toward your daily total.

And let's face it. No matter how busy you are, there is nobody who is so busy that he doesn't have moments in his day that could be filled with mini-bouts of exercise.

the paper left over. Some stuff—canceled checks, receipts, insurance policies, warranties, instruction manuals, personal papers—you need to keep, and you'll need to set up a permanent filing system to do that.

But most people keep a lot more of this kind of stuff than they really need. Yes, you probably want to keep your bank statements, canceled checks, credit card statements, insurance payments, utility bills, and mortgage payments for at least a year, after which you can archive them. But you don't need to keep the stub from every bill you pay. Remember that every check you write is a record of payment. The rest is often superfluous.

To really get your paperwork under control, here are a few points to keep in mind.

BEWARE OF SENTIMENT. Don't think that just because you have set up a filing system, you should keep every piece of correspondence. Once you have answered a card or letter, toss the card or letter. If you're sentimental, just remember that sentiment has its price, and in just a few years you can end up with boxes upon boxes of cards and letters that neither you nor your children nor your children's children will ever want to read.

Schechter says that people often tell her that they just can't get rid of stuff.

"I say, 'Yes, you can. If I held a gun to your head, you could easily get rid of it. But you do not choose to get rid of it.' "

SAY GOOD-BYE TO OLD NEWS. Catalogs, magazines, and newspapers have fairly short life spans of usefulness and are rarely revisited. Toss them on a regular basis, or they'll turn your house into a landfill. We once knew a fellow who would never throw out an issue of the *New York Times* until he had read every word of it. Not surprisingly, given how much there is to read in any day's *Times*, his apartment was furnished with stacks of newspapers going back to the last decade.

CLIP NOT, WANT NOT. If you're into using coupons, you may want to examine whether they're really saving you that much. Remember, your time is worth something. If you spend an hour every Sunday morning clipping and organizing coupons from the newspaper and add another half-hour or so to your shopping by trying to match coupons to items, you may not be saving all that much, Schechter says. You might better use that time for a long bike ride around the reservoir.

Everything in Its Place

Of course, a lot of us don't just get lost in our paperwork; heck, we have to search for our car keys every morning. The solution to this problem is painfully simple: If you always put things in the same place—your car keys in a bowl by the door, for example—then you'll always know where they are.

But some of us resist even that much organization. Schechter has a theory to explain this; she says that people who do this suffer from "treasure hunt syndrome."

"My theory is that they like the adrenaline rush that they get when they find something," she says. "Why else would they not do something that is as simple as putting something back in the same place, in a logical place?"

Making It Sacred

We've discussed a lot of ways to put extra time in your days. If you follow even a few of these suggestions, you'll easily have the few hours a week it takes to nail down a pretty good exercise program.

But time is only part of the equation. Equally, if not more important, is commitment. Exercise time should occupy a place on your calendar as inviolable as any business appointment, as essential as going to the doctor, as lifesaving as dialysis for a kidney patient. You wouldn't skip out on any of these critical appointments just because something else came up, would you?

You should set aside times in your appointment book for exercise and go at those times. Don't be diverted. This is your sacred hour. You have an appointment with yourself, and, after all, who is more important?

It all comes down to you making a choice. "Whether you choose to admit it or not, you are choosing to behave a certain way," Schechter says. "Let's be clear about this. And you have a right to choose not to exercise. But you also have to live with the outcome. If you don't like the outcome, change the choice."

How to Dress Lean
Buying the Right Look

"Society," said the Scottish essayist Thomas Carlyle, "is founded upon Cloth," and "Man's earthly interests are all hooked and buttoned together, and held up, by Clothes."

Carlyle was right, of course. If you have ever run into your boss in the locker room, you know what he means. There is something disconcertingly egalitarian in finding the both of you reduced to the same unprepossessing flesh.

Clothes define us. They tell our fellows who we are. If you doubt this, try getting into a four-star restaurant wearing a "Stud Monkey" T-shirt, or try getting out of a biker bar while wearing a seersucker suit and a boater.

We do judge a man by the cut of his clothes. A good outfit has the power to lift a man up from the shuffling masses, to transform the humblest among us into something that passes for noble. More important, it can alter the bellied into a body that passes for svelte.

This isn't to say that, rather than exercising and watching what you eat, you simply resort to camouflage. You still have to keep working out, and you still have to have the courage to walk through a world of trash food without succumbing to its blandishments, but, hey, as long as you're changing your life, you might as well change your wardrobe.

To help you do this, we have gone to the tailors, fashion directors, and wardrobe consultants—those people who have the gift of garb—and asked them: How should a man dress so that he will look his leanest?

The Seven Dudly Sins

Clothiers have long understood that a man's duds, carelessly chosen, can make him look tubby. Wearing the right duds, however, will reduce his apparent size, says Stan Tucker, fashion director for Saks Fifth Avenue in New York City. "You really can dress lean," he says. "It's when you don't pay attention to the details that you accentuate your body weight."

To help you look your leanest, we have compiled a list of fashion faux pas—what we call the Seven Dudly Sins—that can add substantial bulk to your frame. Remember that the flip side of every one of these don'ts is a do. If you do the do's, you can, without losing an actual ounce, lose pounds in the eyes of your beholders.

1. The Sin of Tightness

Men don't like admitting that they're overweight, even to themselves. Which is why there is a tendency, when buying off the rack or getting fitted for a new set of clothes, to shrink the truth a bit.

"Sometimes a customer will come in, and you'll say, 'What's your waist?' " Tucker notes. "And he'll say, '34.' And then you measure him and say, 'The tape measures 38.' 'I am not,' he'll say."

The problem with tight clothes is that they put your diameter on display. If you wear a suit, for example, that hugs your love handles—what Tucker calls your inner tubes—it will show them off.

"Wearing tight clothes will accentuate fat anywhere on your body," Tucker says. "A man who is overweight should not wear anything tight. They should be a bit looser, or they should fit him better."

So rule number one is to get someone to fit you, says Sheree Crosier, manager of the Personal Touch service at the Dallas branch of the Nordstrom chain of specialty retail stores. "Regardless of what size you are, the most important thing is to get someone, a professional, to fit you so that you're getting the right size," Crosier says. "Because men do have a tendency to want to get into the last size they purchased."

2. The Sin of Brightness

"A lot of people who are overweight have a tendency to wear clothes that call attention to them," says Tucker. "That's one of the biggest mistakes."

So forget the loud plaids and anything that resembles neon.

Go for dark solid colors like black, brown, or navy blue, advises Martin Greenfield, chairman of Martin Greenfield Clothiers in Brooklyn, New York. These colors will actually make you look smaller than light, bright colors will.

If you must have patterns, select very subdued ones. You might, for example, have a glen plaid suit, but a plaid in which the pattern is just a slightly different tone than the background—so much so that you really can't see it without scrutinizing the suit.

3. The Sin of Tiedness

Think of a tie as an arrow, a one-way sign pointing to your gut. The only question, really, is do you want that sign to be a low-profile one or all flashing lights?

"A tie is one of the few pieces of men's apparel that can describe his personality somewhat," says Tucker. "And if you're very large and it's a garish tie, well, this brings attention directly to your middle. That's the first thing people see."

As with all your other clothes, your ties should be subtle and used as an accessory. Patterns are fine, but only if they don't buttonhole the eyes of passersby. "You don't want your tie to stand out so much that that's all they'll see," Crosier says.

4. The Sin of Wideness

Nothing says, "Behold my belly!" like a big, wide belt with a big brass buckle.

"You see these truck drivers, and many times they have a large beer belly accentuated by a belt with a large buckle," says Tucker. "It's somewhat of a phenomenon, I guess."

Obviously, your choice should be a narrower belt with a simple buckle. It will hold your pants up without drawing all that attention to your midsection.

5. The Sin of Stripedness

Unless your body is model-lean, horizontal is a thing that you never want your clothes to be. This is because horizontal lines running across your body emphasize your width, whereas vertical lines call attention to your length.

Try this experiment at home. Pull out that old rugby shirt, the one with the big, bold horizontal stripes, and put it on. Take a look at yourself in the mirror. See how wide you look? Now, replace that shirt with a solid color or a simple pinstripe. See how much narrower you have suddenly become?

A pinstripe shirt "elongates you," says Greenfield. "You don't want to have too much going across because that makes you bigger."

6. The Sin of Hipness

Also known as the Sin of the Low-Slung Levis, this is what happens when you drop your pants several degrees of latitude below your equator.

"Many men who are overweight have a tendency to wear their trousers below their stomach," Tucker says. "All it does is accentuate their stomach—unfortunately, it's just hanging out there."

Wear your trousers at your waist (and not down around your hips), and you will look leaner, Tucker says.

7. The Sin of Tweediness

Fat fabrics make you look fatter. If you're a guy who favors knobby tweeds or wide-wale corduroys, you're going to look a little knobby and wide-whale yourself.

"They will make you look heavier because they look heavy themselves," Tucker says.

Instead, go for a much finer weave of wool in your suits and for thinner fabrics, generally. "Save your tweeds for a sport jacket," Tucker says.

"Heavy tweeds are excellent for thin people," Greenfield adds. "Those are beautiful fabrics to wear, but you have to be built for them."

Suiting Up

Of course, there's more to dressing lean than knowing what to avoid. How, for example, do you buy a suit so that it fits you properly?

To begin with, don't buy it off the first rack you find. "The worst habit I find with men is that they never take time to shop for themselves," says Greenfield, who has been a tailor for more than 50 years and has made clothes for presidents Dwight D. Eisenhower, Lyndon Baines Johnson, Gerald Ford, and Bill Clinton.

"A woman will spend twice as much time or 10 times as much time when she goes shopping. She

Details Make the Man

Dressing so that you look your best can have a tremendous impact in how people perceive you. Not only because you will look more poised, professional, and self-possessed but also because you will feel that way, too. And when you feel that way, you're going to act that way.

The most important thing that you can do is pay attention to the details, says Sheree Crosier, manager of the Personal Touch service at the Dallas branch of the Nordstrom chain of specialty retail stores. "It's like detailing your car," she says. "You can have an old car, but if it's detailed really nicely, it'll look like a brand-new car. It's the detailing that sets you apart from other people."

So how do you detail yourself?

Obviously, the first thing that you need to do is put together a wardrobe that fits you properly and that you feel comfortable in. But dashing duds don't mean a thing if you don't take proper care of them.

For example, "sometimes men don't take the time to have their shirts laundered, and they'll look wrinkled," Crosier says. "They're going to look 100 percent better in a laundered shirt than if they're trying to press it themselves . . . unless they're really good at it."

Even when you're dressing casually, Crosier says, you should try to "look like you are put together. Make sure that things are tailored properly, pressed, and laundered."

If these seem like silly, trivial matters, remember that the man who attends to them will always look better than the man who doesn't. "All of that is going to be much more important in the whole look than anything else," Crosier says.

knows everything they have in the store. But men are very impatient," Greenfield says.

This is particularly bad news if you carry a lot of your weight in your belly—a body type Greenfield refers to as portly.

"If you're portly," he says, "you can't buy a suit ready-made because people don't carry it. So the first thing that you should do is have somebody make up clothing for you, not select from the pieces that are hanging in the store. Because you're doing yourself no favor."

Whether you're buying a suit off the rack and having it altered, or having it built from the ground up, here's what experts advise for getting the best fit.

BE YOURSELF. When you show up for a fitting, there is a natural tendency to show yourself to advantage—by standing straighter than you usually do, for example, or pulling in your gut a few inches.

Don't give nature a helping hand. A good suit is fitted not only to your size, shape, and posture, but even to your habits. "When you're having a custom suit made, and you carry your wallet in your hip pocket, sometimes the tailor will say, 'Take that wallet out.' No. Don't take that wallet out," Greenfield says. "Because you want the suit to fit and to cover up that wallet."

Just as your tailor can cover that wallet, so, too, can he cover your gut. "I want to cover up so that he should show no stomach," Greenfield says.

GO WITH THE STYLE. Many heavy men won't wear a double-breasted suit because they worry that all those extra buttons will make them look fatter. This is only true, Tucker says, when the suit in question is a "six-on-one," which requires that you button only one button.

"If you have a large stomach and you button the jacket, as you should, and it is a six-on-one, it has a tendency to gape open. So I would say that's not the correct silhouette for you. You should not buy the double-breasted six-on-one," Tucker adds.

Instead, he says, go with a double-breasted six-on-two (where you can button the middle button, better covering your middle) or a single-breasted two-button suit.

KEEP IT CLOSED. Wearing your jacket unbuttoned may give you extra breathing room but at the expense of how you look. "If you keep it unbuttoned, which no one should do anyway, it will make you look larger. It will not be flattering," Tucker says.

DRAW THE EYE UPWARD. To achieve a longer, leaner look, Crosier advises getting a suit with an extended shoulder. "That's going to draw attention up to the shoulders and away from the midsection."

TRY A SINGLE VENT. As a rule, Tucker says, a jacket with a single vent at the back works well for men who are large in the belly, but "it depends upon the person and his derriere. Some people's rear end protrudes, and when it does, it will open that vent. And that makes you look fat and makes the suit look as if it doesn't fit."

Look at your back, he says, to make sure that when you button your jacket across your stomach it doesn't pull the vent open.

CONSIDER PLEATED PANTS. "Some men will tell you, 'I don't like to wear pleated trousers because they make me look fat,'" Tucker says. "That, to me, is not true. When you really look fat is when you wear a flat-front trouser because you really do see the fat. It's very much evident. It's like having on a swimsuit."

Greenfield, on the other hand, doesn't recommend that heavier men wear pleats. But if they do, they should get pleats that face the pockets because they stay flatter. "The traditional pleats that face the fly, you have to know when you sit down you have more goods in the front."

BEWARE THE TIGHT ARMHOLE. Fashion fluctuates between tighter and looser armholes in suits, but for the sake of your fit and comfort, make sure that yours are loose enough that your suit doesn't bind and pull whenever you try to move.

Downsizing

No matter how well-tailored your suits are, there may come a time when they no longer fit because you have managed to drop some weight. "If a person loses 5 pounds, that's one size," says Greenfield. "It's 1 inch. If a person loses 10 pounds, it's 2. What is a size? A size is an inch. An inch around your waist. An inch around your chest."

Should you rush out and have all your suits retailored? Not right away. While your goal is to lose weight and keep it off, life is filled with setbacks. The last thing that you want is to have your suits retailored for the new, thin you, only to take them back to the tailor six months later because you gained the weight back.

"I beg them not to take in, at least for one year, the old clothing," Greenfield advises. "Don't do anything until you know you're going to stay there."

Of course, once you have succeeded, then it's time to celebrate. "The first suit I'll make you is going to be fitted to your body so that you're going to look unbelievable," Greenfield says. "I'm going to make you look fitted, slim, and when you walk out, you'll look like a million dollars. Everybody will say, 'Hey, you look so young.'"

How to Act Lean
Slim Tricks of the Stage

As any actor will tell you, the "truth" is whatever he can persuade the audience to believe.

A talented actor can change his appearance and persona to fit any role. How else could an aggressive, charismatic actor like Ernest Borgnine convincingly portray the painfully shy lead in the Academy Award–winning film *Marty*?

What works on the stage can also work for you. Since truth—or at least peoples' perceptions of it—is in the eye of the beholder, there is absolutely no reason not to *act* leaner than you really are.

Of course, nothing short of a corset will make you look leaner if you're as big as a barn. There are limits to the powers of stagecraft. John Candy could never have played Clint Eastwood.

Still, professional actors have a number of techniques for making themselves look taller and leaner, says Charles Werner Moore of the University of Connecticut, who has taught acting for nearly 40 years. Some of his students have included George Peppard, television producer Steven Bochco, René Auberjonois from *Star Trek: Deep Space Nine*, and Gates McFadden, who played Dr. Beverly Crusher on *Star Trek: The Next Generation*.

So how do you act lean? Here are some secrets from stage and screen.

PUT YOUR LEGS TO WORK. "If you take a look at some actors who aren't that tall, you'll see that the one thing they do is take very long steps. Striding out really does amazing things. It makes you look taller," Moore says. "If you know the old movie *The Bridge on the River Kwai*, take a look at Alec Guinness walking,

and you'll see precisely what I mean."

STAND STRAIGHT. Nothing says plump like a posture that slumps, says Moore. "Don't slump. One does naturally, but not when one is trained to use the body as an artistic instrument. You have to train yourself to stand up straight."

THINK UP. Since it's natural to slump a little bit, you may have to remind yourself to pull yourself upright. In classes on stage movement, students are taught "to feel as though somebody were lifting you by your hair. In other words, to think up," Moore says.

GET STUCK UP. Attitude alone can affect how you carry yourself, and this in turn affects how others see you. "It's a matter of what would be considered arrogance in most people," Moore says. "You have to carry yourself as though you were smelling something bad. You're somebody, in other words."

And that, he says, will give people the impression that you're taller and leaner than you actually are. "If you think of yourself as a little bit better than others, you might look a little leaner. You look more authoritative, which enables you to stand up and look down at other people."

Laurence Olivier, for example, was well under 6 feet tall, but he carried himself as though he were 6-foot-2. "It's a matter of training and keeping in shape and standing up as though you were somebody," Moore says.

AMAZE WITH GRACE. Speaking of keeping in shape, this is much more important than you might think. The key physical quality of any good actor is *ambidextrous grace*, which Moore defines as being able "to move like a halfback, just as well to

Using the Beat

Having a passion for music will not make you appear lean. But it very well could help you become lean. Studies in the Department of Physical Therapy at Springfield College in Massachusetts have shown that people who exercise while listening to music tend to exercise longer than those who don't, says Linda Tsoumas, Ph.D., chairman of the physical therapy program.

In one study, researchers asked students to pedal a stationary bike at 70 revolutions per minute. They found that men who pedaled while listening to tunes stuck with it an average of 29 percent longer than those listening to the sound of their own panting. Similarly, women listening to music pedaled 25 percent longer than women who did not.

It didn't appear to matter what music the students listened to, she adds. Whatever they wanted to slap in their portable stereos did the trick.

In other words, you're likely to work out longer if you have a song in your heart—and if you get to pick the song.

the right as to the left, and to be very flexible."

Many of the great performers—like Jackie Gleason, to name just one—lugged around considerable amounts of weight. But because they were graceful and quick on their feet, they never looked as heavy as they really were.

Even if you're not in perfect shape, you can substantially improve your physical grace just by adding stretches to your usual workouts. Or sign up for a weekend or evening dance class; ballet would be ideal. The training that you'll get in dance will add tremendous fluidity to your movements, which will make you appear much leaner than you really are.

"In basketball, you have these great lumbering monsters who move incredibly," Moore says. "Even though they're so big, they can move beautifully."

TAKE A BOW. It's not always easy to feel lean, particularly when your pants' size isn't going down as fast as you would like. But if you have been working out and have successfully sweated off some pounds, you have every right to feel a little taller and a little better than most people. Remember that only about 15 percent of Americans are working out vigorously, so you're in some elite company.

"All this work that you've put into making yourself leaner is not going to do anything for you unless you change in your mind your self-perception—to know that you look good and to act that way," Moore says. "You should bring it into your way of looking at yourself and in how you move."

SCENARIO 1: Seasonal Blues

AGE: 44

WEIGHT: 215

EXERCISE ROUTINE: Lifts weights at the gym three times a week and runs 5 to 6 miles a day the other days.

LIFESTYLE: He's an acquisitions editor at a small publishing company, meaning he has a desk job. Usually eats lunch at his desk because he uses the lunch hour to work out. Eats pretty healthfully, with occasional indulgences in ice cream and other sweets. Drinks moderately, usually no more than two drinks a day.

WEIGHT GOALS: Would like to lose 10 to 15 pounds.

PROBLEM: While he is able to stick with his workout program pretty faithfully through the spring and summer months, he finds himself fighting a growing lethargy as fall wends into winter. Often, it seems as though it's all he can do to just get out of bed in the morning. Moreover, as the days get shorter and colder, he finds himself struggling with overwhelming cravings for chocolate and fettuccine Alfredo. As a result, all his hard-earned fitness gains and weight loss tend to get lost every winter, and he ends up with about 10 new pounds to lose each spring.

Just about everybody gets weary of winter. All those cold, dark days make a body want to curl up in a cave and gnaw on a plate of pasta.

But for some, the problem is a lot more serious than just a seasonal slowdown. This guy is clearly suffering from a condition called seasonal affective disorder, or SAD, in which the body essentially reacts to the cold and dark by shutting down, says Norman E. Rosenthal, M.D., director of light therapy studies at the National Institute of Mental Health and author of *Winter Blues: Seasonal Affective Disorder: What It Is and How to Overcome It*.

Symptoms of SAD include depression, extreme lethargy (you just don't want to get out of bed), and irresistible cravings for sweets and starches. Indeed, some people will put on as much as 40 pounds in a winter, and, although they may lose most of that weight the following summer, they never quite lose it all. It's as if each winter deposits another layer of sediment on their frames until one day they wake up and realize that they're 50 (or more) pounds overweight.

Still, there is a solution for a man like this, says Dr. Rosenthal. For one thing, he has half the year locked. Spring and summer, he has the will, the drive, and the energy to eat lean and exercise, and he can really shed those pounds. It's the other half of the year that he needs to worry about.

Perhaps the best way for him to control his weight and cravings, and to muster the energy to stick with his workouts, is to plug in a light box, says Dr. Rosenthal. These are specialized light sources that consist of a battery of fluorescent tubes in a box, which are placed on a table or desk and which provide anywhere from 2,500 to 10,000 lux of light. By spending a certain amount of time each day sitting in front of one of these boxes, people with this condition may find that they can get through the winter without feeling blue, famished, and fatigued all the time.

When combined with exercise and the proper diet, a light box could make it possible for this man to lose weight in the winter. Turning on the lights will do more than lift his mood, Dr. Rosenthal adds. "Light therapy reduces the amount of carbohydrates taken in and the appetite in people who are seasonal," he says.

Before investing in a light box, however, this man might want to try some simpler (and less expensive) remedies. Keeping his house well-lit, for example, could play a small role in raising his winter spirits. Even though the intensity of room lights can't match the output of specialized units, the extra rays may be helpful.

An even easier thing would be for him to make it a point to get outside on bright days. He could take a walk. Throw a stick for the dog. Work on the car. Even though winter rays are often weak, at best, research indicates that getting as little as an hour of sunlight a day can help folks beat the seasonal blues.

SCENARIO 2: There Is No Time

AGE: 35

WEIGHT: 185

EXERCISE ROUTINE: Doesn't have one.

LIFESTYLE: He works as a shipfitter in a shipyard. Usually chugs a cup of coffee for breakfast and grabs a sub for lunch. Dinner usually consists of something microwavable in front of the tube with a couple beers to wash it down.

WEIGHT GOALS: Needs to lose about 20 pounds.

PROBLEM: He feels that there simply isn't room in his life for exercise. He has to be up at 5:30 every morning just to make it into work (he has to punch the clock at 7:30). He only gets half an hour for lunch, so he usually grabs something fast from one of the street vendors near the shipyard. By the time he gets home at 5:00, he's tired and ravenous, too tired and too hungry to work out.

Clearly, this is a guy who has allowed his work schedule to take over his life. And he compounds the problem with his eating habits. He wouldn't feel so tired and hungry when he gets home in the evening if he began his day eating a good, solid breakfast and packed himself a decent lunch and a couple healthful snacks to get him through the rest of the day. If he would do this instead of skipping breakfast and eating junk food for lunch, at the end of the day he would probably have the energy that he needs to do something besides crash in front of the television, says Pat Harper, R.D., a nutrition consultant in the Pittsburgh area.

He's paying for his drinking, too. If he's drinking more than one or two beers a night, he's drinking too many, says Arthur L. Klatsky, M.D., who has done extensive research on the subject of alcohol and health and is senior consultant in cardiology at the Kaiser Permanente Medical Center and the Division of Research Group in Oakland, California. Besides being bad for his health, all those beers dump a lot of calories into his system (one beer has about 146 calories). That, combined with the chips he probably eats with the beer (8 grams of fat for every 10 of them), is just adding ballast to his hull.

The bigger issue, though, is that this guy's numbers aren't adding up. He says that he doesn't have time to exercise, yet he gets home at 5:00 and goes to bed at 10:00 or 11:00. It would appear that he has 5 to 6 hours a day to do with what he will. Even if we throw a few family responsibilities into the mix—let's say that he has a wife and children—he still ought to be able to find an hour a day to burn off some flab.

Right now, the biggest time-eater in his life, aside from his job, is his nightly ritual of watching television, says Harriet Schechter, co-author of *More Time for Sex: The Organizing Guide for Busy Couples* and founder of The Miracle Worker Organizing Service in San Diego, which, since 1986, has helped thousands of people (and businesses) organize their lives.

The first thing that he should do, Schechter says, is take a hard look at how he is spending his time each evening and then ask himself if this is how he really wants to spend it. He needs to recognize that he is making a choice, and if he doesn't like what's happening to him as a result (his exploding love handles, for example), then there is nothing preventing him from making a different choice.

"If he says, 'I can't exercise, but I feel bad about being out of shape,' well, these are contradictory statements and emotions," Schechter says. "And that's what makes people crazy. I think it's much healthier to say, 'Well, you know, I'd really like to be in shape, but I don't like to exercise, and, therefore, I'm not going to choose exercise, and, therefore, I'm going to live with the fact that I'm out of shape. And I'm not going to feel bad about it.' "

This man knows, however, that he is overweight and that he is not feeling very good generally. If he would just take the first step and start exercising even a little, the improvement in how he feels would likely be dramatic enough to keep him going.

"My theory is ultimately for every person if something bothers you enough, you will change it. If it doesn't bother you enough, you won't do it," Schechter says.

SCENARIO 3: The Frequent Flier

AGE: 42

WEIGHT: 190

EXERCISE ROUTINE: Enjoys tennis—when he has the chance to play. Tries to run—when he has the chance to do it.

LIFESTYLE: He gives seminars nationwide on using computer software. In the course of any average week, he is likely to be in three different cities on either or both coasts, with a couple stopovers in the heartland in between. He spends more time in the air than he does on the ground.

WEIGHT GOALS: He wants to lose about 10 pounds.

PROBLEM: This guy's life is so zooey, it's extremely difficult for him to keep control of anything. Most of his meals are taken from little tin trays at 20,000 feet or in hotel bars while doing business. Given his schedule, it's difficult for him to find time to work out.

This may be an extreme example, but there are lots of men who live lives similar to this. The issue here is one of control; the only way that he is going to lose any weight is by being extremely well-organized.

Since he spends so much of his time in airports and on planes, he has a lot less control over what is set in front of him than he would have in his own kitchen. But if he stays flexible and plans ahead, he can still stay in charge of the situation, says Margery Lawrence, R.D., Ph.D., associate professor in the Department of Nutrition and Family Studies at St. Joseph College in West Hartford, Connecticut.

"He has to put thought into it and plan ahead," says Dr. Lawrence. "Sometimes two days' worth of planning ahead."

For example, if he knows that he is going to have a 2-hour layover in Chicago, he may want to pack some low-fat, healthful snacks. After all, many of the meals and snacks in airport terminals are coronary-bypass specials. "If you're really planning ahead, you have the right kinds of snacks around," says Dr. Lawrence. "Like bags of bite-size carrots and celery."

Other healthful—and, just as important, easily packable—snacks might include bagels, graham crackers, and dried or fresh fruit. Eating a few of these can make it easier for him to resist the salted peanuts that they toss at him when he's in the air.

If he is going to be eating a meal on the plane, he should take advantage of the fact that many airlines offer special low-fat meals to those who have the foresight to order ahead when they make their reservations.

And when he gets to the hotel restaurant, he has to be ever vigilant, looking for the lighter fare. He should search out the salad bars and the leaner menu offerings. And he shouldn't let the guys that he sups with lure him into ordering the chocolate mousse.

On the exercise front, he can use that 2-hour layover to burn some flab. Just strolling around the terminal will burn twice as many calories as sitting on his bum reading a magazine (which is what most of us do when we have 2 hours to kill in an airport).

And when he makes hotel reservations, he should be looking for hotels with exercise rooms and pools—and he should use them. In the event he gets into town after the pool or exercise room has closed for the day, he should feel free to avail himself of the endless stairwells so handily available in most hotels. He can burn 250 calories in half an hour just by walking up and down the stairs a few times.

Again, though, he should really be planning ahead so that he knows what his day in Miami, Pittsburgh, Toledo, or Canarsie is going to be like. And he should pencil exercise time into his schedule for that day—a half-hour jog before breakfast, for example, or an afternoon tennis match—and he should treat that time as if it were a terribly critical business appointment. Which, if he really wants to get into shape, it is.

SCENARIO 4: Getting the Right Attitude

AGE: 40

WEIGHT: 210

EXERCISE ROUTINE: Nothing more than an occasional walk around the block or playing the occasional round of golf.

LIFESTYLE: He sells cars, which means he spends a lot of time sitting behind a desk or walking around the lot. Because his income is based on commissions, he often works days and evenings to "make his nut," leaving himself little time for anything else. He eats a lot of fast food—breakfast at a diner on the way to the dealership, for example, and frequent take-out lunches and dinners.

WEIGHT GOALS: Wants to lose about 20 pounds, but ultimately has a hard time believing that it's possible. As a result, the whole idea of losing weight makes him depressed.

PROBLEM: Obviously, at least part of this guy's problem is his lifestyle, but that's just a symptom of his real problem, which is the way he perceives himself. To bend a line from Rodney Dangerfield, he don't give himself no respect. He tells himself, "I'd look a lot better if I lost some weight," but he doesn't feel good about himself the way that he is now. And because he doesn't feel good about himself, he can't seem to muster the willpower to get up and go to the gym.

This man is experiencing the classic catch-22 of weight loss. How does a guy get started on a program when he doesn't feel good about himself to begin with? Put another way, why should he take up exercising when, in his heart of hearts, he knows that it won't do him any good because nothing does him any good, and this is just one more thing that he'll probably fail?

The first thing that this man needs to do, says Daniel Kosich, Ph.D., a senior consultant for the International Association of Fitness Professionals and author of *Get Real: A Personal Guide to Real-Life Weight Management*, is get a change of attitude.

A negative or conditional attitude such as "If I lose 20 pounds, then I'll like myself" is self-defeating, Dr. Kosich says. If this man doesn't like himself now, there is no way that he is going to be motivated to make the changes he wants to make.

Instead of thinking, "I'll like myself once I lose about 20 pounds," he needs to tell himself, "I like myself now, and, because I like myself, I'm going to take care of myself, and that means I'm going to exercise and lose some weight," says Dr. Kosich.

Losing weight is not so much about willpower, Dr. Kosich says, as it is about accepting yourself for who you are and building on that.

Conversely, if this man bases his self-respect on achieving long-range goals (like losing 20 pounds), "what it does is set a paradigm that really makes it difficult to achieve the long-term goal because he's not looking at this as a pleasurable part of his lifestyle," Dr. Kosich says. "You know, it's like, 'I have to eat right, I have to exercise because I want to get to this weight, but it's not really something I like to do.'"

What this man needs to do is change his focus. If he tells himself, "I'm doing this because I really care so much about myself right now that I'm going to take care of myself and get healthy," then he knows that he's doing good things for himself—not tomorrow, not next month, but today. "It's not like when he gets to a certain point, then he's going to feel good about who he is," Dr. Kosich says.

The truth is, all men find it easier to stick to weight-loss programs when they focus on how they are improving their health rather than merely counting the pounds. And they find it easier still, of course, when they take up activities they enjoy, be they walking, lifting weights, or playing hoops. This is a reinforcing attitude that makes them feel better the longer and more often they are successful. Men who focus on how much weight they still have to lose have a harder time because the rewards—which they measure only as pounds lost—are always deferred.

SCENARIO 5: Living the Good Life

AGE: 55

WEIGHT: 190

EXERCISE ROUTINE: He runs several miles every morning and plays an hour or more of hockey or tennis two or three times a week.

LIFESTYLE: Works nights on a newspaper in a fairly sedentary job. Not a big eater, but eats sensibly as a general rule. Does have a weakness for good steaks, cheap hot dogs, tortilla chips and salsa, and vanilla ice cream. He also indulges in a couple shots of scotch after work sometimes or on nights off.

WEIGHT GOALS: This is a really fit, muscular guy who is not far off the mark for weight, but who, in spite of all his exercise and modest eating, has just a little bit of a belly. He might be able to get rid of it if he lost 5 to 6 pounds.

PROBLEM: In order to lose those 5 to 6 pounds, he would have to give up or cut back on some of the things he loves: the hot dogs, the tortilla chips, the ice cream, the scotch. And he figures, "Well, what's the point of living then?"

This man has a perfectly valid question: What is the point? If he wants absolutely flat abs and is willing to give up those few things that give him pleasure in order to do it, then the solution is simple enough. But he may find the price of those flat abs is a fairly flat life.

He ought to start by asking himself whether he wants flat abs for any reason other than simple vanity, says Daniel Kosich, Ph.D., a senior consultant for the International Association of Fitness Professionals and author of *Get Real: A Personal Guide to Real-Life Weight Management.*

Not that there is necessarily anything wrong with vanity. "It's nice to say that you shouldn't care so much about appearance, but the fact is that people do. It's something that is part of our culture. And it's okay to want to look good; just keep it in perspective," Dr. Kosich says. "For a lot of people, the image that they have in their heads about what they ought to look like or what they can look like is probably off the mark."

This guy just needs "to understand what kinds of expectations he can have based on what he's willing to commit to," Dr. Kosich adds.

If he recognizes the sacrifices that he will have to make to achieve a washboard look, and if he thinks that it's worth it, then he should certainly go for it, says Dragomir Cioroslan, head coach of the U.S. Weightlifting Federation and the 1996 U.S. Olympic weightlifting team.

For starters, he's going to have to cut back on his treats. Scotch, steak, and vanilla ice cream are all enormously high in calories, and if he thinks he can burn off those calories just by adding a little extra exercise into his day, he's going to find that belly very persistent indeed.

Research has shown that people who increase their calorie-burning activities without changing their eating habits often end up eating more to make up for the calories that they're burning.

Besides, he's already plenty active. Although doing exercises specifically targeting the abdominals, like doing crunches every morning after his run, will make those muscles more prominent, it won't have much effect on the extra padding at his waist.

What he really needs to do is whittle away at the problem by whittling away at his pleasures. This doesn't mean giving up steak and scotch. It does mean having them a little less often and in smaller quantities. Instead of two shots of scotch, he can enjoy—and that means really enjoy—sipping just one. Ditto for the steak: Why get a 16-ouncer when the 12-ounce steak will still satisfy his craving for good meat?

Whatever he ultimately decides to do, he has to be realistic. While making these sacrifices will make his gut leaner, they won't necessarily make any big improvement in his health, says Dr. Kosich. That little pad of fat over those rippling abdominals is not a great health problem. The issue may be one of vanity. The question he has to ask himself is "Is it worth it?"

SCENARIO 6: Family Problems

AGE: 34

WEIGHT: 280 and counting

EXERCISE ROUTINE: None

LIFESTYLE: This is a man whose job—working in a medical laboratory—is not physically demanding, and he spends virtually all his spare time at a desk. His body often hurts; he has knee and back pain and often feels fatigued. Even small amounts of physical exertion have him puffing. His eating habits are ultra high-fat, high-cholesterol: lots of spareribs, beef burritos, double-cheese pizzas, and premium ice cream.

WEIGHT GOALS: He knows that he needs to lose at least 80 pounds.

PROBLEM: This man is a heart attack waiting to happen, and if he doesn't change his habits, he's not going to make it to a ripe old age. When friends or doctors have suggested that he might want to try to lose some weight, he has explained that he can't do it because almost everybody in his family, including his parents, is fat.

While genes may play a role in the size of one's jeans, the issue is considerably more complicated. What our individual genetic packages do is make some of us more susceptible to obesity than others. It doesn't make being obese a foregone conclusion.

Put another way, it's not genetics that make most people fat; it's what those people do with their particular genetic packages. Take identical twins, two people with identical sets of genes: Place one on a program of low-fat, healthful meals and regular exercise and let the other take all his meals at the local sub shop, and it's a safe bet that the latter will get fatter.

This isn't to say that it's going to be easy for this man to lose weight. There is no question that for some men, losing weight is hardly a challenge, while for others it is exceedingly difficult, and metabolism can play a role in this.

The fact that his parents are also obese may be due less to any genetic proclivities than to the fact that they are no less sedentary than their son and share the same types of eating habits. Indeed, he is probably more likely to have a weight problem because he inherited his parents' lifestyle rather than because he inherited their genes.

That said, there are lots of things this man could be doing to get thinner, including very small lifestyle changes that would encourage more healthy choices. For example, he could start keeping a lifestyle diary, says Joanne Curran-Celentano, R.D., Ph.D., associate professor of nutritional sciences at the University of New Hampshire in Durham and nutrition research coordinator at the Center for Eating Disorders Management in Dover, New Hampshire. Since he apparently pays little attention to what he eats, it would be a good wake-up call for him actually to log what goes into his mouth on a typical day.

While he is at it, it would be a good idea for him to keep track of the amount of activity that he has in his day, Dr. Curran-Celentano adds. This way, he may finally recognize what his friends and doctors have already noticed: that he needs to take up some calorie-burning activities as well as get his eating under control.

Once he recognizes the need for exercise, he will be more likely to get motivated to make some changes. Since he is extremely out of shape, obviously he has to start slowly, maybe with some easy walks around the block. Those aches and pains that he has been experiencing are a product of his being overweight and out of shape, and even an easy walking program will help ease some of the discomfort.

Since he's starting from almost ground zero, however, the operative word is *slow*. If he tries to push himself too hard too fast, there might be some unpleasant consequences in store, like a heart attack. In fact, he would be well-advised to check with his doctor even before he puts on his walking shoes.

SCENARIO **7**:Becoming Active Again

AGE: 65

WEIGHT: 172

EXERCISE ROUTINE: None

LIFESTYLE: Retired after 40 years of pushing papers in the claims department of a major insurance company, he recently had a heart attack. Now he spends his mornings reading the paper and puttering about the house and, as often as possible, spends his afternoons putting about the country club. He eats fairly well, thanks to his health-conscious spouse, who feeds him lots of fruit, vegetables, carbohydrates, and fiber, which may explain how, after a long and sedentary life, he has managed to stay relatively thin.

WEIGHT GOALS: He is not terribly overweight for his height, maybe 10 pounds or so, but it's all on his belly, and he would like to "redistribute" that weight.

PROBLEM: Aside from golf, he hadn't exercised regularly since he graduated from the college rowing team. Before his recent heart attack, he had become aware of the fact that his drives weren't as long as they used to be and that he was more weary after a walk around the course than he used to be.

This man is paying for a lifetime of leisure. Even though he eats fairly well, he hasn't kept his heart or any of the other muscles in his body in shape. There is now an overwhelming body of evidence that such idleness leads to serious illness. A simple lack of regular physical activity is considered the cause of death for an estimated 250,000 Americans each year.

Moreover, he has just learned that just because he is not obese doesn't mean that he can't suffer from heart disease. There is a strong link between heart disease and belly fat—and he has a belly.

Fortunately, even after having a heart attack, it's not too late for him to shape up. The best thing that he can do is to get himself into a (doctor-monitored) program of regular exercise, in which he will do both aerobics and light weight lifting.

"Improving your aerobic fitness, muscular endurance, and muscular strength will tie in to improving your health, longevity, and quality of life," says Brian Wallace, Ph.D., chairman of sport fitness at the U.S. Sports Academy in Daphne, Alabama.

This man should begin a very light intensity cross-training program in which he will alternate between short intervals of aerobic exercise (say, 6 minutes on a stationary bike or treadmill) and time spent walking and stretching, recommends Dr. Wallace. Each time he does the routine, he should increase the number of minutes on the bike or treadmill a bit, keeping it within a comfortable range. After about three weeks of this, he can add some light weight training to start building up those muscles.

As he increases the duration of his aerobic workouts and increases the amount of weight he is lifting, his muscles (including his heart) will get stronger, and this will help him stay more energetic than if he goes back to his sedentary ways.

He will increase his chances of succeeding if he enlists the aid of his health-conscious wife in keeping with the program, adds J. P. Wallace, Ph.D., associate professor of kinesiology and director of the adult fitness program at Indiana University in Bloomington. In fact, both partners in the marriage would benefit by encouraging each other to exercise. Dr. Wallace has done research showing that married couples are more likely to stick with an exercise program if each spouse supports the other in the effort.

Even men who have suffered something as frightening as a heart attack, says Dr. J. P. Wallace, won't stick with the program if their wives don't support them.

"If the woman really doesn't support the man's efforts to go to rehab and to change his diet, it won't be done," says Dr. J. P. Wallace. "So the adherence of the man really depends on the adherence of the woman."

Part IV

The World of Aerobics

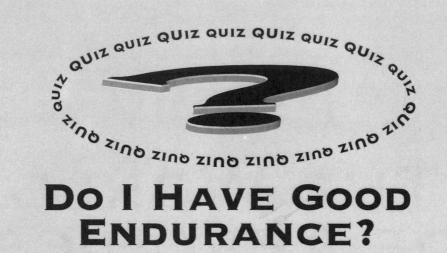

QUIZ QUIZ QUIZ QUIZ QUIZ QUIZ QUIZ QUIZ QUIZ QUIZ QUIZ QUIZ QUIZ QUIZ QUIZ QUIZ QUIZ

DO I HAVE GOOD ENDURANCE?

When it comes to rating ourselves on endurance, few of us err on the side of modesty. Indeed, most men view their physical prowess—along with their looks and sex appeal—in the same clear-sighted fashion that Ross Perot once viewed his chances of becoming president.

Which is why an unfortunate number of men, including those who can barely make it to the car without wheezing, think of themselves as being aerobically fit—although this belief suggests that they're not getting enough oxygen, to say the least.

There are a number of tests for determining aerobic fitness and endurance, most of which require machinery designed by NASA, and which involve simple, everyday language like *anaerobic threshold* and *maximal oxygen uptake*.

Here is an easier way. Take this quiz to see how your aerobic fitness really measures up.

1. What's my resting heart rate?

The heart is a muscle, and, as with any muscle, exercise makes it bigger. (The average heart is roughly the size of two fists put together; a conditioned heart can be 10 percent bigger.) As your heart gets bigger and stronger, it becomes more efficient, so it doesn't have to beat as often. "A larger, stronger heart can pump out more blood with each heartbeat," says Herman Falsetti, M.D., an Irvine, California, cardiologist in private practice who specializes in fitness tests. "That can really pay off in the long run."

The great thing about using your resting heart rate as a measure of your aerobic fitness is that you can actually see it improve, often in a fairly short time.

When checking your resting heart rate, do it in the morning before getting out of bed. With your fingertips, find the carotid artery (the large artery just to the left or right of the Adam's apple). Count how many times it beats in a minute. Here's the breakdown.

- **70 to 90 beats a minute: an average, untrained heart**
- **60 to 70 beats a minute: a mildly conditioned heart**
- **50 to 60 beats a minute: the heart of a regular exerciser**
- **40 to 50 beats a minute: the heart of an elite athlete**
- **28 beats per minute: You're either catatonic or five-time Tour de France champion Miguel Indurain.**

2. Can I do the step test?

An even simpler test of aerobic fitness, says Dr. Falsetti, is simply to walk up a flight of stairs.

If you can walk up three flights of stairs easily with no shortness of breath, consider yourself aerobically fit.

If you can walk up one flight of stairs but not without wheezing or seeing stars, you had better lace up your walking shoes, says Dr. Falsetti.

3. What's my time on a 1.5-mile run?

If you have been exercising regularly for six to eight weeks and want to check your aerobic progress, try this test: Run 1.5 miles—either on a track or on a route that you have clocked yourself—as fast as you comfortably can. Assuming that you're between 30 and 40 years old, here's the measure.

- **14 minutes or slower: This is your wake-up call.**
- **12:01 to 13:59 minutes: You're in fair shape, but you need to exercise more.**
- **10:46 to 12 minutes: Consider yourself average.**
- **9:46 to 10:45 minutes: Congratulations, you're above average.**
- **9:45 or faster: You're in great shape.**

Note: Running 1.5 miles all-out involves tough effort, so if you're not already in pretty good shape, you may want to check with a doctor before doing this test.

4. How's my recovery?

Now that you have just finished a run, this is an excellent opportunity to check your recovery time. As with resting heart rate, this test gives a quick, accurate measure of your overall aerobic fitness.

As soon as you hit the finish line—this can be after doing the run or after completing a brisk 1-mile walk, a 10-mile bike ride, or a half-hour swim—measure your heart rate for 1 minute. Write down the number. Rest 1 minute, then check your pulse again.

The more quickly your heart slows down, the fitter you are—which explains why, 2 minutes after a hard run, elite athletes can smile at the camera and talk in complete sentences, whereas the average man would have to be interviewed while lying on his back and frothing at the mouth. Here's what to look for.

- **If your pulse rate drops 10 to 20 beats a minute, you're in fair shape.**
- **You're in good shape if your pulse drops 30 to 40 beats.**
- **You're in very good shape if it drops 50 to 60 beats.**

5. Do I remember my wedding night?

Cast your mind back to that first night of wedded bliss and ask yourself which of the following statements applies to you.

- **I came to bed wearing a thong.**
- **I came to bed wearing boxers that looked like a thong.**

Since the health of the exterior invariably reflects the health of the interior, this is perhaps the simplest (and all too often, the most unnerving) gauge of your current fitness. "Compare your weight today with what you weighed when you got married," says Dr. Falsetti. "Often your marriage weight is your best weight. Unfortunately, most people gain about 5 pounds a year for every year they're married."

Needless to say, if your navel has gone south, your endurance has certainly followed it.

The Role of Aerobic Exercise
Lighting the Fat-Burning Furnace

If you stop the next passing runner and ask him to define aerobic exercise, chances are you'll get a blank look, followed by the sort of waffling that resonates throughout IRS offices and during election years.

"Ummm, yes, why certainly, aerobic exercise has much to do with the heart and lungs, and there's sweating involved, and every day there are new studies with titles like 'The Effects of Exercise on the Cardiovascular System of Male Cynomolgus Monkeys' that prove how wonderful aerobic exercise is for you."

This is all true. But this sort of hazy thinking is precisely what tends to derail most exercise programs. Exercise without focus is like driving without a map: fine if you want to meander, not so good if you want to get somewhere fast. To get the best results from aerobic exercise—sound health, a lean look, the best fitness you can grab in the time you have—you have to know what it is. Don't think of it as dull physiology. See this knowledge as inspiration. Because once you understand the basics of aerobic exercise and the wonders it can bring, you'll wonder why you didn't dive into it sooner.

The Breath of Life

First, a note on nomenclature: While the terms *aerobics* and *aerobic exercise* are often used interchangeably, they really aren't the same thing. Aerobics generally refers to aerobic dance—leotards, loud music, mirror-covered walls, and so forth. Aerobic exercise, by contrast, means any activity that gets your heart pumping and keeps it pumping. Running is great aerobic exercise. So is biking, shadowboxing, jumping rope, or even, for that matter, aerobic dance.

Aerobic is derived from two Greek words meaning "air" and "life." Aerobic exercise is effort that requires an enhanced flow of oxygen to supply energy. You breathe in. The oxygen spills from your lungs into your bloodstream. Your heart pumps it to your muscles. There, the oxygen is used to break down carbohydrate, fat, and protein into the energy that your muscles need to move. You run, leap, pivot. And breathe some more.

So what exercise isn't aerobic? Examples include lifting a barbell, throwing a ball, jumping, even doing a short sprint. These exercises don't rely on your heart and lungs; they are mostly about short bursts of muscular strength. In these cases, the muscles being exercised rely on the oxygen and glucose that are immediately available to them to meet the challenge you present. For an exercise to be aerobic, it must put continuous demands on muscles, enough to force the heart and lungs to deliver a heightened stream of oxygen for the muscles to keep churning.

By strict definition nearly any exercise performed faster than sitting in a chair is aerobic; your heart and lungs will ratchet up a notch for even small efforts. But to produce a real benefit for your body, there needs to be some real effort involved, which is why the Leisure World Boccie Club won't be storming the Olympic medal stand any time soon. Effective aerobic exercise, the stuff that taxes your heart and lungs and burns calories, generally occurs when you exercise at roughly 40 to 80 percent of your maximum effort.

You need to raise your heart rate to a level that burns sufficient calories and taxes your cardiovascular system, but not so high that you can't suck in enough oxygen to fuel your working muscles. As a rule of thumb, you're exercising at a good pace when you're able to talk at the same time. If you're overdoing it, there won't be enough oxygen to fuel your muscles and limbs, and your lungs will feel as if they are being grilled on a spit. At this point you either throttle back or pitch forward on your face.

Marvelous things happen inside your body when you start up a regular aerobic exercise program. Your lungs become stronger and more efficient, enabling you to take in and dispense more oxygen. Your heart becomes stronger and more efficient, too, pumping more blood and oxygen with each beat. More capillaries are formed to ferry the oxygen to the muscles. Enzymes in the muscle fibers become more active, and your muscles are better able to use oxygen to burn fuel. Perhaps most enticing, the metabolic machinery in the muscles slowly improves its ability to burn fat. In other words, you improve two ways: inside and out.

Lean for the Long Haul

The great thing about aerobic exercise is that it produces stunning transformations in the heart and lungs in as little as a few days or weeks.

"The human body is a remarkably adaptive machine," says John Duncan, Ph.D., professor of clinical research at Texas Woman's University in Denton. "Just a few weeks of training can produce cardiovascular, muscular, and nervous system adaptations that make the body markedly more efficient."

Fine. But as men interested in fitness, we are concerned with deeper issues. Pushing our limits. Gleaning lessons in fortitude, perseverance, and self-destiny. Making sure that our physiques don't resemble a beanbag chair.

It's okay to be superficial. If you don't care about your looks, you're either Dennis Rodman or deceased. But if you're looking to burn calories and

---

Unexpected Benefits

Solid aerobic fitness is good for everything from clogged arteries to depression. Important stuff, certainly, but there are more satisfying benefits to be had. Like self-esteem. Beating the competition. Not having to take guff from anyone—including uppity boatmen who should know better than to try to buffalo a lifelong exercise nut.

Enter Tom Warren, a retired San Diego restaurateur who, at 53, has dedicated a large amount of his life to exercise. This is a man who once did 400 sit-ups in a sauna—on a bet. (The prize was a bottle of beer. A cold beer may not mean that much to you, but it's not Warren's tastes that are the point of this story.)

Back in his younger days, Warren was vacationing in the Bahamas when he boarded a ferry carrying a group of fellow tourists from Paradise Island to Nassau. The ferry operators, treating the tourists like cattle, rudely ordered them around.

"Lighten up," said Warren.

"Quiet down," said the operators.

That's when Warren took decisive action. First, he grabbed back the dollar fee from one of the ferrymen. Then he jumped overboard and swam the mile to the island.

Not only did he make it alive, he got there ahead of the ferry, to the amazement of the slack-jawed and suddenly humbled operators.

"To be physically independent," says Warren, "is real important to me."

---

lose weight, there's nothing better than aerobic exercise. Equally important, aerobic exercise will keep that weight off—unlike slick diet schemes that advertise by trotting forward clients who have lost 30 pounds but decline to show you those same folks three months later because they return to looking like the Michelin Man. Aerobic exercise, combined with a smart diet, is the most effective way to ensure that lost weight stays that way.

This reduced fat has an impact beyond how you look in your Skivvies. Excess fat has been linked to heart disease, diabetes, high blood pressure, and certain cancers.

What's more, recent discoveries have led experts to believe that the vilest fat, the stuff most responsible for this carnage, is the intra-abdominal fat resting out of sight beneath your abdominal muscles.

"A lot of people are concerned with what they look like, and external body fat certainly plays a role there. But from a health-risk standpoint, it's intra-abdominal fat that you really should be concerned about," says Gary Hunter, Ph.D., professor of exercise physiology at the University of Alabama in Birmingham. "Not only does exercise make you leaner but it also makes you extra leaner in the place where you don't want fat."

Unfortunately, shedding fat via exercise is a slow process. When you start an aerobic exercise program, your heart, lungs, and muscles may acclimate quickly. But your metabolic machinery—the body's ability to remove fat from cells where it's stored, carry it to muscles, and then burn it up—adapts far more slowly.

Yes, aerobic exercise greatly improves your body's ability to burn fat and shed pounds, but it can take months before the fat-burning machinery is up and running full bore; there are no shortcuts. Unfortunately, most men either (a) don't realize this, (b) don't have the patience to wait weeks and maybe months for noticeable results, or (c) have seen one too many "Lose 5 Inches a Day from Your Waist!" headlines in supermarket checkout lines. This may explain why many well-intentioned exercisers eventually reduce their exercise to stuffing themselves into their pants.

Don't get discouraged. It takes time to build momentum, but once your system is in tune, you will quickly notice the difference. "Fat loss is a matter of dislodging the fat, transporting the fat, and using the fat—and all three of those take time to physiologically develop," says Ralph LaForge, director of the lipid disorders training program for the San Diego Cardiac Center Medical Group.

Adding Years

While you wait for the pounds to peel away, you can take solace in knowing that aerobic exercise will deliver plenty of other benefits. Dozens of studies have looked at the link between exercise and aging and all have reached the same conclusion—regular aerobic exercise can extend your years.

Stanford University's landmark study of nearly 17,000 Harvard alumni showed that men who burned 2,000 calories a week by walking 3 miles a day had a 28 percent lower death rate than fellow alums who exercised less or didn't do anything at all. More specifically, the researchers found that men who exercised regularly could expect to add about two years to their lives.

That life will be a better one, too. Aerobic exercise relieves depression, anxiety, and stress. It can improve your sex life and foster creativity—a potentially fortuitous one-two punch. It can help ease the sting of minor illnesses; research has shown that the immune systems of regular exercisers can quash colds and flus more quickly. It also reduces the risk of major health problems like heart disease, high blood pressure, colon cancer, and diabetes. No other form of exercise confers as many benefits.

"Basically, aerobic exercise affords you the opportunity to turn back the hands of time," says Dr. Duncan.

Easy Gains

Right about now you're probably thinking, "Right. All I have to do is give up my job, family, and all other interests in exchange for a fanatical exercise regimen and the personal life of moss."

True, it wasn't long ago that exercise physiologists poked their heads out of their labs to issue exercise prescriptions so time-consuming that no reasonable guy with a real life could possibly do them. But studies show that moderate activity provides the same health benefits as vigorous stuff. For basic health, the Centers for Disease Control and Prevention in Atlanta and the American College of Sports Medicine, which is headquartered in Indianapolis, recommend 30 minutes of moderate-intensity physical activity—easy walks, casual bike rides—a day. If you can't grab that exercise in a single 30-minute chunk, shorter bouts totaling 30 minutes will work just as well.

For losing weight, the American College of Sports Medicine recommends burning 1,000 to 2,000 calories a week—about 200 calories a day over and above what you normally burn.

"We used to tell people that they had to go out there and work and sweat to get any kind of benefit from exercise, but we've since found out that that isn't true," says Dr. Duncan.

THE RIGHT QUANTITY
A SMORGASBORD OF CHOICES

How much exercise do you need?

On the one hand, you have the minimalists, folks who would convince you that sound fitness and breathtaking weight loss can be achieved by snarfing cocktail peanuts and making periodic trips to the john. At the other extreme are the compulsive-obsessives, those who assure you that these same benefits can be had only by suffering horribly for whopping amounts of time.

Between these two poles is an abundance of well-intentioned but often contradictory advice. Sorting out how much exercise you need can be more difficult than exercising itself.

The simple answer is obvious: There is no one right answer. The menu of aerobic choices and intensities is a long one. What you ultimately choose depends on your current level of fitness, how much weight you hope to lose, and other, more practical realities, like how much time you can steal for yourself.

The American College of Sports Medicine, which is headquartered in Indianapolis, recommends that you burn roughly 1,500 calories—about half a pound of fat—a week, over and above the energy you use for generally getting about. But how you burn these calories doesn't really matter.

"There is no magic exercise," says Ralph LaForge, director of the lipid disorders training program for the San Diego Cardiac Center Medical Group. "If you used up 1,500 calories gardening each week, you'd have no less fat loss than if you burned that 1,500 calories on the StairMaster."

The amount of exercise needed to shed those 1,500 calories also is difficult to answer in a single sentence. It depends on the type of exercise you do and how hard you do it. In a bit we'll look at a few specific exercise options. For now, the important point is this: Plenty of people are convinced that what they do and how long they do it are the only ways to lose weight, and they'll be the first to tell you so. You can ignore them.

Health versus Weight Loss

If you're serious about losing weight, you need to face some sobering realities—foremost, that weight loss doesn't come quickly. There's a big difference between giving your heart and lungs a bit of a workout and actually losing a few pounds.

The truth is that you can exercise aerobically by walking around the room for a minute, but you don't need a degree in exercise physiology to realize that this won't have a tremendous impact. Doctors recommend getting at least 30 minutes of moderate activity—mowing the lawn, doing housework, raking leaves, and walking up stairs—most, if not all, days of the week.

Can you burn calories with this little effort? Certainly. Any movement burns calories. Can you lose much weight? Certainly not. A leisurely 10-minute walk burns calories, but only about 3 to 4 calories a minute—an impractical approach when you consider that a 6-ounce serving of fries weighs in at about 540 calories or that you need to burn 3,500 calories to lose a pound of fat.

"When it comes to losing weight, there are no shortcuts," says LaForge. "You can get good general heart health with as little as 20 minutes of moderate exercise three times a week. But losing weight requires either more time or more intensity."

Upping the Ante

For serious weight loss and fitness, you will need to move beyond the aerobic minimum, but not as far as you might think.

How much time do you need to invest if you want to lose weight? While it's true that burning calories can be accomplished in virtually any fashion and that gardening will do, if you're looking to lose weight by yanking rutabagas, you'll have to set aside the better part of the day. Why? Because easy activity burns calories at a snail's pace. Assuming that your time is valuable, you'll need to be more efficient with your calorie burning.

The "right" quantity of aerobic exercise, then, can be measured three ways: how long, how hard, and how often you exercise.

It would be unwise to see this as an invitation to extremism. Exercising long, hard, and often will certainly shed the most fat. On the other hand, it will produce burnout, breakdowns, and injuries far sooner. For the long haul, good, solid weight loss is best achieved by exercising for a reasonable time in a comfortable fashion.

"In general, you'll get the most effective fat burning, in terms of weight loss, in aerobic sessions that last from 40 to 90 minutes, exercising at a moderate pace, say, 50 to 65 percent of your maximum heart rate," says LaForge. (To approximate your maximum heart rate, subtract your age from 220. This number has an error of plus or minus 15 beats per minute, he says.)

Obviously, this is a guideline, not a use-this-or-consign-yourself-to-fatdom decree. Assuming that you have a real life—a job, kids, and a wife who would like to see you more than 5 minutes a day—finding 40 to 90 minutes of free time isn't always possible. Besides, doing the same workout at the same pace every day will bore you to cement.

When deciding how much time you're going to spend on aerobics, you have to consider your interests and lifestyle as well as your current level of fitness. Here is what experts advise.

KNOW THYSELF. Weight loss is an intensely personal thing. While study after study has shown that aerobic exercise sheds pounds, those same studies also show that people slough off that fat at dramatically different rates, even while doing the same amount of exercise. Sure, it would be great to lose 20 pounds in time for your high school reunion, but unless your genes decide to cooperate, it may not happen.

"People have to have realistic expectations," says Jack H. Wilmore, Ph.D., professor in the Department of Kinesiology and Health Education at the University of Texas in Austin. "Not everybody is going to be able to get down to where they're extremely lean. There are some people who are just genetically designed to carry more fat, and no amount of exercise can change that."

EXPECT THE BEST—AND PREPARE FOR THE WORST. It happens to everyone: You cut back on desserts, stop eating fatty foods, and attend aerobics classes three times a week. Almost instantly, it seems, you're shedding a lot of weight very quickly. "Easier than I thought," you tell yourself, as you phone in a pizza order and blow off your workout for the night, enjoying the prospect of an easy victory ahead.

Uh-oh. Those early losses may have felt great, but they're misleading. Within a few weeks the needle on the scale invariably seems to stop moving—or, worse, is actually creeping upward. What went wrong?

Researchers are very familiar with this phenomenon. For many people, the heavier they are, the faster they will lose weight. Lean folks don't lose quite so quickly, for the highly scientific reason that they have less fat to lose.

Ultimately, there are no shortcuts. Whether you're heavy or lean, you need—along with a diet short on snack cakes—to exercise aerobically a minimum of three days a week, 30 minutes at a pop.

FORGET THE SCALE. While weight is a pretty good measure of how much fat you're burning, it can also be deceptive. It's not uncommon for men actually to gain weight when they start an aerobic program. Yes, they're losing fat, but they're gaining muscle at the same time, and muscle weighs more than fat.

If you're new to exercise and find that you're losing weight at a snail's pace—or, what seems worse, actually putting on pounds—don't quit in disgust or panic and triple your training. The muscle that you are adding will make you look better. Plus, once the fat-burning mechanisms in those muscles are up and running, that muscle will help burn even more calories, muscle being much more metabolically active than fat.

START SLOWLY. It's true that intense exercise burns calories faster than long, slow stuff. But if you are 40 pounds overweight and haven't exercised since the Ford administration, speedwork on the track is not for you. Start slowly. Begin by building your cardiovascular health. Taking 10-minute walks before breakfast, at lunch, and again before dinner will do it. Then work your way up slowly to roughly an hour of long, slow distance—a brisk walk, a moderate run or bike ride—three to five times a week.

This pace may seem overly cautious, especially since you're undoubtedly anxious for results. But caution is critical. You won't lose chunks of weight instantly, but you will lose it over the long haul if you can avoid injuries that can put an end to all your good intentions.

"Men want to get back into shape quickly," says Herman Falsetti, M.D., an Irvine, California, cardiologist in private practice who specializes in fitness tests. "They go hard from the beginning, and a week later they're injured and finished."

FOLLOW THE 10 PERCENT RULE. It's a natural human tendency to overestimate our abilities while underestimating our weaknesses. But when you're trying to lose weight—and stay uninjured—it pays to be careful.

For every year that you have let yourself slide, says Dr. Falsetti, figure that you'll need to add a month of easy-effort workouts (say, running, biking, or swimming at roughly half-speed) three times a week to get back into shape. As a general rule, don't increase your training time or mileage by any more than 10 percent a week, he advises.

For example, if you have worked yourself up to running 4 miles on Monday, Wednesday, and Friday, and you're looking to increase that weekly mileage, in the next week you would add no more than about a half-mile to each run. This may seem paltry, but if you're making a comeback from a fairly sorry state, it's also smart. Your heart and lungs might be capable of a bigger jump, but their supporting cast of muscles and ligaments need to be brought along more gently.

If you're already fairly fit but moderately overweight or if you're fit and lean and trying to stay that way, well, there's a whole smorgasbord of options open to you, options we'll address later in this book.

Finding Time

Everyone whines about being short on time, but anyone with a core of honesty will admit that he spends at least a certain portion of each day doing nothing more important than picking lint out of his navel. Unless your daily calendar resembles the Pope's, odds are you can find time for exercise. (Even the Pope makes time for a morning walk.) Sometimes you just have to be a little creative.

To be sure, some folks take the urge to exercise to rather extreme lengths. Like the businessman who hopped from his train when it pulled into the station so that he could get in a half-mile jog—but then found himself in a mad sprint as he tried to catch the departing train. Or the triathlete who, faced with a morning fishing trip and an afternoon wedding, carted his stationary bike onto the boat, lashed it to the deck, and mounted up and spun away. Or the fellow who spends idle airport time standing on one leg. "Builds up your knee and ankle muscles," he says.

Fortunately, there are easier ways to work exercise into your daily schedule.

- **Set the alarm to go off earlier.** Few of us can honestly own up to scheduling conflicts at 5:00 A.M.
- **Skip rope or ride a stationary bike in front of the TV.** This can be an impressive exercise arena since Americans watch about 30 hours of TV a week.
- **Set aside reports during the day**—then read them at night while spinning on the stationary bike.
- **Take the stairs.** When Robert Fulghum, best-selling author of <u>All I Really Need to Know I Learned in Kindergarten</u>, is trapped in hotels on long promotional tours, he has been known to don sweats and tromp up and down the stairwell.

  This isn't without risks, of course. On one occasion, Fulghum, dressed in black sweats and padding the stairwell late at night, was collared by a hotel security guard and hauled, protesting, to the front desk. (Fortunately, he was promptly freed.)

DO LESS—MORE OFTEN. If you're having a bad day—and 30 minutes of uninterrupted time is as likely as shared intimacies with the Cowboy cheerleaders—you can still get a great aerobic workout. Research has shown that three 10-minute bouts of exercise provide about 95 percent of the cardiorespiratory benefits of a continuous 30-minute session. The same approach works for weight loss, too. A calorie burned is a calorie burned, whether it's burned in three 10-minute bouts or a 30-minute block.

So don't worry about cutting your workouts short now and then. "If there's any one secret to exercise, it's regularity," says John Duncan, Ph.D., professor of clinical research at Texas Woman's University in Denton.

UP THE INTENSITY. While most weight-loss plans advise exercising at a moderate rate for 40 to 90 minutes, there are ways to speed the pace—namely, by boosting the intensity of the effort. (For more on intensity, see The Right Quality on page 119.) Let's just say that the time-crimped are by no means weight-loss–impaired.

For example, while you can burn 220 calories by exercising 30 minutes at 50 percent of your maximum capacity, you can boost that burn to 332 calories by exercising for 30 minutes at 75 percent of your max. In other words, upping the intensity can allow you to burn about 50 percent more calories in the same amount of time.

STAYING THE COURSE. There's no question that aerobic exercise is a great way to lose weight. Once those pounds are off, however, it's not necessarily that hard to keep them off.

When you're lean and in good shape, you can often maintain that happy state by exercising three to five days a week, 20 to 60 minutes at a time, at 55 to 90 percent of your maximum heart rate—right where the American College of Sports Medicine says your workout should be. In fact, if you're careful with your diet, you may even be able to slack off a bit.

But always keep an eye on the scale. After all, a large tub of popcorn (for example) adds 864 calories to your waist. While you can maintain general health with 30 minutes of moderate activity a day, that's not enough to strip off a lot of surplus as well.

Reaching the Peak

The great thing about aerobic exercise is that the same workouts that have you losing weight are also the best workouts for solid cardiorespira-tory fitness—a dandy combination that allows you to breeze through three sets of tennis and doff your shirt without embarrassment during the proceedings.

To achieve good, solid heart and lung fitness, experts say, you need to work large muscle groups. These are the muscles used in running, cycling, cross-country skiing, and other sports. They require lots of oxygen to fuel their movement, thus taxing—and in the long run, strengthening—your heart and lungs. Again, you don't need to spend huge amounts of time. Getting out three to five times a week, 20 to 60 minutes at a pop, is all it takes—assuming, of course, that you're pushing your heart to 55 to 90 percent of its maximum rate.

Better still, this decidedly rational time commitment is enough to whip you pretty close to peak shape. For years, men interested in serious fitness have been driven mad by a simple question: If some exercise is good, isn't more better? The answer is yes, but only up to a point.

"Most people really don't need to train that hard to reach a physiological peak. They just have to train consistently," says Jack Daniels, Ph.D., professor of physical education at State University of New York College at Cortland.

"We've blown the mega-mileage thing clear out of proportion," he adds. "You need to realize that as you increase training, there's a curve that's going up, yes, but it's flattening off all the time. The more you train, the smaller and smaller the additional benefits are."

The real question, then, isn't how much exercise do you need, but how much exercise do you want.

"It's really up to you," says Dr. Duncan. "You just have to decide 'Well at what point am I happy? At what point does this make me feel the best?' That's the amount of exercise that's right for you."

In short, when you're exercising to lose weight, you can turn a deaf ear on the endless nattering about the latest exercise regimens, the most exciting gadgets—both of which are usually being offered by someone who is trying to sell you something. All you really have to do is choose the workouts that you like best—and stick with them.

THE RIGHT QUALITY
THE SECRET TO SUCCESS

Quality is your exercise ace in the hole. It can sculpt a heart that thumps like a bass drum and lungs with the capacity of a Hoover vacuum.

And here's the kicker: It can save you a heck of a lot of time. That's critical, because unless you are 18, single, and working part-time at Wendy's, time is one thing that you probably don't have a lot of. High-quality aerobic exercise makes it possible to shave a couple hours off your weekly workouts while still getting high-quality results.

When experts talk about "quality" aerobic workouts, what they usually have in mind is intensity—that is, pushing yourself so that your heart rate is elevated to a degree sufficient to work the heart and lungs and, over time, strip blubber from your midsection. The activity itself doesn't matter; you can get a quality aerobic workout by running, swimming, circuit training, speed golf, or anything else that gets you huffing and puffing for an extended period of time.

Just how extended that period of time is depends on the intensity of your workout. For example, you can get a quality aerobic workout by bumping your heart rate to a relatively leisurely 40 to 60 percent of its maximum capacity—but only if you keep it up for 60 to 90 minutes. A pleasant way to go, perhaps, but only if you can afford that kind of time.

A quicker way to ignite the aerobic burn is to boost the intensity. If you push yourself aerobically so that your heart is beating at 85 percent (or above) of its maximum capacity, you can wrap up an aerobic session in as little as 20 to 30 minutes.

High-intensity workouts are fast and effective. And because they don't take a lot of time, you can work a large variety of them into your usual workouts. Of course, they also require special handling since they involve pushing your heart, lungs, and muscles harder than you may have pushed them before.

Boosting the Burn

Unfortunately, when it comes to losing weight, quality aerobic exercise is often ignored, and for one simple reason: misinformation.

The biggest single myth regarding weight loss is that fat is burned most efficiently at slow speeds maintained for long periods of time—a long jog, for example, or during a long-distance bike ride. Which may explain why a lot of would-be exercisers give up after about three weeks, believing as they do that the only way to shed pounds is to jog, say, the length of Georgia.

It is true that the longer you exercise, the more calories you'll burn. But when you go long and slow, you're burning those calories at a snail's pace. This is where intensity comes in. Stroll along at 40 percent of your maximum effort, and you'll burn 3 to 4 calories a minute. Jog, and you'll burn 8 to 10 calories a minute. Run hard—at, say, a 6-minute-mile pace—and you'll burn roughly 20 calories a minute.

So much for going it long and slow.

"Yes, long, slow distance works for weight loss," says Ralph LaForge, director of the lipid disorders

The Heart of the Matter

Many men think that exercise should be a simple affair. You pound, you sweat, you shower. The only time they give any thought to their heart rate is when it goes through their skull.

To wage a really effective war on fat, you need to use, and understand, your heart rate. Because your heart rate can tell you precisely how hard you're exercising and whether you're exercising at an effective fat-burning level. The traditional measure—"I'm sweating, so I must be burning fat"—just doesn't cut it.

Perhaps the simplest formula is to subtract your age from 220. This tells you (roughly) your maximum heart rate, allowing you to figure out lesser efforts from there. If you're 40, for example, your max heart rate is roughly 180 beats a minute. If your goal is to exercise at 60 percent of that, just do the math: $180 \times .60 = 108$ beats a minute.

Of course, not every 40-year-old has the same maximum heart rate, any more than every 40-year-old has the same shoe size. To get a more accurate number, one that's based on your actual heart and level of fitness, try this.

1. **To get your resting heart rate, take your pulse before getting out of bed in the morning, counting the number of beats in a minute.**

2. **To get your target heart rate—the one you want to achieve during any given exercise, do this formula: (220 − age − resting heart rate) × percent effort + resting heart rate.**

   It looks complicated, but here's how it shakes out. Assume that you're a 40-year-old man with a resting heart rate of 60 beats a minute. You want to exercise at 60 percent of your max. Your heart rate should be . . . $(220 − 40 − 60) = 120$. And $120 \times 0.60 = 72$.

   Then $72 + 60 = 132$ beats per minute—your target heart rate.

   You'll notice that this second method gives a higher target heart rate than the simpler 220-minus-age method given above. In other words, if you're fit and using the simple formula to calculate your effort, you're not pushing as hard as you should be.

training program for the San Diego Cardiac Center Medical Group. "But if you're fit enough to up the effort to 50 to 70 percent of your max or higher, you'll burn more calories in less time."

A Word of Caution

This is not an invitation to be a perpetual firebrand. Whatever your aerobic activity of choice, be it biking, jogging, or boxing, trying to make every session your personal best is neither smart or realistic.

Only a sadist or someone who owns stock in Ben-Gay would recommend going all-out all the time, since high-intensity aerobic efforts always carry a risk of injury. Your heart and lungs may be in great shape, but overdoing it can cause the supporting cast—the muscles, ligaments, tendons, and other structures that hold you together—to produce a symphony of popping that will have Orville Redenbacher standing at attention.

Indeed, if you're new to fitness, high-intensity workouts shouldn't be a consideration at all. You need to condition your muscles first with slow, easy exercise—a minimum of three months'

worth, three to five days a week—before you start doing harder work.

Even if you're already fit, doing high-intensity, high-quality workouts has its drawbacks. First, you have to sustain it: You won't burn many calories if you sprint out the door and, 30 seconds later, fall on your face. The truth is, even for conditioned athletes, high-intensity workouts—exercising at 85 percent of your max and above—put a lot of stress on muscles and connective tissue. It's a great way to burn fat, but it's also a great way to burn out.

The hard stuff hurts. Go hard too often, and you'll quickly find your interest in exercise waning. It's hard to lose weight when you spend all your time telling yourself that you'll certainly get around to a really, really hard workout—sometime next week.

Most experts advise pushing really hard no more than one day a week. In other words, these super-high-intensity workouts should be just a small part of your overall workout plan. The rest of the time, you'll still be doing quality workouts, but at a slightly lower pace—say, at 60 to 70 percent of your max—for a slightly longer time.

Getting the Most

You can lose a lot of weight without resorting to hard-core, lung-splitting stuff. Ideally, high-quality aerobic workouts will maximize the calorie burn while minimizing the time you spend doing it. Here's what experts advise.

ALLOW FOR BREAK-IN TIME. Whether your ultimate goal is to burn a little fat or go Olympic, it's critical to start small and build slowly. Moving too fast doesn't make you fit. It makes you injured. You won't lose a lot of weight when you're hobbling around the house like an old war hero.

According to guidelines from the American College of Sports Medicine, which is headquartered in Indianapolis, a baseline workout plan consists of 40 minutes to an hour of moderate aerobic exercise, three to five days a week. That's a great foundation, and once you build up to that, you'll continue to make considerable fitness and weight-loss gains over the next six months.

BUMP THE PACE—BUT JUST A LITTLE. Every aerobic workout plan has a plateau phase, at which time the early, exciting gains—or, when you're talking about weight, losses—start to flatten out. At this point it's time to make some changes, if only to keep yourself from getting bored.

For example, if you have been riding a stationary bike for 40 minutes at 50 percent of your maximum effort, all you have to do is tweak the intensity so that you're cruising at 60 percent of your max. Assuming you're already in pretty good shape—and by this time you probably are—upping the intensity a few notches will be a productive challenge.

GO FOR THE BURN. When you're in shape and ready for a change of pace, add a few high-intensity sessions into your schedule. The goal here is to push yourself to at least 85 percent of your maximum heart rate. Doing this once a week does more than burn a lot of calories in a short amount of time. It pushes your heart, lungs, and overall metabolism to the next level, which will help you get in even better shape later on.

WATCH THE TIME. When you're pushing yourself to the max, you don't want a long workout. As a rule, experts say, high-intensity, high-quality workouts should be limited to about 5 to 10 percent of your total weekly effort.

For example, if you typically run 30 miles a week, you might consider putting in a day of in-

An Exercise Sampler

Contrary to what many men believe, you don't need long, slow exercise in order to burn large amounts of fat. Yes, that stuff works, but so do more intense (and less lengthy) approaches. Each of the following eight exercises, says Ralph LaForge, director of the lipid disorders training program for the San Diego Cardiac Center Medical Group, is great for burning fat. You can focus on doing just one, or you can mix and match all eight.

1. Do 60 to 90 minutes of variable terrain walking at a leisurely pace, at 40 to 50 percent of your maximum heart rate.
2. Walk/jog on flat ground for 40 to 50 minutes, alternating a fast walk at a comfortable pace with an easy jog, at about 55 to 65 percent of your max.
3. Cycle for 60 to 90 minutes at 40 to 65 percent of your maximum heart rate.
4. At the gym, spend 15 minutes on a treadmill, 15 minutes on a stationary bike, and 15 minutes on a stair-climber, all at 50 to 70 percent of your max.
5. Jog at 60 to 70 percent of your maximum heart rate for 35 to 50 minutes.
6. Do aerobic step exercise or aerobic dance for 40 to 50 minutes at 50 to 70 percent of your max.
7. Swim without stopping for 45 to 60 minutes. Switch strokes occasionally to work different muscles. Swimming is among the most difficult sports, so it's really not important to shoot for a maximum heart rate. Besides, it's pretty hard to check your heart rate mid-swim in the water.
8. Ride a stationary bike for 40 to 60 minutes at 50 to 70 percent of your max.

tervals at the track—maybe running hard 220s with an easy 220 jog in between, with the hard-running time totaling less than 3 miles.

AIM FOR INTERVALS. When you're pressed for time but still want a serious calorie burn, consider interval training. This consists of alternating hard efforts with short periods of "active rest," in which you keep moving but essentially take it easy. Interval training can provide a substantial calorie-burning workout in as little as 20 to 30 minutes.

For example, a 30-minute run (at an 8-minute-mile pace) would burn about 505 calories. The same 30 minutes spent doing intervals would burn about 10 percent more, or 560 calories.

How you do intervals is entirely up to you. Here are a few things that you might want to try.

- **Ride hard on a stationary bike for 2 to 4 minutes, spin easily for 2 to 4 minutes, then go hard again.**
- **For a 30-minute run, run hard for 2 to 4 minutes, then cruise at an easy pace for 2 to 4 minutes, then pick up the pace again.**
- **When running for distance, try alternating 110-yard sprints with 110-yard easy jogs, switching back and forth for a total of 20 minutes. Or you can simply pick up your pace over the last half-mile of a 5-mile run, or throw in short, hard bursts throughout the run—by running hills, for example, or by sprinting to that stop sign 50 yards ahead, easing off until your heart settles down, then taking off again for that distant stand of trees.**

The interval format works whether you're rowing, running, swimming, or riding a mechanical bull. It is important, however, always to keep the work-to-active-rest ratio roughly at one-to-one. You need to rest long enough to recover, but not so long that your heart rate drops to easy-chair levels—it's the elevated effort that burns calories.

The great thing about intervals is that they're fast. Given a 10-minute warm-up and 10-minute cooldown (crucial when you're doing hard stuff), you can get a superb calorie burn in as little as 30 minutes.

MAINTAIN THE EXCITEMENT. Boredom is perhaps the main reason that many men fall off their exercise and weight-loss plans. Doing long, slow runs—or even fast ones—month after month requires remarkable diligence—plus the ability to ignore the fact that your exercise program has the pizzazz of glue.

The advantage of higher-intensity, high-quality aerobic exercise is that it gives you the ability to periodically boost the benefit of your usual workouts while at the same time throwing some excitement into the mix. In other words, it's a fast way to transform a workout that was formerly as exciting as watching mud dry into something far more interesting and more beneficial, too.

"Variety helps you stick with exercise, and quality can offer that variety," says LaForge. "And sticking with exercise is the key to weight loss and fitness."

CROSS-TRAINING
BRINGING YOU INTO BALANCE

Despite its scientific pedigree, cross-training is just a spiffy word for mixing up your exercises. The best way to achieve solid weight loss and sound fitness while maintaining a grip on your sanity (ever listen to someone who runs seven days a week?) is just such a varied attack.

"If you want to gain all the benefits of exercise—and there are lots of them: strength, endurance, health, a lean look—you'll have a much better chance of covering all the bases by doing different activities," says Jack Daniels, Ph.D., professor of physical education at State University of New York College at Cortland.

The term *cross-training* is often defined as combining different types of exercise: for example, stretching, aerobic, and resistance exercises. But any time you mix up your workouts—cycling plus running plus speed walking, for instance—you're cross-training.

Cross-training isn't complicated. You can do it simply and effectively without a personal trainer or without a pair of sneakers so expensive that they ought to speak four different languages and do your taxes. More important, it has wide-ranging benefits.

Mixing up your exercises brings more muscles into play. This will make you stronger and less prone to injury—and few people lose weight nursing a muscle pull. This whole-body muscle zap will make you look better, too, enabling you to avoid the funhouse-mirror look of the zealous cyclist with Terminator thighs and a taffy torso.

From a practical standpoint, cross-training provides you with more options—and fewer excuses. Pool closed? Go for a run. Run snuffed by a fresh dump of snow? Grab the cross-country skis. Stuck in a strange city whose traffic is outdone only by its crime rate? Bang out some calisthenics in your hotel room.

If your goal is to get lean while enjoying a tremendous range of exercises, sports, and workout times, then cross-training is definitely for you. "If you want to build a sound fitness base and burn fat, cross-training works really well," says Herman Falsetti, M.D., a cardiologist in private practice in Irvine, California.

The Aerobic Attack

With the exception of steering clear of onion rings, snack cakes, and other high-fat (and fattening) foods, the most efficient way to excise surplus calories is with regular aerobic exercise. By alternating among a variety of aerobic choices—everything from cycling and swimming to in-line skating—you'll whip your heart and lungs into shape, while at the same time working (and balancing) muscles in every part of your body.

THINK BIG. It's a simple rule, so it should be easy to remember: The more muscles involved in an exercise, the more calories burned. When you're looking to burn fat, go after the big muscle groups—the kind you work by running, swimming, cycling,

Cross-Training: The Downside

When it comes to exercise, more is almost always better than less. But while cross-training is a great way to work muscles that you didn't even know you had, it's not necessarily the best choice when you're trying to put the sharpest possible edge on your athletic talents.

There is an exercise concept called specificity, which means, in short, that specific exercises work specific muscles—and the specific nerves that fire those muscles. If your goal is to medal in the 400-meter high hurdles, you won't gain much benefit from duckpin bowling.

But the truth is, many elite athletes do use cross-training—not to gain a competitive edge, necessarily, but to give their bodies and minds a break. The rest of us aren't priming for the Olympics in any event. So the issue of specificity, while of academic interest, isn't of tremendous concern.

Despite what the single-sport zealots tell you, you're not losing anything by mixing exercises. "Aerobically, you're getting roughly the same benefit," says Herman Falsetti, M.D., a cardiologist in private practice in Irvine, California. "And you're avoiding the potential for injury in the process."

cross-country skiing, rowing, tennis, basketball, and so on. Table tennis certainly has its intrinsic values, but unless you're a member of the Chinese national team, weight loss isn't one of them.

START EARLY. You don't have to be a seasoned athlete to take up cross-training. It's also a superb way to ease back into shape. Mixing up exercises eases the initial shock to unfit muscles. Start a fitness program with running only, and you put a lot of repetitive stress on some pretty fragile muscles like the calves and Achilles tendons. But if you run one day and bike the next, your calves and hamstrings get a rest on cycling days, and your quadriceps get a break when you run.

Better yet, get off your feet entirely—alternate running or biking with a day of swimming. It's not only great exercise but it's also a wonderful liquid balm the day after a bike ride or run—stretching out the muscles and freeing them from the stress of gravity.

MIX IT UP SLOWLY. It's a painful scenario: A long-time cyclist decides to do some running. He sets off hard. Calf muscle makes a sound like the peeling away of Velcro. Cyclist spends many weeks rehabilitating.

Whether you have just started exercising or have been buffing your butt for longer than you care to admit, it's critical to take up new exercises slowly. Even if your heart and lungs aren't the limiting factor, your muscles and tendons are—and if you don't coddle them, you'll have problems.

"If you're coming back from time off or you're starting something new, going straight into hard effort will set you up for a tendon or ligament injury," says Mark Plaatjes, a Boulder, Colorado, physical therapist and world-class marathon runner. "You'll have better results if you're patient and build things slowly."

When you're taking up a new sport, Plaatjes recommends no hard effort for at least four to six weeks. In the meantime, take it slow and easy. (If you're working too hard to carry on a conversation without gasping for air, you're pushing too hard.) Build endurance and condition the muscles first. "Don't worry about speed," he says. "Just go slow and have fun."

SPLIT UP YOUR WORKOUT. There's a male mystique that says you always have to finish what you start. If today is your running day, you run. When you start on the exercise bike, you finish on the bike. While this sort of single-track thinking may get you through business school, it isn't as productive when it comes to aerobic exercise.

You can sidestep fatigue to a degree by doing two different aerobic exercises during the same workout. Shifting the onus to a different set of muscles in mid-workout will let you push harder just a bit longer, and pushing harder helps maintain a higher calorie burn.

Calorie burn varies from person to person, but generally if you spend 15 minutes on the treadmill exercising at 70 percent of your maximum ability, and then hop to the cross-country ski machine for 15 minutes at the same intensity, you'll burn roughly a third more calories than you would if you ran on the treadmill at 50 percent effort for 30 minutes.

"You might not be able to sustain that effort every time just because you switch activities, but as a rule you will be able to benefit both psychologically and physiologically by changing things up," says Wayne Westcott, Ph.D., national strength-training consultant for the YMCA, the American Council on Exercise, and the National Academy of Sports Medicine.

The same mix-it-up approach can be applied outside the club as well. Run to the pool. Or toss a pair of in-line skates into a backpack, ride your bike for 15 minutes, then hop off and skate.

DO WORKOUTS WITHIN WORKOUTS. Technically, cross-training involves the mixing of different sports and exercises at different times. But we'll be creative for a moment and suggest that you mix things all at the same time.

Remember, the more muscles you involve in your exercise or the more you tax those muscles, the more calories you'll burn. So innovate. Carrying a pair of 3-pound dumbbells as you run can increase the amount of calories burned by as much as 20 percent. Wear swim fins in the pool; it will make those big, oxygen-hungry muscles in your legs work harder and gobble more calories.

Obviously, you don't want to take this too far—using dumbbells while riding a bike will likely bring trouble—but, really, the only limit is your imagination. It doesn't take big changes to get results. For example, during speed hikes in the Colorado mountains, businessman Gary Scott, of Colorado Springs, gets his upper body involved by stabbing at the trail with ski poles.

LOCATION, LOCATION, LOCATION. We have said that there are no hard-and-fast rules when it comes to mixing routines, but here's a recommendation that really should be a rule: Make it convenient. If you take up a sport that can only be done, say, in a fitness park across town and only between the hours of 5:00 and 6:00 A.M., you won't be doing it long. "It has to be convenient so that you'll do it," says Dr. Falsetti. "If you have to drive 15 miles across town to exercise, you're not going to do it."

BE REASONABLE. Yes, cross-training is the best route to well-rounded fitness, but this doesn't mean that you should take up an exercise routine that requires its own appointment book. The sporting goods industry would certainly like it if we all incorporated boxing, volleyball, running, cycling, aerobic dance, and judo into our exercise week, but this is neither practical nor wise. You need to engage in a specific exercise with some regularity.

Why? Because repetition brings conditioning. If you're only running once every two weeks, you'll be starting almost from scratch each time, and you'll certainly never get in good enough condition to work hard enough to burn serious calories.

Though this isn't written in stone, experts generally advise picking two aerobic exercises that you like and then mixing them through the week—say, cycling on Monday, Wednesday, and Friday and running on Tuesday, Thursday, and Saturday (because each exercise stresses different muscles, alternating them like this give those muscles a day off to recover). Even God took a day off to rest. You should, too.

Building Muscle

That weight training could be used to lose weight might seem ludicrous, since even recreational lifters add bulk to their frames, and serious lifters look like sides of beef. But in recent years experts have found that weight training is an extremely effective tool in the battle to burn fat, particularly when combined with aerobic workouts.

Though sorely outnumbered on most of our frames, muscle cells are far more metabolically active than fat cells. A pound of muscle can require 35 to 45 more calories just to get through the day. Fat cells are an overfed aunt picking through the leftovers. Muscle cells are Jenny Craig enrollees given the go-ahead at an all-you-can-eat buffet.

"Adding more muscle to your frame actually helps to burn fat more effectively throughout the day," says Harvey Newton, a certified strength and conditioning specialist and the executive director of the National Strength and Conditioning Association in Colorado Springs, Colorado. "You won't find too many people who disagree that weight training is part of the total weight-loss package."

Particularly when combined with aerobic workouts, cross-training in the weight room works a larger variety of muscles than by doing the same lifts over and over again. That means existing muscle cells grow, and that, of course, means more fat burned.

When you're trying to lose weight, experts say, it's a good idea to combine three days a week of aerobic exercise with two days of weight training. While two days of weight training isn't enough to promote substantial strength gains, it's more than enough to provide muscle mass to achieve the metabolic burn that you're looking for.

WORK THE BIG GROUPS. If you spend much time in the gym, you've almost certainly seen the big guys spending what seems like an inordinate amount of time working on small parts of their anatomy—doing wrist curls, say, or heel raises. But when you're trying to lose weight—unless you're also auditioning for the role of Popeye—doing isolated dumbbell curls isn't your best bet.

Instead, focus on lifts that hit big muscles and big groups of muscles. "The more muscles and joints involved in a lift, the more caloric expenditure," says Newton.

There are lots of these big muscle groups to work on. Doing lunges, for example, works the glutes, quads, and hamstrings; bench presses are good for building the chest, shoulders, and triceps; lat pull-downs do the shoulders, back, and biceps.

DO THE CIRCUIT. A great way to combine lifting with aerobic exercise is circuit training. It works like this: Select six to eight big-muscle lifts that will give your whole body a workout. Do 12 to 15 repetitions of each exercise. Rest 30 seconds between exercises. After you have done all the exercises, rest up to 2 minutes. Then repeat the circuit.

"Lifting this way drives the cardiovascular system to a higher level and then keeps it there because you don't allow enough time for recovery," says Newton. "Because your cardiovascular system is elevated, you're burning more calories."

One important note: When doing circuit training, you'll want to substantially reduce the weights that you normally lift. As a rule, experts say, plan on lifting 40 to 60 percent of your current max. If you're new to weight training, you'll want

to build a strength base first: three days a week of lifting for two to three months should do it.

STAND AND MOVE. To boost the calorie burn just a little more, concentrate on standing lifts. For example, do standing dumbbell military presses as opposed to those performed seated. Standing lifts burn slightly more calories because you are working to support your own weight, too. Add some movement to those standing lifts—say, by doing lunges instead of taking a seat on the leg-extension machine—and you'll up the caloric burn yet again.

A Quick Stretch

Cross-training, by definition, is a whole-body approach. Which brings us to the uncomfortable matter of stretching. Experts tell us that stretching is a crucial part of a fitness plan, especially since, as we age, we stiffen up faster than roadkill. We nod our heads in somber agreement, then ignore stretching entirely. Who has time to do it?

We'll deal with stretching in the Flexing and Stretching section, beginning on page 335. For now, we'll leave you with something to chew on, courtesy of Bob Anderson of Palmer Lake, Colorado, author of *Stretching*.

"One of the signs of aging for most of us is a gradual loss of range of motion, a creeping rigor mortis, if you will," says Anderson. "Ironically, it doesn't take much effort at all to maintain quite a bit of flexibility throughout your life. Five to 10 minutes of stretching a day will do it. At 30, stretching may not seem like much of a concern. At 50, 60, 70, and 80, you'll be glad you stuck with it."

BOXING
KNOCK OUT CALORIES

Exercise physiologists have measured boxing's caloric burn, and it's impressive—up to 1,400 calories an hour in the middle of a round, roughly twice the burn of hard running. Which is why you rarely see a fat boxer.

"Boxing is a total-body workout and an incredible calorie burner," says Tom Virgets, Ph.D., of Atlanta, an exercise physiologist who left a teaching career to train professional fighters such as Tommy Morrison and Donovan "Razor" Ruddick. "Cardiovascular fitness—you have to have it; muscular strength—have to have it; muscular endurance and flexibility—you have to have it."

Boxing has other advantages, too, explains Dr. Virgets. Done correctly, a boxing workout (as opposed to an actual fight in the ring) rarely causes injuries. Boxing stresses (and sculpts) the body in well-rounded fashion, so you don't have the overuse injuries that are common to repetitive motion sports like running. It also fosters practical skills that aren't gained by humping away on the stair-climber. "You'll develop balance, agility, speed, power, and hand-eye coordination," Dr. Virgets says. "Add those components, and you put boxing in a category of its own."

The idea of boxing as a fitness and weight-loss tool escaped the public for years, possibly because the public wasn't keen on having its face caved in. But these days there are plenty of clubs and boxing gyms where you can use boxing's proven tools—hitting the heavy bag, jumping rope, shadow-boxing, and so forth—without risking your bridgework.

Indeed, most clubs don't offer "boxing" at all, but instead refer to the workouts as boxercise or aerobox. Don't be put off by the cute names. While these activities involve no real boxing—that is, there is no glove-to-face contact—you'll still get an excellent workout. Do it regularly, and you will muscle up your shoulders, harden your stomach, trim your hips, firm your legs, and flare your lats. In short, you'll look like someone you would want to avoid in the ring.

"You look at any middleweight boxer; if you work hard enough, that's the look you'll get," says Mike Wareing, owner of Wareing's Gym in Virginia Beach, Virginia. "Definition, not bulk. Lean, light, and aerobically fit."

Getting Started

Boxing is not a complex sport. There are four punches—jab, cross, hook, and uppercut. The exercises and equipment are simple. Unlike certain exercise machines that require physics training to operate, heavy bags and jump ropes are easy to use.

Still, when you take up boxing as exercise, you do need to know what you're doing. Hit the heavy bag with a poorly thrown punch, and you could hurt your shoulder or break your wrist. More important, you also need to remember what you aren't doing.

"These boxing training programs teach you how to punch and give you great exercise, but you're not by any stretch of the imagination learning to be a fighter," says Wareing. Hitting a

Getting into the Ring

As an exercise physiologist, Tom Virgets, Ph.D., of Atlanta, understands the full benefits of boxing for fitness. But as a boxing coach, trainer, and former fighter, he hesitates to recommend life in the ring. "The rewards are great, but the punishment can be terrific," he says.

But for some men, the allure of boxing doesn't end with jumping rope. They want to get into the ring and fight.

The first thing that you need to do is find a boxing gym. Dr. Virgets recommends calling U.S.A. Boxing, the governing body for amateur boxing, at (719) 578-4506, which can put you in touch with a gym in your area.

You have to be careful of which gym you pick, Dr. Virgets adds. The litmus test is simple: "You want a gym that has your interests in mind and will protect you, let's say, from just being someone's punching bag."

At a good gym, the instructors will make sure that you do plenty of work before you ever get in the ring. In fact, some may require you to get a medical checkup beforehand. Because if you're not in good shape, you're the one who is going to pay. They will teach you how to throw punches and combinations of punches. They will teach you how to bob, weave, and slip the punches that will be thrown at you.

Most gyms supply all the equipment, although you'll probably have to pop for hand wraps and a form-fitting mouthpiece. Because, make no mistake about it, when you get in the ring, you're going to get hit.

To some extent, good conditioning will help soften the blows. Dr. Virgets especially recommends neck exercises, which can help keep your head from spinning around like a gyroscope when you take a punch. But once you get in the ring, you have to expect some pain. "Boxing takes an ungodly amount of courage, and the only way that courage is developed is through practice, and that means getting hit," he says. "It's not for everyone. In fact, it's for very few."

menting that with running or weight training on their own. Other people are more serious, doing a boxing workout five to six times a week. Wareing recommends doing at least an hour of boxing drills, one to three times a week. But how often you work out isn't nearly as important as the quality of that workout. To get the most from boxing without getting hurt, here's what you need to know.

JOIN A GYM. With the right equipment and some basic knowledge, you can get a good boxing workout in your garage. But a gym offers some things that your garage doesn't: qualified instruction, equipment you don't have to buy, and the camaraderie of like-minded people. Most people find that the cost of a gym is offset by the benefits.

If you do decide to teach yourself, pick up a training video or book, says Dr. Virgets. There are plenty to choose from. If you can't find anything in your area, check the ads in boxing magazines like *Boxing Illustrated* and *Ring.*

GET EQUIPPED. Obviously, when you join a gym, you don't have to invest much in the way of equipment. All you really need are hand wraps—strips of cotton that look like an elastic bandage, which you wrap around your hands to keep them from getting scraped when you hit the heavy bag.

Boxers who actually get in the ring wear protective headgear and mouthpieces, but since no one is throwing punches at you, you won't need that protection unless the heavy bag takes an unfortunate swing.

If you're doing some of your workouts at home, here's what you'll need to buy.

- Jump rope
- Bag gloves. These weigh about 12 ounces and provide padding and wrist support for hitting the heavy bag.
- Heavy bag. A quality heavy bag weighs 70 pounds and is made of canvas, nylon, or leather. Leather bags are the most durable and, thus, the most expensive, but you can save yourself some money because canvas and nylon bags work just fine.

  Most of them need to be hung from a fairly substantial beam. Or you can buy a freestanding heavy bag, which sits on a round, weighted base.
- Speed bag. Less essential than the heavy bag, the speed bag is used to develop hand speed and coordination.

heavy bag and jumping rope will get you in great shape. It won't help you survive in the ring against Mike Tyson.

Most people who take up boxing for exercise use it as part of a cross-training program, coming into the gym two or three times a week and supple-

WORK INTO IT SLOWLY. Boxing workouts (and boxing matches) are ruthlessly efficient conditioners and calorie burners for a simple reason: Boxers expend a lot of energy while getting very little rest.

Consider that a professional bout consists of 3-minute rounds with a minute rest between each round. Most boxing workouts are patterned on this rigorous model. For instance, you might go three 3-minute rounds on the heavy bag, with a minute rest between each round.

"It's the short rest that's essential," says Dr. Virgets. "That keeps your heart rate up and the calories burning."

Actually, the 3-minutes-on, 1-minute-off pattern is what you will eventually build up to because in the beginning you'll find that whopping away on the heavy bag for 30 seconds will turn your arms to noodles. So start by hitting the bag for 30 seconds, then rest a minute, recommends Dr. Virgets. As you get fitter, hit the bag for a minute, rest a minute. Hit the bag for 2 minutes, rest a minute.

CHECK YOUR PULSE. While we're on the subject of rest, it's important to note that for some people, and virtually all beginners, a minute's rest may not give you enough time to fully recover. Make no mistake, you *need* this recovery time. Without it your muscles will quickly build up lactic acid and get sore and heavy. It's hard to throw punches when your arms have turned to stone.

On the other hand, you don't want too much rest since this will slow your training. This is where taking your pulse comes in handy. "When your pulse drops to 120 to 130 beats a minute, then go again," says Dr. Virgets.

WATCH YOUR FORM. There's a tendency, especially when you get tired, to begin flailing away without paying close attention to your moves. Be careful. Sloppy punches are more likely to break your wrist than dent the bag.

Planning Your Workout

There are as many boxing workouts as there are personal injury lawyers. If you're new to boxing, but are still fairly fit, Wareing suggests this beginner's workout: Start with 1 to 2 miles of running. Then do three 3-minute rounds of jumping rope, two sets of 30 sit-ups, three sets of 15 push-ups, three sets of eight pull-ups, and three 3-minute rounds of shadowboxing. Then do two 3-minute rounds on the heavy bag (punching slowly to conserve energy), followed by one (or more) 3-minute rounds of jumping rope. "In the beginning you really need to pace yourself," he says.

PUSH YOURSELF HARDER. Once you have the core workout down, it's time to really get strenuous. "Throw more punches and increase the number of rounds you do," says Dr. Virgets. "And if you really want to make it tough, decrease the rest interval, too."

For example, while a beginner might throw 60 punches at the heavy bag in a 3-minute round, an experienced boxer will throw three times as many. As you get fitter, try adding 30 punches to each 3-minute round, suggests Dr. Virgets. For example, start with 60 punches, then work up to 90, then 120 and so on. The faster and harder you hit, the more intense the exercise.

Since boxing is so rigorous, pushing yourself too hard too fast will surely put you down for the count. It's good to extend your limits, but you don't want to end your workout feeling as though you are the punching bag. "Intensity is always good, but stay within your means," says Wareing. "Consistency wins out over intensity every time, and it's hard to be consistent if you're hurt."

CALISTHENICS
THE ULTIMATE IN CONVENIENCE

Most of us got our first taste of calisthenics in gym class, where the coach used them to fill time between slam ball and wrestling. After that, for most of us, calisthenics fell out of our lives.

Which is unfortunate. Properly done, calisthenics—exercises in which your body weight provides the resistance—are a superb way to whip yourself into shape. "You can get some outstanding benefits from calisthenics," says Harvey Newton, a certified strength and conditioning specialist and the executive director of the National Strength and Conditioning Association in Colorado Springs, Colorado. "You'll increase your strength and your muscular endurance, and you'll get some increased flexibility. And if you do them right, they'll burn a few calories along the way, too."

Calisthenics offer another benefit as well. In a world that is forever throwing curve balls (or excuses) at our exercise ambitions, calisthenics are the perfect antidote. You don't have to hover on the periphery of the weight room, as guys three times your size hog the equipment, or try to get a decent workout in hotels that have a single multistation weight machine that looks like it has been maintained by baboons with sledgehammers. With calisthenics you can get a solid workout anywhere, anytime. "They're effective, convenient, and cheap," Newton says. "You always have your body with you."

The Basics

You banged off calisthenics without a thought in high school, but back then you had acne, too. The point is, your body has changed. To get the full benefit of calisthenics without killing your back or knees in the process, here are a few things you may want to try.

ALWAYS START SLOW. Calisthenics sound tame, until you find yourself dangling under a pull-up bar, trying to get your chin over the top. (Don't be embarrassed—anyone who isn't still in high school will be dangling right beside you.) Don't waste time (or motivation) committing yourself to high numbers of repetitions. If five chin-ups—or push-ups, back extensions, or anything else—seem to be your max, then five is what you do.

DO LESS, BUT DO THEM RIGHT. "Don't sacrifice form for number of repetitions," says W. Keith Prusaczyk, Ph.D., a research physiologist at the Naval Health Research Center in San Diego who works with the calisthenics-reliant Navy SEALs, some of the fittest folks around. "An exercise is designed to work a specific muscle group. If you alter your form, you're altering the amount of stress on those muscles and defeating the purpose of the exercise."

ALLOW FOR RECOVERY. If you do calisthenics regularly, always take at least a day off between routines. Your muscles need time to recover, and not only for comfort: It is during the rest phase that individual muscle fibers get larger and stronger.

Building a Program

There are hundreds of calisthenic wrinkles, but most people want to keep it simple. Here are two programs, courtesy of Harvey Newton, a certified strength and conditioning specialist and the executive director of the National Strength and conditioning Association in Colorado Springs, Colorado, that provide a solid, whole-body workout.

Beginning Program

Step-ups. Stand in front of a chair or a bench. Step up, then down, alternating feet each time. Do 12 to 15 repetitions per foot.

Crunches. Lie on the floor on your back, cup hands behind your ears, elbows out, with your legs bent and on a bench. Lift your head off the floor and try to touch your ribs to your pelvis. Do 15 to 20 repetitions.

Lower back extensions. Lie facedown on the floor, arms against your sides. Raise your head so that your shoulders are 6 inches off the ground, then lower. Do 12 to 15 repetitions.

If this is too easy, make it harder by doing a "superman." Lie facedown with your arms in front of you. Simultaneously lift your chest, arms, and legs off the ground.

Push-ups. Get in the push-up position, with your hands about 2 feet apart. Lower yourself until your chest touches the floor. Pause at the bottom, then push up. Repeat. Do 12 to 15 repetitions.

Pull-ups. Using an underhand grip on the bar, pull yourself up until your chin is over the bar. Be sure to keep your back and legs straight. Do 12 to 15 repetitions.

Advanced Program

When you can easily complete three sets each of the exercises above, don't bother adding more sets. Instead, make each exercise more intense. At the same time, add 2 to 3 minutes of jumping rope between exercises.

Step-ups. Use a chair that makes you step higher. Better yet, instead of alternating legs, do a complete set using one leg, then switch to the other.

Crunches. Place a 5-pound weight plate across the top of your chest, holding it in place by crossing your arms.

Lower back extensions. Use the superman described above but wear shoes and hold a small book in each hand.

Push-ups. Do them slowly: 5 seconds down, 5 seconds up.

Pull-ups. Do them slowly: 5 seconds up, 5 seconds down.

Putting Them to Work

It's true that calisthenics, done correctly, build muscular endurance and aerobic stamina and burn plenty of calories at the same time. It's also true that doing calisthenics the way that most people do them will hardly get you breathing hard. Doing a set of 10 push-ups, then swaggering around the gym for the next 5 minutes is not a calorie-burning exercise.

"You have to keep moving. That's the key," says Ed Burke, Ph.D., associate professor of exercise science and an exercise physiologist at the University of Colorado in Colorado Springs. "How many calories you burn depends on the intensity. If you want to get the most benefit from calisthenics, you have to make the exercises hard and then move quickly from exercise to exercise to ensure that your heart rate stays up."

THINK IN MULTIPLES. The more muscles you involve in an exercise, and the bigger those muscles are, the better your workout is going to be. Exercising big muscles, and lots of them, requires you to expend more energy and thus burn more calories.

Push-ups and pull-ups are good upper-body exercises that bring lots of muscles into play. For the legs, step-ups provide an excellent, multimuscle workout while giving the heart an extra kick. "The leg muscles are large muscle groups that are far from the heart," says Newton. "When you start working the legs, your heart really has to work hard, and that gets the calories burning fast."

KEEP MOVING. No one burns calories just standing around. To burn a lot of calories, you need to get your heart rate up between 60 and 80 percent of its maximum rate (to roughly estimate your maximum heart rate, subtract your age from 220) and keep it there for as long as you can. The only way to do this is to keep the rest between sets short.

Mark De Lisle, a former Navy SEAL, has designed a hellishly difficult calisthenics program with no more than 15 to 30 seconds' rest between exercises. Some of the routines are truly brutal, but that's not the point here. Any kind of calisthenics will be made harder and more effective by keeping the rest times short.

MAKE USE OF YOUR DOWNTIME. Rather than standing around between sets, keep your heart blasting by doing something aerobic. After each set of push-ups, for example, jump rope for 2 to 3 minutes. Or jog in place. Or hop on the stair-climber, a treadmill, or a stationary bike. Then do another set of calisthenics. "If you keep moving, that ensures more calories will be burned," says Dr. Burke.

INCREASE THE DIFFICULTY. Minimizing rest time is one way to get the most from calisthenics. The other is to make the calisthenics harder. For example:

- Do pull-ups with a dumbbell clasped between your feet, says Newton.
- Wear a diving belt (to which you can attach little weights that look like bricks from Fort Knox) when doing pull-ups and dips.
- To increase grip and arm strength, use a thicker pull-up bar. Or wrap tape around the bar you have.
- Do push-ups slowly—5 seconds down, 5 seconds up—which will make them a heck of a lot harder. So will putting your feet on a step, weight bench, or chair, says Newton; elevating your legs forces your arms to move more weight.

PUSH YOUR MUSCLES HARD. Most people do calisthenics in a hit-and-run fashion. They pump out a set of pull-ups until their muscles scream. Then they quit and gratefully flee to another exercise.

"That's just what you don't want to do," says De Lisle. Additional stress, not rest, is what makes muscles stronger. De Lisle recommends doing pyramids, in which you gradually increase stress on an already-stressed muscle. For example, you might do two push-ups, rest 15 seconds, do four push-ups, rest 15 seconds, then do six push-ups. Then you go back down: six push-ups followed by four followed by two. "You'll get tremendous benefits doing it this way," he says.

TAKE THEM BY SURPRISE. The problem with any kind of exercise, calisthenics included, is that eventually you reach a plateau. That is when your muscles, which are remarkably adaptable, get used to the exercise and so stop progressing. Plateaus are common for the simple reason that most people change their exercise routines about as often as Rush Limbaugh changes his mind.

"Variety is crucial," says Newton. "Your muscles need to be shocked if you want to keep making gains."

It doesn't take major changes to shake muscles out of their rut. Change the order of your calisthenics. Shorten (or occasionally lengthen) the rests that you take. Throw in completely new exercises. Make minor adjustments to your current lineup (for example, by reversing your grip on the pull-up bar). Indeed, most experts recommend throwing small changes into your routine every time you exercise.

CROSS-COUNTRY SKIING
MAKING THE MOST OF WINTER'S BURN

The cold months are often a time of repose, if only because there are so many things to do other than exercise—most of them involving buffet tables buckling under the weight of holiday birds, fruit-cake, and similarly "healthful" fare.

Which is why the bird songs of spring are often interrupted by the gasps of merrymakers who, looking down, can no longer see their feet.

This is an unfortunate and wholly unnecessary state of affairs because winter offers the chance to engage in the most ruthlessly efficient calorie-in-cinerating exercise of all: cross-country skiing.

The numbers tell the story. Even at a comfortable pace, cross-country skiing can easily burn 20 calories a minute. That's the caloric equivalent of a heated volley with Andre Agassi or a full-court scrimmage with the Chicago Bulls. In an hour, a 155-pound man will burn between 1,000 and 1,500 calories.

Time: That's another great thing about cross-country skiing. Even if you are moderately fit, you can ski for an hour or more, whereas a succession of full-court turnovers will send even the fittest athlete to the sidelines. "Cross-country skiing burns the most calories per minute and the most

calories total because you can sustain the effort," says Jim Stray-Gundersen, M.D., assistant professor of orthopedics and physiology at the University of Texas Southwestern Medical Center at Dallas. "It's the best exercise there is."

The reason cross-country skiing is so efficient is that it works almost every muscle you have. "It's one of the few sports where your upper body and lower body both come into play," says Gordon Lange of Park City, Utah, head coach of the United States cross-country ski team. "You're using muscles in your chest, arms, stomach, back, hips, and thighs. They're all working all the time. Even when you're going slow, all those muscles are still firing, and they're burning calories every time they fire."

One more word from Dr. Stray-Gundersen—based not on his expertise as a physiologist but on his experience as a cross-country skier since the age of three: "Gliding along over a snowy track, feeling really comfortable in the middle of winter, it's incredible fun," he says.

Getting Ready

Even though cross-country skiing is a relatively gentle sport—it doesn't abuse your joints or muscles the way running, basketball, and soccer do—it can still be a tough workout. If you are totally out of shape when you start the day, you are going to

Cross-country's beauty is also its biggest drawback. Namely, you need snow. But the Jamaican bobsled team managed without it, and, if necessary, you can, too.

Cross-country ski machines. There is a host of ski machines on the market, and your health club probably has one or two. We won't get into a buyer's guide here. We will tell you this: The calorie burn on a machine comes close to the real thing.

That said, don't think that clacking away on a machine while watching Christmas specials will prepare you for the trails. "Machines stack up well as far as calorie burn, but they can't teach you how to ski," says Jim Stray-Gundersen, M.D, assistant professor of orthopedics and physiology at the University of Texas Southwestern Medical Center at Dallas.

Here is another, more serious drawback to machines. If you are like most men, even the best-designed equipment will eventually bore you to stone. "Being out in the country is much more rewarding than just being able to stop your watch after 40 minutes and say, 'Well, I did it,' " says Gordon Lange of Park City, Utah, head coach of the United States cross-country ski team.

Roller skis. Substitute the city for woods and pavement for snow, and you have roller skis. These are simply narrow skis about 3 feet long with a wheel in the front, another in the back, and a cross-country ski boot on top. Add ski poles to reach forward, plant, and drive yourself forward, and you'll essentially be mimicking all the movements of the real thing.

While you can roller-ski on any hard surface, blacktop is best. The smoothness lets the wheels roll easily, and the slightly soft texture allows you to dig in with your poles a little bit. On cement, by contrast, the pole tips tend to skip.

Roller skiing has the advantage of being accessible and a lot of fun. But there is one caveat: Pavement is a lot less forgiving than snow, so wearing a helmet is a must.

feel pain at the end of it.

A few weeks before heading for snow, Lange says, it is a good idea to start getting your muscles ready. He recommends finding terrain that mimics the ground that you will ski on—in a word, ups and downs. Get in some hiking time and speed-walk the uphills. To get your upper body conditioned, bring along your ski poles. Take long strides and kick off with your feet, while planting and pushing off the ground with your poles. (To protect your equipment, use old poles.) Mountain biking will also help get your legs—and your heart and lungs—into shape. (For more information, see Mountain Biking on page 138.)

Hitting Your Stride

If you have never cross-country skied before, it can seem both intimidating and confusing. Intimidating because it appears to be the province of svelte Norwegians with hearts the size of basketballs. Confusing because there are numerous specialized cross-country skiing styles like classic skiing, backcountry skiing, skating, and more. In addition, the average skier has more equipment than a Desert Storm strike force. It is hard to know where to start.

Don't be overwhelmed, and don't spend a fortune on gear, Lange advises. "It's really a simple sport," he says. "Anybody can do it."

GET EQUIPPED. As a beginner, you don't want to get bogged down in equipment decisions. But there are a few things that you will need—specifically, skis and poles.

Traditional cross-country skis are narrower and longer than downhill skis, a design that allows you to cross ungroomed terrain without sinking into the snow. Which size you get depends on your height. The old rule was that a cross-country ski should stretch the distance from the wrist of your upstretched arm to the ground. This made for a long and ungainly ski, and beginners were forever crossing their ski tips and plunging forward on their faces.

Today, most cross-country skis are shorter and more manageable. But before plunking down a large chunk of change, Lange says, rent different types and try them for yourself. When you find a set that feels right, then you can make the investment.

Incidentally, when you're ready to buy, bring along the gloves and socks that you'll be wearing. This will help ensure that the poles and boots will be the right fit.

DRESS FOR THE WORST. Wearing the right clothes to stay warm would seem like a no-brainer. Nonetheless, rescue teams regularly pluck human snow-cones from the backcountry after they ventured out wearing jeans and a sweatshirt.

"Winter weather can change dramatically, and

you need to be prepared," says Lange. "You always want to have enough clothes to be prepared for the worst."

There are two approaches to dressing for cold. One is to start light, then add layers when you get cold. The other is to start bundled up, then strip layers as you heat up. Both approaches are fine. The important point is that wearing clothes in layers allows you to adjust to changing conditions.

This said, there are a few immutable rules for dressing for cold. Wear a synthetic material from the ski shop against your skin, something that wicks away sweat. The worst thing you can do is wear a T-shirt, which quickly will become soaked with sweat. No matter how uncomfortable cold is, it's a lot worse when you're wet.

Unless you are already an experienced skier, you can expect to spend a lot of time wallowing in the snow. A wool sweater or a cotton sweatshirt will suck up moisture and keep it there. With dryness in mind, make sure your outer layer is waterproof.

Finally, get good gloves since frostbite starts at the extremities. Also, you should wear a hat. Without one you will lose 25 to 40 percent of your body heat through your head.

PACK IN SOME FOOD. You are going to be burning a lot of calories, and if you don't replenish that energy, you are going to be exhausted long before you get back to the car. The same goes for water. You will be sweating buckets out there, and getting dehydrated can be even more uncomfortable—and dangerous—than going hungry.

GET USED TO FALLING. You are going to be doing a lot of it. There is no escaping the fact that skiing involves propelling yourself across a slippery surface on inherently unstable supports. Which is why beginning cross-country skiers generally spend a lot of time on their backs waving their skis in the air.

The good news is that falling on cross-country skis isn't nearly as hazardous as it is with downhill skis. For one thing, you are usually not moving very fast. More important, since skiing cross-country requires a walking motion, your heels aren't locked to the ski. This is why cross-country skiers avoid the ugly ankle breaks suffered by downhillers, who are grafted to the ski as solidly as if they had stepped into buckets of wet cement.

PICK YOURSELF UP. It wouldn't be fair to leave you thrashing in the snow without a quick word on how to get up. After taking a tumble—

and after spending a contemplative moment or two admiring how cold snow gets—roll over on your side. Put your skis together, pointing the tips in the direction you are facing. Then reach for the tips with both hands. This draws you forward and into a good position for rolling over and onto your knees. Then plant a pole on each side and stand up.

THINK ABOUT LESSONS. The quickest way to cut through the confusion and get off on the right foot is to get good instruction. Most ski areas offer lessons, usually in a package deal that includes rental equipment and a few hours of instruction.

Skiing for Fitness

The great thing about cross-country skiing is that you get a solid workout even when you take it slow. When you are ready to push things a little harder, though, here are some workouts to try.

GO LONG AND SLOW. Even at a leisurely pace, cross-country skiing is a ruthless calorie-burner. There really isn't much need to push harder. In fact, it may be counterproductive. Because if you push hard, you won't be able to go far. "Go long and slow," advises Dr. Stray-Gundersen.

Here's the math. Ski comfortably for an hour, burning 15 calories a minute, and you'll use 900 calories. Ski harder—say, at a 20-calorie-per-minute pace—for 30 minutes, and you'll use 600 calories.

Lange coaches some of the country's best skiers. Despite their awesome levels of fitness, he generally has them skiing long and slow, keeping their heart rates below a pedestrian 150 beats per minute to develop endurance.

TAKE A SHORT CUT. Obviously, not everyone can afford to merrily ski away an entire afternoon. When you are short on time but still want a tough workout and calorie burn, you have no choice but to boost the intensity.

Here's a simple, 40-minute workout: Warm up with 10 minutes of slow, easy skiing, Lange says. Then charge the hills. "Every hill you come to, kick it into high gear," says Lange. "Come up and over the hill hard, then cruise until you get to the next hill." Do this for 20 minutes, then cool off with 10 minutes of easy skiing, and you're done.

ALTERNATE THE PACE. If there aren't good hills where you're skiing, then you may want to play with intervals. For example, alternate 3-minute bouts of hard skiing with an easy minute of slow recovery.

IN-LINE SKATING
CAN THIS MUCH FUN BE EXERCISE?

Once, at a San Francisco restaurant, Eddy Matzger—in-line skating's most decorated racer—consumed a seafood salad, rack of lamb with potatoes and string beans, linguine with calamari, 1¼ loaves of bread, a glass of wine, a slice of cheesecake, and a cup of coffee.

Only when Matzger was dabbing his mouth with a napkin did he admit to his dinner companion that he had also eaten a good meal before coming to the restaurant. "Being an in-line skater," he said, "will turn you into a metabolic hummingbird."

Experts agree. In-line skating taxes the hips, the butt, and all the leg muscles—big muscles that force the body to gobble a lot of calories. And unlike running, it won't splinter your knees; there is virtually no impact when gliding on wheels.

Of course, the main reason people take up in-line skating is that it's a lot of fun. "The biggest reason people don't exercise is because they find it boring," says John Porcari, Ph.D., an exercise physiologist and executive director of the La Crosse Exercise and Health Program at the University of Wisconsin in La Crosse. "With in-line skating you can do something that's fun and still get a great workout at the same time."

Staying Alive

Before going any further, it's important to acknowledge that in-line skating isn't the easiest—or safest—sport around. According to the U.S. Consumer Product Safety Commission, in 1995 there were approximately 105,000 in-line skating injuries that required treatment in emergency rooms. Most injuries, of course, were relatively minor. Some—like concussions and broken bones—weren't.

We don't want to scare off potential skaters, but we'd like merely to note that no one has ever accrued fitness gains while stretched out in traction. Most in-line skaters get by without serious problems, but they're the ones who skate smart. If you use your head, you probably won't smash it. Here are some things to keep in mind.

DON'T EXCEED YOUR TALENTS. "Only go as fast as you're comfortable with stopping," says Joel Rappelfeld, founder of the Roll America In-Line Skating School in New York City and author of *The Complete In-Line Skater*. "Always stay within your comfort zone."

WEAR PROTECTION. Keeping your body intact isn't all mental. Wearing a helmet, wrist guards, and knee and elbow pads is essential. This is not the time to penny-pinch. Buy a quality helmet that offers rearward-impact protection; many head injuries result when skaters fall over backward.

Just as important are good wrist guards. When you're going out of control, the natural tendency is to throw your hands in front of you, which explains why about 28 percent of hospital visits for in-line skating injuries involve the wrists.

GET INSTRUCTION. If you have the natural balance of an Olympic athlete, you can skip this part. But if, like most mortals, you're not entirely steady when you first put on wheels, getting lessons will save you some tumbles.

PRACTICE SMART. When you get your first pair of in-line skates, you're going to want to charge outside and have at it. Do so, but do it on a level surface away from traffic. (A tennis court or empty parking lot works well.) You don't want to be learning to brake and turn when you suddenly arrive at the bottom of Nosebleed Hill—and realize it empties into four lanes of fast-moving traffic. Though judging from the injury statistics, a surprising number of people do so.

Getting Fit

While it's up to you to set the pace, here are a few strategies for getting the best burn every time.

GET LOW. To skate vigorously, you have to skate low. It's the long, powerful strides, like those of a speed skater on ice, that build fitness and burn calories. "The longer stride is a lot more work, so it burns a lot more calories," says Rappelfeld.

In the beginning, tucking low won't be easy, and your screaming back and legs will let you know it. So build up to it slowly. You may want to crouch low for a minute, then stand and roll easily to recover. As you get fitter, you'll be able to stay down longer.

USE YOUR UPPER BODY. Good skaters don't let their legs do all the work. They're constantly moving their arms—not just to balance themselves but also to gain momentum. At the same time, of course, it burns more calories.

SKATE LONG AND SLOW. While you can burn a lot of calories doing a fast dash, some of the best in-line skating workouts involve a relatively slow pace maintained for a long time. Researchers at the University of Wisconsin Performance Laboratory in Madison found that in-line skaters needed to cruise at 8 to 12 miles an hour for at least 20 minutes to get a substantial cardiovascular workout. Don't try to go too fast. In-line skating looks easy, but if you push at more than 60 to 70 percent of your max, you probably won't make the distance.

GO EVEN SLOWER. Very slow. The best in-line skaters will sometimes glide along at barely a snail's pace, bent extremely low. Super-slow-motion skating, in which you're moving so slowly that you're almost on the point of falling over, is one intense workout.

When skating slow, concentrate on maintaining perfect technique. Stay low and propel yourself with a long push followed by a long glide. Don't try to do it for more than a few minutes at a time. Because there's so much muscle tension, slow-motion skating works your legs like a weight workout. It's intense. Plus, it fosters good habits.

Having Fun the Hard Way

Plenty of people have decreed that getting fit is a matter of monastic dedication and rote regimen. Pity for you if you believe them.

Eddy Matzger certainly doesn't. Matzger, who holds the in-line skating world record for 10 kilometers (16 minutes, 19 seconds), is a poster child for free expression. He implements a flexibility and innovation in his training that makes Dennis Rodman's hair look monotonous. "Why shouldn't it be fun?" he says.

Here are a few training options from the exercise fringe, all courtesy of Matzger.

- Join up with a group of cyclists but leave your skates on. "Skating in a pace line with cyclists is a rush; you can really get your heart rate up for a long period of time," he says.
- Shoulder a backpack. "Fill it with anything you want, preferably something heavy."
- Fill an inner tube with sand and carry it around your waist. "It weighs about 40 pounds. That's definitely going to make you sweat more. Guaranteed," Matzger says. "Now that you have these radial tires, though, it's getting harder to find a tube."
- Dispense with the U-Haul. The last time Matzger moved, he did it all on in-line skates. He made about 60 trips—one of them with a solid oak kitchen table on his back—covering some 96 miles.

TAKE A SHORTCUT. Obviously, not everyone can take the afternoon off for a leisurely skate. When time is short, intensity has its rewards. With a training technique called intervals—high-speed bursts separated by brief rests—you can get a tough workout quickly.

Try skating hard for 30 seconds, resting for a minute, then skating hard for another 30 seconds. Repeat this three or four times. As you get in better shape, you can slowly add intervals, lengthen them, and shorten the rest period.

Another way to do intervals (which is emphatically not for the faint of heart) is on hills. Charge uphill for 30 to 60 seconds, then skate back down, resting for 2 minutes before going up again.

For those who don't relish speeds that send their cheeks flapping behind their necks, uphill intervals are a boon. "You can be kicking butt and getting a great workout and still be going only 5 miles an hour," says Rappelfeld.

MOUNTAIN BIKING
TAKE A RIDE ON THE WILD SIDE

No doubt, cycling is a fat burner. A 165-pound man cycling down the road for an hour at a fairly leisurely 13 miles an hour will burn about 690 calories, about the amount in a half-pound of cheesecake.

Stationary bikes aren't bad either. Riders in a Tufts University study in Medford, Massachusetts, lost 19 pounds of fat and added 3 pounds of muscle by riding regularly for three months.

But for many men, traditional riding—either in the gym or on the streets—is about as dry as these statistics. Which may explain why nearly 10 million Americans now own mountain bikes, and why more and more folks are hopping on the fat-tire bandwagon.

Mountain bikes are fun. They don't have those pointy little seats that turn your butt numb. And they allow for something extra that many forms of exercise don't provide. "Terrific adventure," says three-time Olympic cyclist John Howard, of San Diego. "Going off-road, you can escape from traffic and see things you wouldn't normally see."

Even if you are less interested in adventure than in losing a few pounds, mountain bikes are still a great choice. In traditional cycling, your legs do all the work; your upper body just sort of sits there. But when you are riding your mountain bike over rugged trails, your upper body comes into play constantly—jerking the bike over logs, for example, or pulling away from sheer free falls that suddenly materialize inches from your front wheel. And of course, the more muscles you get hopping, the more calories you will burn.

Here's another factor. There is a tendency, when riding on the road, to slip into a pace that resembles a casual plod, especially if the road is flat. On nature's trails, the route is rarely a smooth one. "It's varied terrain and that forces you to use a lot more energy," says Howard. "Off-road your wattage is consistently higher."

And energy expenditure equals calorie burn.

Rules of the Off-Road

Many people who own mountain bikes never venture beyond city streets, and that's okay. The bikes perform well on asphalt; the fat tires ride smooth, and the bikes have more gears than the traditional road bike, making it easier to get up hills. They make for a fine commute.

But they are designed to go off-road (the true mountain bike enthusiast would argue that they nearly cry to do so), and nature's trails, though they can be wide and groomed, aren't usually lovingly tended by road crews. The demanding terrain unique to mountain biking requires off-road smarts and technical skills. When you are just starting out, here is what the experts advise.

LOOSEN UP YOUR WALLET. There is a huge number of mountain bikes on the market, along with a ceaseless stream of new, high-performance doodads (shock absorbers, special handlebars, and so forth) to put on those bikes. What equipment do you absolutely need, and how much should you spend?

We will keep the equipment advice short: Don't

scrimp. If you buy the cheapest bike that you can find, you may find yourself lying down on the trail—with parts of your bike bouncing around you. These days, you can get a solid, dependable bike for about $500. Don't spend more than that if you are just getting started. And don't accessorize now; lots of riding will let you know what kind of gear you really need.

CHECK THE SEAT. Before taking your new wheels for the maiden voyage, take a minute to check and, perhaps, adjust the seat. This is critical. For one thing, having the wrong seat height—too low or too high—is terrible for your knees. Plus, sitting at the wrong height means that your bike won't handle as well as it should—and at that point knee injuries could be the least of your worries.

The easiest way to adjust your seat is to have the guy at the bike shop do it. Ask him to mark the post so that you can readjust it in the future.

BEWARE OF DOWNHILLS. There are lots of technical skills that you will need to develop as a mountain biker, but because of the potential for serious carnage, none are more important than mastering the descent. "People tend to go downhill fast before they develop their skills," says Ned Overend of Durango, Colorado, six-time mountain bike national cross-country champion and 1990 world cross-country champ. "They end up crashing and hurting themselves. You have to develop the downhill skills before you develop the speed."

Getting downhill effectively—and safely—isn't complicated. Here are the basics.

- **Move your weight further back on the seat (or off it entirely). This puts weight over the rear tire, giving invaluable traction.**
- **Look way down the trail so that you can see what is coming. Don't focus on the 6 inches of trail right in front of you.**
- **Use the front brake lightly. It has far more stopping power than the rear brake; jamming it down at high speeds will send you over the handlebars. It is better to use the rear brake more, while feathering the front brake for precise control.**

GET INSTRUCTION. While mountain biking generally is neither difficult nor dangerous, coping with trails requires a bit more experience than taking a spin to the corner convenience store. It is helpful, before taking your first dive, er, drive, to get some key tips—like how to brake and shift,

Inside Tips

Many off-road lessons are learned the hard way. Granted, being stranded 20 miles from nowhere ensures that you will probably remember a spare tube the next time. But there is no sense in needless suffering. Here are a few tricks that you should know ahead of time, all courtesy of Tom Hillard of Morgan Hill, California, downhill coach for the professional Specialized Mountain Bike team.

Use clip-in pedals. These are shoes that are designed to clip your feet to the pedals and, equally important, allow you to unclip quickly. If your feet aren't clipped to the pedals, you can't generate maximum power or maximum control on your bike.

Experiment with tire pressure. Hard tires are jumpy and skittish, and work best on paved or hard dirt roads. Soft tires give you more purchase on the loose dirt and rocks common on trails, making you less likely to take a spill.

Check your tire location. Most tires are specific for front or back use, says Hillard. In addition, they should be aligned properly (check the arrow located on the sidewall). Since rear tires provide much of the grab when climbing and breaking, they will need to be replaced more often than those on the front.

how to ride around (and over) obstacles, and all the other nuances that will make life easier and potentially less painful. "It's a lot like learning to ski for the first time. There are some important fundamentals, real simple things that you need to learn initially to avoid falling down," says Howard.

A fun way to learn the ropes, though certainly not the cheapest, is to attend a school or camp for personal instruction. You can find ads for camps and clinics in mountain bike magazines. Or check in at your local bike shop. They stay on top of the scene and will be able to steer you to qualified instructors in your area.

RIDE WITH FRIENDS. If you're not ready to commit to a camp, which can be pricey, joining a group of mountain bike riders is a great alternative. You can find out about bike clubs at your bike store. Most clubs have riders with a range of abilities, and most of the more experienced riders are happy to help with basic skills.

It is important, though, to find a club with

At first glance, cycling garb might seem to include an unnecessary number of silly, and potentially embarrassing, accoutrements: gloves, tight Lycra shorts, form-fitting jerseys. Small wonder cyclists rarely stray far from their bikes.

Actually, most of this stuff serves a purpose, though not all of it is necessary, says Tom Hillard of Morgan Hill, California, downhill coach for the professional Specialized Mountain Bike team. Here is his take on some of the most common gear.

- **Lycra cycling shorts.** The seams are placed with riding in mind; your gym shorts, by contrast, can put a seam in the tenderest of places. And because Lycra shorts are tight, they don't ride up on you. A man who is indifferent to these benefits and takes a long ride over rough terrain will soon discover the true meaning of chafing.

  If you don't like the tight elastic waistbands, you can buy shorts "bib tight"—basically, Lycra shorts held up by suspenders.

- **Cycling gloves.** Some riders like them because the padded palms ease some of the pressure between your hands and the handlebars. Without gloves, your hands can fall asleep.

  A helpful hint: Tilting the nose of your bike seat up just slightly reduces the tendency to rest heavily on the handlebars, which will help keep your hands from going numb.

- **Cycling shoes.** Regular tennis shoes work fine, but because the soles are softer and more flexible than cycling shoes, you lose a little force every time you

pedal. This may seem like a small thing, and it is if you are riding for 30 minutes or less. But if you are riding longer, you will start wasting substantial amounts of energy. Plus the constant flexing of your soles will make your feet ache.

- **Cycling jerseys.** Good ones are made of materials that wick away sweat, keeping you from getting soggy. Some are windproof in front; others zip down to allow on-the-move cooling. Jerseys also have pouches that let you carry extra water, tire tubes, bananas—you name it. If you are willing to forgo all that, a T-shirt works just fine.

- **Helmets.** Absolutely, positively, yes. If you don't wear one, a head-banging spill (a very real possibility on rugged trails) could render you dumb as a cashew. Though if you're riding without a helmet now, you're dumb as a cashew already.

  Short of a full suit of armor, a helmet is the best protection you can wear. To make it still better, affix a small sticker listing your name, blood type, allergies, and other important medical information.

- **A razor.** Serious mountain bikers keep their legs shaved because they often get leg massages, and a massage is far more pleasurable without the constant pinching of hairs. Smooth gams also come in handy if you crash. Picking gravel and dirt bits from raw patches of skin is unpleasant enough; adding body hair to the mix makes it worse. That said, a majority of riders—at least among the men—get by without slick legs. Your choice.

people whose skills suit you. Many clubs have beginner rides, and if you are a beginner, that is where you want to be. Where you don't want to be is on the advanced ride—riders hammering hard and fast over rough terrain, leaving you gasping and alone on the trail—or, worse, flying over the handlebars. "Riding with experts will only make you frustrated and will slow you down in the long run," says Howard.

Training Basics

As we noted earlier, mountain biking is a great sport not just for adventure but also for shedding pounds. To get a great workout every time, here are a few more tips to keep in mind.

KEEP THE WHEELS SPINNING. Beginning bikers tend to ride in too high a gear, as though the mere act of shifting upward confers superior benefits. Give your shifting hand a rest. What you want is to find a gear that lets you spin at 80 to 90 revolutions per minute (you can count the number of pedal strokes or you can buy a cyclometer to do it for you). This pace gives your heart and lungs an excellent workout while maximizing the efficiency of your pedaling and reducing the risk of knee damage.

SKIP CRUISE CONTROL. Biking is hypnotic. There is a tendency to slip into a comfortable speed and just stay there. But when you are riding for fitness, you have to shoot for a pace that is a little uncomfortable. "Calorie burning is a function of the speed or intensity you're maintaining," says Edward F. Coyle, Ph.D., director of the Human Performance Laboratory at the University of Texas in Austin. The faster and harder you go, the more you'll burn.

PICK A REASONABLE PACE. While pushing yourself is good, coughing up your lungs is not. "Going flat out isn't good because you overtax the body," says Howard. Experts agree that you will gain more benefits—in terms both of weight loss and heart/lung health—from a lower-effort workout than one that takes everything out of you.

Keeping your rides between 60 and 90 percent of your maximum effort will give you everything that you need in terms of conditioning and weight loss, without the dangers of running yourself into the ground, says Dr. Coyle.

Rides to Try

Although you will burn plenty of calories by freestyling—indeed, much of mountain biking's beauty lies in its decided lack of formality—you may want to occasionally increase the caloric burn by following a more formal workout plan. Here are a couple to try.

The group challenge. Here is a fun workout to try if you are riding with a group, either on the trail or on the road.

First, form a pace line, with the riders strung out single file and close together, with just a few feet between tires. For a minute or two, the person at the front of the line does a "pull." This is tough stuff, since you are breaking air for all your tailgating fellows. You should be in a fairly large gear, which will strengthen your leg power and your wind.

After your stint at the front, drop to the back of the line. Now, sucked along by the draft—a wind-free vacuum created by the riders in front of you—the ride gets easier. At this point you shift down to an easier gear, forcing you to spin faster. This spinning will really get your heart working. As each rider drops back from his turn at the front, you will slowly move up in the line (still spinning fast in the easy gear) until you are back at the front.

The hill interval. This one is ugly but effective, and you need to be in pretty good shape before trying it. (It's a favorite of Ned Overend, whose nickname, "The Lung," gives an idea of what it's going to take out of you.)

Find a fairly long hill, say, 2 to 4 miles long. After warming up for 20 minutes on a level surface, start your intervals. Riding up the hill, take it easy for 3 minutes, then push hard for 3; ride easy for 5 minutes, then ride hard for 5; take it easy for 3 minutes, then hard for 3. Finally, cool down with an easy 10-minute ride on level ground.

"Because it's all on the hill, you're forced to recover while you're still climbing," says Overend. "It's a really tough workout in a short amount of time."

RUNNING
MAKING THE MILES COUNT

Many people have tried running, and many people have hated it. The roots of this displeasure can be traced to the running boom of the 1970s, when running proponents, caught up in a near orgiastic buzz, loudly pronounced that the best approach to running was longer, faster, and harder, and they did exactly that—until they succumbed to debilitating injuries and were suddenly consigned to a lifetime of more forgiving activities like lawn darts and weenie roasts.

But if you do it correctly—meaning, with moderation—running doesn't have to mean pain, discomfort, and the potential for large orthopedic bills. More important, its potential for weight loss and fitness gains is impressive. For example, running at a sedate 12-minute-mile pace burns roughly 10 calories a minute. Kick that up to an 8-minute mile, and you'll burn 15 calories a minute. That's 600 calories burned in a 40-minute run.

"The most important concept is to stay below the threshold of fatigue and soreness," says Jeff Galloway of Atlanta, a former Olympic runner who has been running for 39 years. "Running is great exercise, it's a great fat burner, and it's convenient. But you have to be smart about it."

The Mantra of Moderation

Smart running means ignoring people who say that you won't get any benefits unless you're spitting your lungs up. Even the best runners intersperse hard training with plenty of slow running and outright time off to allow for recovery.

Running puts a lot of stress on your body. Each time your foot strikes the ground, it hits with a force equal to three to four times your body weight. Runners who ignore this fact and consistently push themselves to fatigue do so at their peril.

BEGIN WITH CAUTION. If you're out of shape and burning most of your calories at the buffet table, you'll need to start slower than if you're already active but not running.

"The really important thing is to monitor your soreness," says Galloway, author of *Galloway's Book on Running.* "If you're sore, you're doing too much, and you need to back off."

He recommends that out-of-shape runners start with 30 minutes of walking, three times a week. When this starts feeling comfortable, kick up the pace, but still limit the walk to 30 minutes. Then add some jogs to that 30 minutes.

ADD TIME TO YOUR ROUTINE. A lot of us are already running, though not much. Typical is the runner who notches 2 to 3 miles in 15 to 30 minutes. That's not a bad workout, but if you want to really burn fat, you need to increase the time to a minimum of 45 minutes.

FOLLOW THE 10 PERCENT RULE. If your normal run is 20 minutes and one day you decide

Cutting through the Shoe Zoo

If you've been watching shoe ads lately, you've probably come to the conclusion that it's easier to get a degree from the Massachusetts Institute of Technology than to decipher the claims about the hundreds of running shoes on the market.

Gone are the days when running shoes meant sneakers. Today, you'll find shoes with features ranging from air soles and dynamic reaction plates to Hydroflow cushioning pads, whatever those are. There are shoes for marathoners and shoes for sprinters. There are even shoes for walkers. And as you move up the price scale, you'll find that they're increasingly loaded with all the high-tech gizmos that your feet could ask for.

While all of these "special" features go a long way toward making shoe manufacturers' bottom lines more comfortable, they won't necessarily do the same for you. More to the point, your feet may not be able to tell the difference between any decent shoe, whether you're spending $60 or $200.

So forget the hype and make life simple. When you're shopping for shoes, the only thing to be concerned about is the fit. You need a shoe that's snug in the back, flexible at the ball of the foot, and has about a half-inch space between your longest toe and the end of the shoe. That's it.

Admittedly, you can't expect to get a pair of quality shoes for less than about $60. If you buy an off-the-rack pair for $15 at a discount store, you'll regret it the first time you take a long run. But if you buy your shoes at a store that caters to runners, just about anything they have in stock is going to work well.

Just be sure to bring along your old shoes. By looking at the wear, salespeople may spot irregularities in your running form (like pronation, for example, in which the feet roll in), and they may recommend a shoe to compensate.

One final tip. When trying on shoes, taking a quick walk between the cash register and storeroom isn't going to give you a real feel for the fit. Take them out for a spin. The foot you run with is different from the foot you walk with. The only way to get a feel for how a running shoe performs is to run in it.

---

to go for 40, you're going to get hurt, not fit. Galloway recommends a more measured approach. Each week, boost your running time by 10 percent. By giving your legs (and lungs) time to adapt, you'll find that you're no more tired after a 45-minute run than when you were doing one half as long.

BREAK IT UP WITH WALKING. There isn't a running cop out there who will bust you for changing pace when you start getting tired. A lot of runners, experienced and beginners alike, will alternate 5 minutes of running, say, with 5 minutes of walking. By allowing time to recover, you'll find it's easy to stay on the move 45 minutes or more, and the run will be comfortable.

Interspersing a run with walking may sound tame, but you lose little and gain much. For example, when you jog for 5 to 8 minutes, then walk a minute, you'll burn 95 calories a mile. Jogging continuously will burn only an extra 5 calories. "It might sound sedate, but a combination of walking and running will turn you into a fitness animal, and it'll keep you at it," Galloway says.

CHANGE YOUR RUNNING PACE. Even if you're beyond the walking/running stage, it's still smart to incorporate easy jogging into your hard runs. Advanced runners often take a slow jogging break every 10 minutes, says Galloway.

DON'T SKIP THE PRELIMINARIES. In a perfect world every run would begin with 10 minutes of light jogging to warm up the muscles, followed by 10 minutes of stretching, says Ed Burke, Ph.D., associate professor of exercise science and an exercise physiologist at the University of Colorado in Colorado Springs. But the real world is not that generous with time, and trying to cram a run plus stretching into a lunch break is impractical. A quick way to prepare your muscles for the run ahead is to jog very slowly for 10 minutes before running, he advises. (If it's cold out or you're unusually stiff, walk for 5 to 10 minutes before taking that easy jog.)

While we're on the subject of saving muscles from unnecessary pain, don't forget to cool down when you're done, says Dr. Burke. Ending a run with a punishing sprint and a screeching halt will leave your muscles wallowing in lactic acid (a by-product of hard exertion), making you sore and stiffer than the Tin Man. Ending your run with a 10-minute jog allows blood to flush lactic acid from your muscles.

Staying Comfortable

Running is a hard sport (if it weren't, it wouldn't burn many calories and you wouldn't be reading this section), and it's crazy not to try to make it easier. Before setting out, here are a few things to keep in mind.

THINK SOFT SURFACES. As mentioned earlier, every time your feet hit the ground, they're generating a tremendous amount of force. To reduce shock to your joints, seek out soft surfaces on which to run.

Cement and concrete are the worst. Blacktop, which has an infinitesimal amount of give, is a bit better. Better still is dirt or grass, or, if there's one nearby, the high school track. These are often made from spongy rubber surfaces such as Tartan, which are very forgiving on the feet.

DRINK OFTEN. This is obvious advice that runners all too often ignore, says Ellen Coleman, R.D., a registered dietitian in Riverside, California. In fact, she says, runners typically replace only 50 percent of the fluids lost during exercise. That's why they're continually confronting thirst, headaches, dizziness, and even vomiting—in short, the various stages of dehydration.

It is possible to lose tremendous amounts of fluids when you run—up to 6 pints an hour during vigorous exercise in the heat. Neglect to replace those fluids, and you might find yourself bent double examining—or worse, soiling—your shoes.

Drink 16 ounces of fluid 2 hours before a run, recommends Coleman. While you're on the road, drink 5 to 10 ounces of fluid every 15 to 20 minutes.

Many runners swear by sports drinks such as Gatorade. While these drinks do replenish carbohydrates and electrolytes, their most important ingredient is water. "Water is the most commonly overlooked athletic aid," Coleman says.

SAVE YOUR LUNGS. The key benefit of running is that it gets you breathing hard, but when you're an urban dweller in a sea of bus exhaust, the equation seems a bit less straightforward.

You can't avoid pollution entirely, but you can time your runs so that it's a little less noxious. On sunny days—when car exhaust and sunlight combine to form ozone—it's smart to run later in the day after the ozone has been depleted or early in the morning before it has a chance to form. Running on cloudy days is good. So is running after a thunderstorm because rain flushes ozone from the air.

Having Fun

Running doesn't have to be drudgery, though every day thousands of runners do their best to make it so. If you're going to stick with running (or, for that matter, any exercise program), you have to shake things up now and then. "Often we develop a sort of teeth-clenching, rigid approach to our exercise," says Bob Larsen, head coach of men's track and field and cross-country at the University of California, Los Angeles. "We need to open our eyes, look around, and remember that we're supposed to be enjoying this."

CHANGE COURSE. Many of us run the same trail in the same direction and at the same time of day—day after day. Why not do things differently? For example:

- If you run the same loop every day, try running that loop in the opposite direction, Larsen says.
- Rather than religiously keeping the same pace and distance, play with the numbers, advises Larsen. Instead of running 5 miles, for example, make it 3—but run a little faster. If you usually run 3 miles, make it 5—but slow your pace to accommodate the extra effort.
- Running in a new place is a great way to get your mind and body charged. Larsen sometimes rises early on Sunday mornings so that he can run in places where runners aren't normally seen. "If you run early enough, you can go right down a major boulevard with no traffic," says Larsen.

RUN WITH FRIENDS. It's fun to have someone to run with. Plus, having a regular running companion means that there's someone who will boot you out of bed on days when you would just as soon blow it off. "They can give you a swift kick in the rear if you're thinking about not getting out there," says Galloway.

GO WILD. Running off-road has lots of advantages. There's no traffic, no yammering toy poodles, and few, if any, people. Plus, dirt and grass trails are more forgiving on your joints, and the terrain's ups and downs offer a challenging workout.

SCULLING
A SLIDING SEAT CAN'T BE BEAT

Here, in scientific terms, is the problem with most men's exercise programs: They hate them.

Which is why, when you talk to scullers, one thing immediately becomes apparent: They love it. And why not? For them, the sport of rowing isn't about exercise—at least, that's not all it's about. "In the fall, to row on a lake or river just full of colored leaves is the most amazing thing," sighs Frederick Hagerman, Ph.D., a rower and director of the physiology laboratory at Ohio University in Athens. "And it's quiet. There's no sound except the birds and the wind."

Since the 1960s, Dr. Hagerman has been researching the benefits of rowing. "Rowing develops terrific aerobic benefits, muscular strength and power, plus flexibility and skill," he says. "Plus if a person is careful to learn the techniques correctly, rowing has an advantage over a lot of other aerobic activities in that rowers suffer less wear and tear on their joints. Actually, virtually none."

It's also, he adds, a great way to remove ballast from your midsection—which is why you're unlikely ever to see a fat sculler. (The fact that the typical shell is only 12 inches wide may have something to do with this.) A single hour of rowing can burn 600 to 800 calories.

NASA commissioned a study to find out whether astronauts would be better off rowing or cycling in space. Dr. Hagerman found that rowing consistently burned 15 to 20 percent more calories than cycling—and no one ever got a flat in a rowing scull.

Along with cross-country skiing, rowing is "probably one of the highest calorie burners there is," Dr. Hagerman says. "These two exercises are in a league by themselves."

A Word of Explanation

Although the terms *sculling* and *rowing* are often used interchangeably, they're entirely different sports. Rowing (as in rowing a canoe or a health-club rowing machine) is good exercise, but it doesn't compare with sculling. Rowing mostly works the upper body. Sculls, by contrast, employ a sliding seat. You use your legs to drive the oars through the water. Indeed, sculling works virtually every major muscle group.

"You're using all the big muscles: your legs, your butt, your back, and your arms. Just about every muscle in your body goes into the stroke," says Clay Felker, an avid sculler who heads the rowing program at Lake Austin Spa Resort in Austin, Texas. "It combines the benefits of weight training, aerobic workouts, stretching, and meditating, all rowed into one stroke."

Getting Your Oars Wet

While most sports are easy to learn on your own, sculling isn't one of them—unless you're willing to exercise by dog-paddling alongside an overturned boat. The average one-person scull is about 27 feet long and 1 foot wide and weighs 30 to 50 pounds. For beginners, they are slightly less stable than certain Middle Eastern regimes.

Rowing at Home

Rowing, as pictured in brochures, always takes place on mirror-smooth lakes licked by a summer evening's sunshine. Real life, however, presents certain obstacles to this view—namely, crappy weather and water conditions that can resemble the chase scene in Moby Dick.

If you find yourself landlocked, an indoor rowing machine is what you need. There are two basic types: those that use a flywheel for resistance and those that use hydraulic pistons, which look like the shock absorbers on your car. Most gyms have the piston version. These are usually occupied by folks frantically yanking away at the "oars" as though a school of piranhas were making its way across the carpet.

"The piston-style rower is basically a weight-training device, like a Nautilus machine," says Frederick Hagerman, Ph.D., director of the physiology laboratory at Ohio University in Athens. "But rowing works the legs. If you're not properly using your legs in a rowing motion, you might as well be doing something else."

He recommends using the flywheel-style machine (often called an ergometer). Because ergometers bring the legs into play and mimic a real rowing stroke, they'll burn lots more calories than piston machines. Indeed, you'll probably burn more calories on an ergometer than you would using the real thing.

"The energy cost is probably a little higher on the rowing ergometer than on the water because the boat moves underneath you but the ergometer doesn't," says Dr. Hagerman.

To try your hand at the oars without getting soaked in the process, here is what experts advise.

FIND A CLUB. Once practiced mainly by upper-crust collegians, sculling in recent years has attracted a wide audience. Most major cities—and quite a few smaller ones—now have rowing clubs.

GET SOME LESSONS. "Rowing a scull is not instinctive at all," says Shirwin Smith, who runs the Open Water Rowing Center in Sausalito, California. "People will try to row a shell like a rowboat, and they'll wonder why it seems awkward and unfriendly and tippy. You just have to know what you're doing."

Many rowing clubs offer one-day lessons without requiring you to join up. Lessons usually last a few hours and cost anywhere from $20 to $100. That may sound like a lot, but it's cheaper than plunking down $1,000 to $2,000—about what you would spend for a cheap scull. "A beginner can get the basics down in a 2-hour lesson," says Felker.

GET THE RIGHT GEAR. Every sport has its gear fanatics—folks who will mortgage the family home to purchase the latest widget—and rowing is no exception. Save your money, advises Mark Miller, who runs the Rio Abajo Rowing Club in Santa Fe, New Mexico. "Bike shorts and a T-shirt work fine, and a pair of tennis shoes or socks to keep the foot straps from pinching your feet."

To make your row a bit more comfortable, you may want to buy multisport shorts. These incorporate the Lycra-tight fit of bike shorts (which prevents painful blisters from occurring in tender places), but without the butt padding.

Whatever you wear on top (a windbreaker, sweatshirt, or T-shirt) should be fairly tight, since anything that billows around the waist is something that the oar handles can snag on. You'll certainly appreciate a pair of water shoes, which protect your feet from cuts and blisters and keep them warm when you're splooshing in and out of the boat.

EMPLOY FINESSE, NOT POWER. Sculling, done properly, is a subtle symphony of technique: the light feathering of the oars, the powerful drive of the legs, the curiously light grip on the oars. A light touch is often difficult for men—who tend to equate rowing with mowing down everything in sight—to achieve. Trying to muscle a scull is both impractical and potentially ugly. "At best, you're just out there slamming around," says Smith. "At worst, you'll go over. Power certainly is part of the equation, but save it until you have your technique down."

GO FOR THE BURN. For beginning scullers, just getting out on the water and working on technique is plenty of mental exercise. But once you have a handle on technique, you can put some power into it, Smith says. Felker recommends doing an hour workout—10 to 15 minutes of warm-up, 30 minutes of continuous rowing at 70 percent effort, and 10 to 15 minutes of cooldown.

To spice things up a bit, Felker will sometimes stop in the middle of the lake, strap the oars together, and do a few sit-ups, keeping his feet anchored in the foot holders.

Most of the time, though, the basics are enough. "Just going out and rowing at a steady pace is pretty much all you need," he says. "I don't make it any more complicated than that."

SPEED GOLF
ADDING GAS TO A SLOW GAME

When you think about aerobic fitness, golf isn't the first thing that comes to mind. After all, the primary action of this contemplative, slow-moving sport consists of squatting, peering, practice swinging, and pants adjusting. Players are often indistinguishable from lawn ornaments—only lawn ornaments rarely launch clubs into the woods after missing 2-foot putts.

In recent years, however, an increasing number of players have begun picking up the pace with a game known as speed golf. By combining speed and finesse, they're able to shoot 18 holes, get their hearts and lungs pumping, and if the gods are smiling, score in the low 70s—and be back in the clubhouse not much later than first light.

Several mornings a week Bob Babbitt, a 45-year-old publisher and sports talk-show host, stands at the first tee of the par-3 Lomas Santa Fe Executive Golf Course near San Diego. He wears running shoes and floral shorts. A fanny pack with half a dozen golf balls is strapped to his waist. He doesn't waste any time getting into position, lining up his shot, or testing the wind. He simply strides to the ball, hauls back his 6-iron, and belts the ball about 150 yards. Almost before the ball hits the ground, he is sprinting down the fairway, carrying only a 6-iron, an 8-iron, and a putter. If he is hitting true, he will finish the hole in under 2 minutes, and then dash on to the next one.

On a good day Babbitt will knock off 18 holes in about 30 minutes, getting a tough aerobic burn. Speed hasn't slowed his game in the least: His top score is a 66.

"Time is your most precious commodity," says Babbitt, president of the newly formed Speed Golf Association in San Diego. "Normally, it takes 3 to 4 hours to play 18 holes. It takes me half an hour. I have 2½ hours on everybody else, plus I've gotten in a great workout."

New Links

While few studies (actually, none) have been done on the aerobic burn of speed golf, a few simple calculations show that it can provide a great workout in a remarkably short time.

For example, Babbitt runs the course at roughly a 7½-minute-mile pace, burning about 17 calories a minute. In the 30 minutes it takes him to shoot 18 holes, he will burn roughly 510 calories—about the equivalent of a 4-mile run.

Contrast that to your typical duffer, who uses a cart and burns about 3.5 calories a minute—about the same as washing the dishes.

Babbitt isn't the only man to bring speed to the links. Thom Hunt, a former American record holder for the 10-kilometer road race, is passionate about the game. So is Steve Scott, who once ran a 3-minute, 47-second mile. Another is Sinjin Smith, who has won more pro beach volleyball tournaments than any other player.

An avid duffer, Smith sees speed golf as a dream come true. "If you want to play the game you

The Origins of Speed Golf

Speed golf got its official start in 1987 when John Bell, head pro at the Rams Hill Country Club, 100 miles east of San Diego, began hosting games. Although a few people were already playing for speed, in most cases they were watching the clock—the score didn't really matter.

"Sure they'd golf fast," says Bell. "But they'd also hockey-puck the ball around the course and shoot a million."

So Bell did the obvious thing and made the score count. Specifically, the score is added to the time it takes to play the round, with the final tally being your score. For example, if you cover 18 holes in 60 minutes, shooting a 98, your total score is 158.

Soon after Bell initiated this more demanding version of the game, he noticed something odd. His assistant pros, young men with considerable stamina, would run the 7,500-yard Rams Hill course in 50 minutes and shoot in the 80s, not far off their normal scores. In fact, the second time Bell played, he covered 18 holes in just under an hour and shot a 73.

"The real deterrent to playing good golf is that we think too much," says Bell. "Speed things up and you have less time to think. And the less we think, the better we're going to play."

love—and also get a workout and save the rest of your day—speed golf is the way to go," Smith says.

Tips from the Top

Speed golf is still in its infancy—by some estimates there are only about 100 active players nationwide—so it's not always easy to find experienced partners to play with or to get advice on playing the game. But if you like the idea of traveling light, moving quickly, and still getting a chance to smell the grass, here are some tips on getting started.

TEE OFF EARLY. Golf is traditionally a genteel sport. Charging full-steam through that slow-moving foursome from the Elks Club won't make you any friends and may get you tossed off the course. "You can't go in the middle of the day, or you're going to kill people," says Babbitt. "You have to be the first guy on the course."

CALL AHEAD. Although many club managers have never heard of speed golf, they're likely to approve your plan—especially when you explain that you'll be paying the full fee while getting off the course in one-fifth the normal time. "I think most clubs won't have a problem with it," Babbitt says.

TRAVEL LIGHT. Since the goal of speed golf is, well, speed, you can't be hauling around a heavy leather, two-car bag. When playing a par-72 course, Babbitt limits himself to three clubs: a 3-iron for driving, an 8-iron for shots to the green, and a putter. Plus, he wears a fanny pack containing extra balls. "You can't waste time looking for balls," he explains.

DRESS FOR SUCCESS. Forget the golf cleats and long, plaid pants. Forget the mushroom cap, too, since it will probably blow off. Most speed golfers don running shoes and shorts. "You don't want to be bogged down by equipment," says Hunt.

TRUST YOUR INSTINCTS. Since time is critical when playing speed golf, you simply can't address the ball in the mannered, leisurely fashion of the traditional game.

"Run up to the ball, line it up quick, take the club back, and hit it," says Jay Larson, who shot a 75 in 39 minutes at the PowerBar Speed Golf Challenge. "Rely on what you know about the game and what you've learned on the practice range, and trust it. Just take it back and swing."

BUT DON'T RUSH. Running too hard can be as detrimental to your score as moving too slowly. After all, your score will surely suffer if your lungs burst. Hunt recommends moving at about 75 percent of your comfortable maximum speed.

FORGET THE LONG DRIVE. When teeing off, it's generally preferable to go for a conservative, accurate drive that drops on the fairway rather than a Daly-esque rip that scorches hairlines on the clubhouse patio or sends you into the rhododendrons to search out your ball.

"Better to hit it short and keep the ball on the fairway," says Hunt. "You don't want to waste time and energy looking for your ball."

STAY CALM ON THE GREEN. Putting is notoriously difficult under the best of circumstances, and employing fine motor skills is doubly difficult when your body is spitting up adrenaline.

"You can't worry about really reading the green and those intricate breaks. You have to just kind of take a general look, make your best bet, and then hit it close," Hunt says.

"Forget long putts," he adds. "Forget short ones, too. You're forever missing putts."

SWIMMING
A WHOLE-BODY WORKOUT

Let's deal with the weight-loss issue right off, because if we don't, you might bypass one of the best exercises around.

Swimming, tradition has it, is not a good way to lose weight—an enduring piece of misinformation that admittedly isn't dispelled by newspaper photos of Hindenburg-size marathon swimmers stumbling from some frigid ocean.

True, when you swim, your body is supported by water, and because you aren't forced to fight gravity, there can be less calorie burn. It is also true that some marathon swimmers won't be modeling underwear anytime soon (actually, it behooves marathon swimmers to carry some fat as valuable insulation against frigid water). And it's true that a 150-pound man swimming at a leisurely pace burns roughly 6 calories a minute. He could burn nearly twice the calories running at a pedestrian 12-minute-mile pace.

But before you turn your back on the pool, consider this. That same 150-pounder can double his calorie burn by swimming faster. Swimming butterfly (the most difficult of swimming's four strokes) burns roughly 14 calories a minute—a better caloric burn than tennis, squash, or soccer. What we're talking about here is intensity, and *that* explains why Olympic swimmers (unlike marathon swimmers) have the sort of body that gets the role of Tarzan.

Swimming offers other benefits that can't be ignored. Because you are supported by water, it's a low-impact sport and thus virtually injury-free. For the same reason it's also a great exercise if you're overweight, since it spares your joints the pounding experienced in gravity-bound sports like running. The varied strokes used in swimming take your joints through a full range of motion that can improve flexibility. Most important, few exercises give you the head-to-toe muscle workout that swimming does.

"You are using almost all the major muscle groups of the body. The legs, hips, abdominals, chest, shoulders, and upper back—all of these muscles are working," says Ernest Maglischo, Ph.D., author of *Swim for the Health of It* and head coach of the men's swimming team at Arizona State University in Tempe. "You can also get tremendous stimulation to the heart and respiratory system. As far as general health goes, swimming is an excellent conditioner."

Getting Started

Here's a likely scenario: Excited by the prospect of all these benefits, man goes to pool. Man dons suit and goggles. Man pushes off the wall and makes for the other end. Man gives self and lifeguard a serious scare.

Swimming, it needs to be said, is not a sport that comes effortlessly. Witness recreational pools, which are typically filled with folks who look like they're more interested in self-preservation than exercise. We're going to show you how to make the transition from thrashing wheezer to graceful swimmer and how to improve even if you're already at home in the water.

GET QUALIFIED INSTRUCTION. Learning to swim may seem like something for preschoolers in water wings. But even if you can successfully navigate from one end of the pool to the other, proper technique is not something that you can learn on your own.

BE PATIENT. We expect to pick things up quickly. Swimming won't be one of them. Learning proper stroke technique takes time, and that takes patience. "People want results right away, but swimming is extremely technical, which is really frustrating for a lot of people," says Michael Collins, head coach of the Davis, California, Aquatic Masters team, the largest masters team in the country.

Newcomers to Collins's program undergo a barrage of stroke technique drills before they even start thinking about conditioning. Don't be intimidated by this, says Collins. Learning swimming's four strokes—freestyle, backstroke, breaststroke, and butterfly—is not difficult. But it is essential that you learn how to do them properly if you want to get the most from the sport.

RELAX IN THE WATER. When you're learning to swim, relaxing is the most important thing that you can do—and the most difficult. "When people are learning to swim, they get nervous and they tense up. And when they do that, they find themselves sinking, and it's just that much harder," explains Collins. "You need to relax and stay loose."

If you happen to be one of those people whose muscles lock into a state resembling rigor mortis whenever you go near the pool, you may want to pick up a pair of swim fins. They make your kick more powerful, which means that they will keep you up and planing across the surface, even when you're tense and tight.

GET THE RIGHT EQUIPMENT. There's not a lot that you have to buy, just a suit and swimming goggles. The choice of suit is yours. You can opt either for a racing suit or your standard beach britches. You might be embarrassed about wearing a racing suit—which, admittedly, reveals areas of your anatomy only your intimates are familiar with—but it's a good investment. Racing suits are light and comfortable. More important, they offer virtually no drag in the water, whereas the pockets of your beach britches will fill with water and drag you to the bottom.

Swimming goggles are a must. Keeping a pool from becoming a virus reunion requires liberal use of chemicals—and many of these chemicals are hard on the eyes.

Occasionally, you'll see swimmers wearing nose plugs or earplugs. Save your money. Unless you're particularly prone to swimmer's ear, the human body is designed to withstand moisture in these particular orifices. In any event, earplugs tend to fall out while you're swimming, and nose plugs make it hard to breathe—and when you're swimming hard, you want to be sucking in all the oxygen you can.

Swimming for Fitness

Swimming looks easy, especially when you watch experienced swimmers glide through the water. But swimming is an extremely demanding sport; for beginners it can be a fight just to get to the other end of the pool.

To achieve solid basic fitness, Collins recommends swimming three to four times a week, logging between 2,000 and 3,000 yards (roughly 1½ to 2 miles) each workout. Most swimmers can get that kind of yardage in about an hour.

If you're fairly fit but new to swimming, experts recommend swimming between 500 and 1,000 yards each workout. (That's roughly a quarter to half a mile.) Then build slowly from there. Swimming is a vigorous activity. You'll be using new muscles, and it's easy to stress them. Shoulder injuries are especially common among overzealous newcomers.

START WITH A WARM-UP. Swimming may be a forgiving sport, but you still want to loosen up before plunging into a high-bore workout. Collins advises swimmers to warm up with a 400-yard swim—200 yards of freestyle, 100 yards of backstroke, and 100 yards of breaststroke—mixing up the strokes to bring all the muscles into play.

WORK UP TO INTERVALS. Although you can get an excellent workout by swimming straight time—doing the same stroke at the same pace for half an hour or so—you'll burn substantially more calories by doing an interval workout. This is nothing more than a series of swims separated by a specific amount of rest (the interval).

For example, you might do ten 50-yard freestyle swims, leaving the wall every minute. Or you might do five 100-yard freestyle swims leaving the wall every 2 minutes.

A typical swimming workout consists of several sets, with roughly 10- to 30-second intervals between each swim of the set, then several minutes' rest between each set.

A Training Sampler

There are countless options for designing a swimming workout. You'll almost certainly want to be doing intervals, but apart from that you can be as creative as you want.

Here is a 1-hour workout for swimmers of all fitness levels, courtesy of Michael Collins, head coach of the Davis, California, Aquatic Masters team, the largest masters team in the country. Pick your level of fitness—beginner (B), intermediate (I), experienced (E), and advanced (A)—and do the warm-up and intervals suggested for your level. If you follow the target distances, here's what you'll achieve.

- Advanced = 3,300 yards
- Experienced = 2,900 yards
- Intermediate = 2,750 yards
- Beginner = 2,000 yards

Warm-Up

(A,E) Swim 200 yards freestyle, 100 yards backstroke, and 100 yards breaststroke.

(I) Swim 200 yards freestyle, 75 yards backstroke, and 75 yards breaststroke.

(B) Swim 100 yards freestyle, 50 yards backstroke, and 50 yards breaststroke.

Interval Set One

Rest 15 seconds between each.

(A,E,I,B) 5 × 100 yards freestyle. All kicking is done on the side, switching sides every 12 kicks with one strong stroke.
1. Swim 100 yards freestyle.
2. Swim 75 yards freestyle, 25 yards kicking freestyle.
3. Swim 50 yards freestyle, 50 yards kicking freestyle.
4. Swim 25 yards freestyle, 75 yards kicking freestyle.
5. Kick 100 yards freestyle kick.
Rest 2 to 3 minutes.

Interval Set Two

Rest 40 seconds between each. Each swim is 200 yards freestyle, then 100 yards backstroke or 100 yards breaststroke.
(A) Swim 7 × 300 yards.
(E,I) Swim 6 × 300 yards.
(B) Swim 4 × 300 yards.
Rest 2 to 3 minutes.

Interval Set Three

This is a sprint set, with 15 seconds rest between each sprint. Swim all four of the strokes. The first sprint should be butterfly, the next backstroke, then breaststroke, then freestyle. Repeat that same order if necessary.
(A) Sprint 12 × 25 yards.
(E) Sprint 8 × 25 yards.
(I,B) Sprint 4 × 25 yards.

The important point is to not allow too much rest during the set—you don't want to fully recover between swims.

MIX YOUR SPEEDS. "A lot of people just condition themselves to swim at one speed because they do the same kind of workout all the time," says Collins. "If you want to improve, you need to learn to swim fast."

It's not that every swim should be a sprint. The idea is to mix things up. Rather than swimming the same half-mile pedestrian plod every day, for example, do intervals instead. And make at least one of those interval sets involve fast swimming. Swimming fast brings more muscle fibers into play, taxes the heart and lungs more, and—nice surprise—burns as much as twice the calories.

Of course, when you're swimming fast, you'll need to rest longer between each swim so that you can really make a quality effort. For example, when doing ten 50-yard swims, you may want to leave the wall every 2 minutes instead of the 1 minute recommended for a slower pace. "You're resting more, but I guarantee you will be beat," says Collins.

An additional point: It's always a good idea to do your sprint sets early in the workout while you're still fresh.

MIX YOUR STROKES. Many swimmers swim nothing but freestyle. If you're one of them, you're missing out. Tossing swimming's other strokes into your workouts will help you hit more muscles and improve your flexibility by bringing different motions into play.

PUT YOUR ARMS AND LEGS TO WORK. Pulling (swimming using just your arms) and kicking (using just your legs) are good additions to any swimming workout. Pulling is a great upper-body conditioner. Kicking hits your legs;

Swimming Free

There's nothing wrong with getting your workouts at the local pool. It's convenient, the water's warm, and there's a concession stand, so you can tank up on soft drinks and snacks while working on your tan.

But when you find yourself getting tired of smelling chlorine and doing the same strokes in the same narrow lane, it may be time to head for open water. Swimming in lakes or the ocean allows you to pit yourself against waves and current. Plus, freeing yourself from the confines of the pool can be a magical experience.

"You notice how the warm sunshine spreads across your back. You hear the calls of waterfowl. You see wavery bands of silvery fish sliding beneath your fingertips," says Lynne Cox, of Los Alamitos, California, a veteran open-water swimmer who has swum some of the world's most treacherous waters, including the Bering Strait (average water temperature during that swim was 43°F).

Before waxing whimsical, though, you need to think practical, Cox advises. Be sure to check with lifeguards or others who know the local conditions well. Wear sunscreen and tinted goggles to ease the sun's glare. You should also wear a brightly colored swimming cap, for two reasons: One, you can lose up to 80 percent of your body heat through your head, and the cap will keep you warm; two, the bright color makes you more visible to boaters, jet skiers, and windsurfers, who otherwise might plow right over you. Apply petroleum jelly around your neck and under your arms to prevent chafing. You can also wear a wetsuit if you want to.

Things aren't as controlled out there as they are at the local Y, so it's important to swim smart. At a minimum, you should be fit enough to swim a mile comfortably in the pool before tackling open water, Cox says. For your first open-water swim, cut that distance in half just to be safe. Finally, if you are swimming alone, swim parallel (and close) to shore. Better yet, find a partner to go with you.

add a pair of fins, and you'll increase ankle flexibility, making your legs work even harder. And because they involve large muscles, kicking and pulling elevate your heart rate almost as much as swimming the complete stroke.

When kicking, Collins adds, don't use a kickboard. Holding on to the plastic foam board raises your upper body and drops your hips and legs down. Good swimming means balancing the hips and head near the surface of the water; having your legs angling down like anchors doesn't accomplish that.

GET A FAST BURN. If you're looking for a tough workout that you can do in minimal time, here's a challenging option, courtesy of John Flanagan, head coach of the Washington D.C. Masters. The key to this workout isn't speed, per se, but reducing your rest periods to the absolute minimum.

Using the stroke of your choice, keep the effort fairly easy—say, 60 percent of your maximum heart rate. But keep the rest period between swims very short, no more than 7 to 15 seconds, depending on the distance you're swimming. For example, if you're doing a series of short swims (say, 50 yards), you may want to rest about 7 seconds between each one. For longer swims of 200 yards, for instance, take 15 seconds between each one.

Keeping the rest periods short allows almost no time for recovery, Flanagan explains. This keeps your heart rate up and banging, giving you a terrific workout in a relatively short time.

"You're training your heart to be a lot more efficient," says Flanagan. "And it doesn't mean more time in the pool. It means swimming more laps in that given time. You can get in a great workout in an hour lunch break."

WALKING
A COMFORTABLE APPROACH TO FITNESS

Walking has never been accorded much respect. Traditionally, it has been considered useful locomotion but ineffective exercise. Worse, it is decidedly lacking in glamour. People shaped like bowling balls walk. Willard Scott walks.

"That was my attitude, too," admits John Duncan, Ph.D., professor of clinical research at Texas Woman's University in Denton. His thinking changed after he did a study comparing walkers and joggers. He found that people who walked 3 miles a day, five days a week, at a 5-mile-an-hour pace garnered the same cardiovascular gains as joggers running at an 8- to 9-mile-an-hour pace. Indeed, jogging at a moderate pace will burn 400 calories an hour; racewalking will burn about 600.

"The fact is, walking is much better exercise than we ever believed," Dr. Duncan says.

Stepping Up the Pace

All walking is decent exercise, and there's no question that taking a 20-minute stroll once or twice a day will provide substantial benefits to your heart and lungs. But when you're trying to lose weight, you want to burn serious calories. That means doing one of two things: walk longer or walk faster.

"A 20- to 30-minute walk at a moderate pace tones muscles and relaxes you. It burns a few calories, but it isn't enough for significant weight loss," says Viisha Sedlak, director of the American Walking Association in Paonia, Colorado. "If you're really looking to shed fat, you have to walk for 45 minutes or longer."

This steady approach may lack glamour, but it pays dividends. Assuming that your diet stays the same, walking 45 minutes a day, four days a week for a year can result in losing 18 pounds.

It's possible to get the same benefits in half the time by picking up the pace. "If you walk a little faster, you can get everything out of walking that cycling, swimming, or running gives you," says Casey Meyers, of St. Joseph, Missouri, author of *Walking: A Complete Guide to the Complete Exercise.*

We've been talking about walking as though it is a complete training program in itself. For many people, in fact, walking is their sole workout. But it's also an excellent adjunct to an overall fitness plan. For example, runners often walk on their easy days, giving their muscles and joints a chance to recover.

Getting Started

Unlike virtually any other sport or exercise, walking is something that everyone can do. You don't need lessons. You don't have to be in great shape. You don't need specialized gear. All you have to do is lace up your sneakers and step outside.

Speaking of sneakers . . .

GET THE RIGHT SHOES. Despite what certain salesfolk might tell you, walking is not rocket science and so does not require space-age gear. Still, having the right shoes can save your feet a lot of unnecessary pain.

"Walking is such a low-impact sport, you really don't need anything fancy," says Sedlak. She advises

Racewalking: A Faster Road to Fitness

If you have only heard about racewalking, you probably imagine overweight "athletes" waddling like ducks, taking mincing little steps and not making a lot of progress.

You'd be wrong. For starters, racewalkers don't waddle; the hips move forward and back, not side to side. Second, it provides an excellent exercise option. If you're serious about walking, fitness, and calorie burn, racewalking is the way to go.

Racewalking at a moderate pace can burn 600 calories an hour. Compare that to jogging at a moderate pace, which only burns about 400. Why does racewalking burn more calories? Unlike running, in which the upper body stays fairly still, racewalking gets most of the upper body—the arms, back, and shoulders—involved. "It can be very strenuous," says Viisha Sedlak, who has been ranked number one in the world among masters female walkers. She is also director of the American Walking Association in Paonia, Colorado.

"But if you want to get the most from race- walking," Sedlak adds, "you have to do it right." Here's how.

Keep your back upright. Walking fast with a bent or swayed back can cause injury because stress is absorbed by improperly aligned body parts. Translation: You'll kill your back or knees. So keep your back upright at all times.

Get the steps down. Racewalking isn't merely fast walking; it has a form all its own. What you want to do is step forward with a straight leg, landing with the heel first. (Walking with knees bent puts a lot of stress on the hips, knees, and spine.)

Stay loose. It's good to swing your arms backward behind the body when racewalking, but be sure to keep them relaxed. This workout is about efficiency, and tensing your arms wastes energy.

Control your hips. You want them to move forward and back with each stride, not side to side. The reason is simple: You want every part of your body to be moving forward; side-to-side movements cost momentum.

getting shoes with a stable heel support and a reasonable degree of impact cushioning. A good shoe will cost at least $50, she adds.

BRING ALONG SOME SOUND. We all have days (actually, quite a few of them) when we would rather put our feet on the couch than on the walking trail. Here's an easy way to combine R and R with a little bit of exercise: Hook up your portable player and catch the news or plug in a music tape while you walk. "Listening to fast-beat music not only makes exercise more fun but the beat also makes it easier to walk faster," says Meyers.

ESTABLISH A TRAINING PACE. While fast walking is great for fitness, your muscles won't appreciate it if you plunge into a 12-minute-mile pace without giving them advance warning. Meyers recommends using the first half-mile as a warm-up. Accelerate slowly until you feel warm and loose. Increase the middle portion of the walk to your maximum pace, then use the final half-mile to wind down.

PLAY WITH SPEED. Walking can quickly become monotonous, which is why many fitness walkers develop their own training regimen. For example, you might want to alternate brisk walking with sudden bursts of speed—say, a 60-yard sprint to the mailbox down the road. Or walk pyramids— that is, go hard for a minute, easy for a minute, hard for 2 minutes, easy for 2 minutes, hard for 3 minutes, easy for 3 minutes and so on, going as high as you like and then coming back down.

TAKE THE UPHILL ROAD. Obviously, walking uphill requires more effort than strolling on a flat surface, which is why the world has yet to see a fat Sherpa. Depending on how fast you walk, walking a moderately steep hill can burn anywhere from 8 to 15 calories a minute.

GO OFF-ROAD. With hills in mind, trails are a great walking option, too. "You'll get a better workout on varied terrain," says Sedlak. If you're out hiking, you're probably carrying a backpack, too, and that can increase the calorie burn even more.

TAKE ADVANTAGE OF WINTER. What's bad for your heating bill can be great for your health. Walking in soft snow can burn up to 20 calories a minute. To get an equivalent calorie burn in the summer, you would have to run at a 6-minute-mile pace. Inclement weather offers other advantages as well—like reducing traffic and, if you're lucky, keeping the neighbor's yappy Pekingese indoors.

PART V
BUILDING A PROGRAM

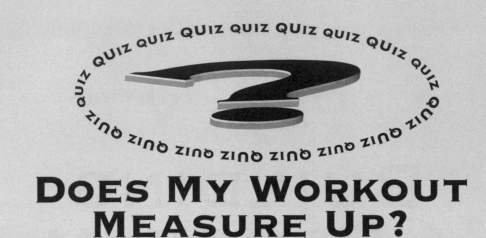

DOES MY WORKOUT MEASURE UP?

Weight lifting has an uncompromising direct-ness to it that's both elegant and brutal. You take a bunch of weight, and you lift it. The stronger you are, the more of it you can lift. In a confusing world filled with ambiguous motives and hidden agendas, it's hard to beat that kind of purity.

Yet lifting weights can also be a long, slow process, and the benefits aren't always immediately apparent. Whether you want to lift pianos or simply to feel less tired at the end of the day, you need guideposts to gauge whether your workouts are working for you the way they should. Here are a few points to consider.

1. Is my workout progressing?

There's a simple axiom in weight lifting: If you aren't getting stronger, or larger, or developing more endurance, you're probably doing something wrong. "The single best test of a workout that isn't doing what it should is a failure to progress," says Art Drechsler, former board member of the U.S. Weightlifting Federation.

There are many measures of progress. Can you bench-press more this month than you could last? Has the size of your biceps increased? Do you rest only 30 seconds between sets when you used to rest 60?

The best way to track your progress is to keep a workout diary, Drechsler says. Keep track of the lifts you did and at what weight, how many sets you did, and how long you rested between sets.

You should also log how you felt during and after each workout—whether a particular lift felt especially worthwhile or worthless, whether you felt invigorated or exhausted, whether you felt great or you had leg cramps.

"What happens over time," Drechsler says, "is that you begin to see patterns develop. You can see that at a certain point you added an exercise and a month later your chest size increased. You become your own best coach because you can monitor your progress very closely."

For this type of system to work, however, make sure your points of comparison are consis-tent. If you're measuring your biceps, always put the tape in the same place. If you're counting push-ups, make sure that your form at the end of the set is the same as it was at the beginning.

2. How do I feel on Monday?

No one goes from whip-thin to Terminator proportions overnight, but you still should see improvement fairly quickly, says Wayne Westcott, Ph.D., national strength-training consultant for the YMCA, the American Council on Exercise, and the National Academy of Sports Medicine. On any given Monday you should be better than you were the previous Monday—either in the amount of weight you can lift or in the number of repeti-tions you can do per set, he says. "I'm tempted to say that you should show improvement in each workout, but in real life too many things can happen for it to be quite that consistent. But week to week, you should be able to detect a small but measurable improvement."

3. How do I look?

For many of us, the less-scientific standards of fitness often take precedence over more-objective measures. Dr. Westcott recommends the ever-reliable mirror test. If your muscle tone looks better today than it did a month ago, then your workout is measuring up.

Another traditional, if less-than-scientific test of fitness: the fit of your clothes. If you've been working out hard, you should be fitting more comfortably into your jeans than you did two months ago. If you've been working on your chest and arms, your shirts should be fitting a little more snugly.

Obviously, you have to be realistic. Significant muscle growth takes at least five to six weeks, while significant weight loss often takes two to three months, says Gary Hunter, Ph.D., professor of exercise physiology at the University of Alabama at Birmingham. On the other hand, you can expect to feel stronger and look better almost immediately after beginning weight training. If you don't, you're doing something wrong.

4. Am I assembled correctly?

While you're looking in the mirror, check yourself for proportion. Do your various body parts fit together in a reasonably harmonious whole, or do you appear to have been stitched together from spare parts? Picture the huge forearms on Popeye: He obviously spends too much time on upper-body work and not enough down below. A well-rounded workout should hit all the major muscle groups, giving your body an overall look of proportion. Men who ignore this rule often find themselves with barrel chests and taffy legs, or hurdlers' legs and toothpick arms.

5. How do I feel?

A key measure of your workout's effectiveness is what it does to your energy level. If it's doing what it's supposed to do, you should feel strong and energetic. On the other hand, if you find yourself feeling wiped out for days on end, you're probably overtraining. "Everybody has a bad day once in a while, but overtraining is the kind of feeling that lasts for a week or two weeks or longer," says Frank Eksten, strength coordinator in the Department of Athletics and visiting lecturer in kinesiology at Indiana University in Bloomington. "Your body is trying to tell you something."

6. Am I getting hurt?

Working out should make you stronger and more flexible, and, hence, less vulnerable to injury. If you find yourself getting hurt on a regular basis, it could be that your workout isn't doing what it should be.

Getting hurt when you lift is an obvious sign that something is wrong, Dr. Westcott says. Either your technique is bad or your judgment is. Either way, watch for persistent soreness in your elbows, shoulders, or other joints. These are warning signs that suggest that a reassessment of your routine is in order.

7. Am I enjoying myself?

The only successful fitness plan is the one you stick with, and the only plan you'll stick with is one that you enjoy. Ideally, whatever you're doing should fit smoothly into your life; if the gym is across town, you're less likely to use it. Your workout should deliver regular improvement, and it should change often enough to stay interesting. Otherwise, human nature being what it is, you'll find plenty of reasons to skip it.

"Working out should be pleasant and enjoyable, not a stressful, have-to-do-it activity," says Dragomir Cioroslan, head coach of the U.S. Weightlifting Federation and the 1996 U.S. Olympic weightlifting team. "If your workout is adding stress to your life, find a better way to work it into your schedule."

HOW TO LIFT
A COMPLETE GUIDE TO GETTING STARTED

For a long time, weight lifters were badly in need of public-relations assistance: They were physically fit but were image-impaired. Most people thought of them as hulking troglodytes who inhabited smelly, clanking dungeons where civilized people feared to tread.

"My father thought that if you spent a lot of time in the gym, you had nothing going on from the neck up," says Todd Edelson, a physical therapist in Montclair, New Jersey, and winner of the 1978 National Collegiate Athletic Association weightlifting championship. "But that whole image has definitely changed."

Indeed it has. Instead of the old torture chamber motif, modern weight rooms feature sleek machinery and fancy decor. In some of them, you're as likely to run into a supermodel or movie star as you are the Incredible Hulk.

The change in image hasn't been all cosmetic. Exercise physiologists have piled up reams of research about the health benefits of strength training. These benefits include lowering blood pressure, reducing bad low-density lipoprotein (LDL) cholesterol while raising good high-density lipoprotein (HDL) cholesterol, keeping blood sugar levels in check, and building stronger tendons, ligaments, and bones.

Research has also shown that there's no truth to the most persistent of weightlifting canards, that lifting makes you muscle-bound. "Lifting weights makes you more flexible, not less," says Harvey Newton, a certified strength and conditioning specialist and the executive director of the National Strength and Conditioning Association in Colorado Springs, Colorado. "You can become stiffer lifting weights, but you can also become stiffer running if you don't do it properly."

In previous chapters we have discussed how important it is for dieters to work out so that the weight they lose is fat, not muscle, and we've discussed how muscle tissue eats up calories a lot faster than fat does. (For more information on the muscle/fat connection, see "Weight Training" on page 29.) Here's another excellent reason for getting into strength training: According to Wayne Westcott, Ph.D., national strength-training consultant for the YMCA, the American Council on Exercise, and the National Academy of Sports Medicine, men who do not do regular strength exercises will lose about 5 pounds of muscle every 10 years. The most effective way to fight that gradual transformation into jelly is to lift weights.

Perhaps the most glorious fact of all is how quickly weight lifting produces results. "If you've ever done weight training, you know it takes very little time to get that toned feeling," says Thomas R. Baechle, Ed.D., professor and chairman of exercise science at Creighton University in Omaha, Nebraska, and co-author of *Weight Training: Steps to Success.* "In 5 minutes in the weight room, I can get my muscles pumped up, and I can feel the difference. That's the excitement of weight training."

We're not claiming that your potbelly will disappear overnight, but tangible, measurable results can materialize a lot faster than you might expect. Dr. Baechle says that novice lifters will see some tightening of flaccid muscles within about two weeks. That's fast. In a study at the University of Maryland, 13 men shed 4 pounds of fat and added about 4 pounds of muscle after weight training for four months. Better yet, almost half the fat lost was from their guts.

If your goal is strictly to lose weight, nothing beats aerobic exercise, adds Alan Mikesky, Ph.D., director of the Human Performance and Biomechanics Laboratory at Indiana University–Purdue University in Indianapolis. But for building strength, lifting can't be beat, and the best belly-flattening strategy of all is a dual attack: aerobic exercise plus strength training. Here's how to get started on the muscle part.

The Workout Ethic

If you didn't have to work for a living, you probably wouldn't. Your muscles are like that, too. They need to be pushed. They get stronger when they're challenged.

Exercise physiologists call this the overload principle, and it's the essence of why weight lifting works. In order to strengthen a muscle, you have to challenge it beyond what it is used to.

This isn't quite the same thing as "no pain, no gain." Pain means injury, and that is not the intent of any training program. "It's more of an exertional discomfort than pain," says Dr. Mikesky. "But let's be honest: There are some things that you just have to work for, and improving strength is one of those things."

Commitment is the first requirement of any successful exercise program, strength training included. If you're ready to pay the price, though, the rewards are tremendous, not only in terms of physical improvement but also in terms of self-esteem. Here's how to get there.

Learning the Basics

Weight training isn't like physics. There's not a lot of terminology you have to learn before getting started. But there are a few concepts that you need to understand.

For starters, every strength-training workout consists of repetitions and sets. A repetition is simply an exercise done once: 1 bench press, 1 repetition. A set means doing the same exercise a certain number of times: 10 bench presses, one

Imagine Success

During a training session five weeks before the 1984 Olympic Games in Los Angeles, a young Romanian collapsed under a 600-pound barbell. He could hardly move, and the 15 years spent preparing for the Games seemed lost.

A team adviser told the young Dragomir Cioroslan, who is now head coach of the U.S. Weightlifting Federation and the 1996 U.S. Olympic weightlifting team, to keep training—in his mind.

Seven hours a day for the next 10 days, Cioroslan mentally worked through his routines. He couldn't get out of bed, but he could imagine the details—the weights, seeing himself walk up to the bar, bracing, contracting, lifting—as though he were actually doing it.

It paid off. He was back on his feet sooner than expected and went on to win a bronze medal in the Games. "You think the mind is not important in exercise?" Cioroslan asks today. "Wrong. It is very important."

As a coach, Cioroslan uses the mental training that he learned to help athletes reach their potential. The same techniques that work for elite athletes will work for you, too.

Before and during every lift, imagine how each muscle is working to complete the movement. "It's very important to focus on what's happening within the muscle, to perceive it," Cioroslan says. "Be the observer and controller of the movement. Is it right? Is it a quality movement? Pay attention. By concentrating mentally you will help your brain send the right impulses to the neuromuscular units to make the muscle contraction effective. There's no question that mental concentration helps maximize the physical effect."

set. In shorthand, a "10-rep set."

One of the great beauties of strength training is that you can customize the number of sets and repetitions to achieve certain goals. Runners who want to build endurance, for example, may do leg exercises requiring high numbers of sets and repetitions but moderate amounts of weight. Conversely, a boxer wanting to increase the explosive power of his punch may bench-press relatively heavy weights fewer times.

We'll get into the principles of repetitions and sets in more detail in the next chapter. For now, just plan on doing between 8 and 12 repetitions

Like any sport, weight training has its own language. Here's a short glossary of terms that you're likely to hear around the weight rack.

Resistance training. Exercise in which a muscle acts against some form of resistance of sufficient intensity to maintain or increase strength levels. Lifting weights is the most obvious form, but push-ups and even pushing your two hands against each other are forms of resistance training.

Weight lifting. It's what most of us call lifting barbells and dumbbells in the hopes of strengthening muscles. But the term weight lifting has a more specific definition in the world of competitive lifting: getting the heaviest possible weight over your head. Weightlifting events include the snatch lift, in which the barbell is lifted overhead in one motion from the floor, and the clean and jerk, in which the bar first is lifted to shoulder height and then raised above the head.

Power lifting. Another form of competitive lifting. Events include squats, bench presses, and the dead lift.

Strength training. Lifting aimed at developing strength, usually in specific areas of the body. Often, the terms resistance training, weight lifting, and strength training are used interchangeably, even though they have slightly different meanings.

Body building. The focus isn't on developing strength but on the size and appearance of the muscles.

Circuit training. This involves moving quickly from one resistance exercise (and one group of muscles) to the next. It's a way to combine cardiovascular and strength training into one workout.

Pyramiding. A way of intensifying the impact of an exercise by starting with a light weight and, in consecutive sets, incrementally increasing the weight. After reaching the top of the "pyramid," the weights are incrementally lowered to complete the workout.

Split workout. A training routine that focuses on one part of the body one day and another part the next. For example, many lifters work the back and biceps one day, then focus on the chest and triceps the next.

Superset. Performing two or more exercises in succession that target a specific muscle or muscle group.

Plateauing. A frustrating phase every lifter periodically reaches, in which progress essentially stops. Plateauing usually occurs because the muscles have grown accustomed to the usual workout and require new challenges to continue growing.

Cycling. Mixing intense workouts with less-intense workouts. Lifters who have plateaued sometimes use this technique to give muscles the opportunity to recover.

The sticking point. The point in a lift where the muscles are strained the most.

---

per set, says Dragomir Cioroslan, head coach of the U.S. Weightlifting Federation and the 1996 U.S. Olympic weightlifting team.

Repetitions and sets are just part of the equation. There is also the weight you lift. Obviously, this will be different for every man, but a reasonable goal is to expend 65 to 70 percent of your energy per set. In practical terms, this means using enough weight so that you can barely finish the last repetition in the set, yet not so much that you can't take a rest and complete another set.

A solid workout involves doing two or three sets, with 8 to 12 repetitions in each set, Cioroslan says. These numbers, however, will be different for everyone. See what feels right—that's probably the number that's right for you. Many people get good results with only one set.

CHOOSE YOUR WEAPONS. There are two basic types of lifting equipment: free weights (the old-fashioned barbells and dumbbells) and ma-chines. Machines are often recommended for beginners because they're easier to learn (they only move in the way they're designed to move), they're safer (no big hunks of metal to drop on your foot), and they don't require a spotter (someone to help out when you're lifting awkward or heavy weights). Machines are also fast and convenient (you don't have to spend time putting weights on barbells), and they offer an easy way to focus on specific muscle groups.

Advocates of free weights, on the other hand, argue that barbells and dumbbells are the superior route to overall conditioning because they exercise your flexibility, coordination, timing, and balance along with your muscles. They also offer a wider variety of exercises, once you know how to use them.

Newton, who was lifting competitively before the new machines were developed, doesn't hold much affection for the new technology. Still, he agrees that they serve a purpose. "There's room for

Setting Up a Home Gym

The first thing you need to start weight training are some weights. There are two basic ways to get them: Join a gym or buy weights that you can use at home. While many men enjoy the social activity that comes from working out in a gym, others are into privacy, are short on time, or simply want to save a few bucks. For them, a home gym is the way to go.

You don't need to spend a fortune to set up a good home gym, says Dragomir Cioroslan, head coach of the U.S. Weightlifting Federation and the 1996 U.S. Olympic weightlifting team. Here is his shopping list.

- **One bar.** An Olympic-style weight bar is 7 feet long, weighs 45 pounds, and costs about $85. You can probably shave a few bucks by getting a standard 6-foot bar, which will work as well.
- **One set of weights.** Weight plates come in increments of 2½, 5, 10, 25, 35, and 45 pounds. Start with two 5s, four 10s, and two 25s. Cast-iron plates are best because they have a larger center hole to accommodate modern bars. Prices start at about 43 cents a pound.
- **Two collars.** These anchor the plates to the bar. Old-fashioned collars use screws, which need to be adjusted each time you load or unload the bar. Newer collars use tension and are easier to use. Expect to pay between $7 and $30 a pair.
- **Four pairs of dumbbells.** Get 12-pound, 15-pound, 25-pound, and 30-pound sets. Basic hexagon dumbbells cost about 44 cents a pound.
- **An exercise bench.** Get one with a rack to hold the weights for bench presses. Make sure it's sturdy—no rocking from side to side. The standard size is about 25 to 30 inches high (it should be high enough that your arms don't drag on the floor) and 4 feet long. These usually cost $100 to $150.
- **A set of squat racks.** These hold the barbell at about shoulder height and are essential for anyone who doesn't have a friendly spotter permanently on call. The racks should be adjustable to your height. They cost about $59 a pair.
- **A hyperextension machine.** This works your lower back, abs, and legs. While it's not essential, it's nice to have. It costs $150 to $350.
- **A full-length mirror.** An important accessory for keeping an eye on your form. It costs about $10.

---

both," he says. The best advice for the beginner? Take some time getting a feel for machines and free weights and use what you're most comfortable with, he says.

GIVE YOUR MUSCLES A BREAK. After you've finished a set, your muscles need time to recover before you ask them to perform again. The amount of rest that you take between sets depends on your goals, says Cioroslan. Basketball players, for example, will do leg workouts in which their sets are only 30 seconds apart. That trains the muscles to respond with a limited amount of rest so that at the end of a hard-fought fourth quarter they can still go up for that crucial last-minute rebound.

For overall conditioning, Cioroslan says, the general rule is to rest 2 to 3 minutes between sets. If you feel that you need more rest, however, take it; putting strain on a muscle that hasn't adequately recovered is more likely to hurt it than make it stronger.

STAY FOCUSED. There's no shortage of distractions in the gym, from the newest magazines in the lobby to the aerobics class in the room next door. Stay focused on your workout, Cioroslan ad-

vises. Not only will this help you get the best exercise but it will also help prevent injuries, which usually occur when you're not paying attention.

AIM FOR THREE. Research has shown that while beginning lifters can gain strength doing as little as two workouts a week, three will produce optimal results. It doesn't have to be time-consuming, Cioroslan says. Once you're familiar with your workout, you can probably finish the whole thing in 20 to 30 minutes a session.

REST YOUR FIBERS. It's important to get at least 48 hours' rest between workouts, Cioroslan says. Research has shown that letting strained muscle fibers recover and rebuild causes strength to improve more quickly. This doesn't mean that you have to take a day off. You can work your legs one day, for example, and your arms the next. On the third day your legs will be ready to work again.

WORK THROUGH THE PAIN. Although lifting weights shouldn't cause pain over the long run, be forewarned that you're going to be sore—significantly sore—when you first start lifting. The discomfort will subside after a few workouts—if you keep working out. "Soreness is a beginner's syndrome," says Cioroslan. "It is not an obstacle. If you interrupt your training routine, the soreness will come back the next time you train. You have to work through it."

GO STRAIGHT TO THE MAJORS. Lifters have come up with an astonishing number of ways for conditioning even the most minute parts of their bodies. "A lot of guys do these elaborate routines that include as many as 20 to 30 exercises and hundreds of repetitions," says Dr. Baechle. "Their workouts take so long that they have to pack lunches and take flashlights in their gym bags. That's not necessary."

A better strategy for getting into shape, Dr. Baechle says, is to develop a basic routine that focuses on the major muscle groups. (Later, you can customize workouts to address more specific problem areas.) The main muscles include the quadriceps (in the front of the thighs), hamstrings (in back of the thighs), the gluteals (in the butt), trapezius and erector muscles (in the back), the abdominals, and shoulder, chest, and arm muscles.

Build a routine around compound exercises, those that work several large muscles or muscle groups at once, Cioroslan recommends. Squats, for example, work the shoulders, lower back, abdominals, arms, and legs. That's a lot of bang for the exercise buck.

BUILD GENTLY. As you get stronger, you'll begin to lift more weight. Indeed, the loads that you can handle will increase in far bigger leaps in the beginning than later on. Don't be in too big a hurry, though. To be safe, Newton says, build gradually. You want to stay in the range of 8 to 12 repetitions per set. When you're ready to handle more weight, increase it by 2 to 3 percent. If you increase the weight too much too fast, you're going to get hurt, not fit.

While it's easy to add small amounts of resistance when using free weights, many weight machines can't be fine-tuned. That's okay, Newton says. Go ahead and increase the weight to the next level. If that's more than the recommended 2 to 3 percent, lower the number of repetitions for a while or stay at the same weight and increase the number of repetitions.

GET THE BLOOD FLOWING. Before pushing muscle fibers beyond what they're used to, give them some advance warning. Frank Eksten, strength coordinator in the Department of Athletics and visiting lecturer in kinesiology at Indiana University in Bloomington, recommends starting a workout by doing 5 minutes of light aerobic activity, such as riding a stationary bike, walking, or jogging in place. After that, he says, spend another 5 minutes stretching gently—and no bouncing, please.

Stretching at the end of the workout is also important to do. "It cools you down and helps maintain and increase your flexibility while you strength-train," he says. (For more information on proper stretching techniques, see the Flexing and Stretching chapter on page 338.)

GET PROFESSIONAL HELP. You don't need any more than a good book or two and maybe an exercise video to learn the basics of strength training, says Art Drechsler, former board member of the U.S. Weightlifting Federation. But if you want personal guidance, you may want to join a gym that includes a trainer as part of the membership. Many gyms do.

If your gym doesn't provide trainers, you may want to hire one, at least for a few sessions. Drechsler says that you can expect to pay a minimum of $25 an hour for their services; one or two sessions will buy you a hands-on demonstration of the equipment and some suggestions for designing a personal workout program.

Focus on Form

In weight lifting, style is substance, especially for the beginner. According to Dr. Mikesky, improper technique in the weight room is the source of many injuries. Before loading on the weights, he advises, take some time to practice each exercise, concentrating on balance and control. Knowing how the exercise is supposed to feel will pay off because bad form makes you more vulnerable to injury. It's worth learning how to get it right from the outset.

Dr. Baechle recommends starting off with light weights—even using a broomstick or a dowel for exercises that use a bar—until you're comfortable with the movements required.

In the next chapter we will get a lot more specific on developing good form for a variety of exercises. But here are a few guidelines for getting started.

SIT STILL. When doing an exercise that requires sitting on a bench or stool, keep your body as still and stable as possible. This is important for two reasons: By holding the rest of your body still, you can focus the full stress of the exercise on the specific muscles being worked. Also, leaning or bouncing has a tendency to throw you off balance, which means you—and the heavy metal you're heaving around—are more likely to hit the floor.

If you're using a machine that has an adjustable seat, take the time to adjust it. If a machine has a belt, there's a reason why the belt is there. Use it.

LIFT SMOOTHLY. Lifting movements should always be slow, smooth, and controlled, says Dr. Mikesky. That's partly to avoid injury and partly to give your muscles more of a workout. One YMCA study found that men who spent 10 seconds lifting the weight and 5 seconds lowering it increased their strength 50 percent faster than those who lifted at a faster pace.

RESTRAIN FROM BOUNCING. You've probably seen more than a few bench pressers bouncing the bars off their chests to gain extra lift. While using momentum allows you to move more weight, it cheats muscles of the load required to grow, thus reducing the benefits. It also signifi-

cantly increases the risk of injury, warns Dr. Mikesky. Lifting slowly and with control taxes muscles to the utmost, and that's what you're looking to achieve.

GO TO THE LIMIT. To get the most out of each exercise, be sure to extend the lift through its full range of motion. Don't, however, lock your arms at the end of a lift. That shifts the stress off the muscles and onto ligaments and bone, says Dr. Mikesky. "Keep a soft bend in the joints that you're working. If you lock the joint, the muscle is unloaded."

BREATHE EASY. There's a tendency to hold your breath while lifting. Don't do it, Dr. Mikesky says. Instead, exhale whenever you're putting out effort (lifting weight against gravity) and inhale when you're returning to the starting position.

GET A GRIP. It may seem obvious, but lots of bruises testify to the importance of wrapping your fingers and thumbs firmly around a barbell or dumbbell before lifting. You don't have to use a pulverizing death-grip, but it should be tight and secure.

How to Design a Workout
Keeping Your Goals in Mind

One of the earliest known fitness experts was a gentleman in ancient Greece named Milo of Crotona.

Milo came up with a rather ingenious method of training for the Olympics: He took a newborn calf and lifted it on his shoulders. He did the same thing the next day and every day after that. The calf kept getting bigger; Milo kept getting stronger. By the time the Games began, he amazed the assembled multitudes by carrying a full-grown bull across the Olympic stadium on his shoulders.

Milo, it's clear, instinctively understood one of the fundamental principles of weight training: that you steadily increase strength by incrementally increasing resistance. He also managed to design a workout that was perfectly suited to his particular fitness goals.

Zeroing in on your goals is a critical first step in any workout plan. Experts call this specificity. It means putting together a workout that directly addresses your specific goals as well as your strengths, weaknesses, and even your time schedule.

Specificity can be taken too far, of course. You don't want to get so focused on fine-tuning a few specific muscles that you overlook overall conditioning. But personalizing your workout means that your goals are always front and center. That means you are more likely to stick with it for the long haul, says Frank Eksten, strength coordinator in the Department of Athletics and visiting lecturer in kinesiology at Indiana University in Bloomington.

Whatever your goals—building leg endurance for bicycling, gaining back strength to prevent injuries, or putting another inch on your biceps to impress your kids—you can customize a workout plan to fit. With the help of our experts, we have put together a five-step plan.

Step 1: Setting Your Goals

Weight training is extremely versatile; it's up to you to customize your program to achieve the goals you have in mind. Are you most interested in how your body functions or how your body looks? If function is most important, think about the activities that you like to do and the movements that make up those activities. For basketball, you will need strong hips and legs, while a strong midsection and shoulders are more important for tennis. You can also use lifting to improve how you look by increasing muscle tone and size. There are three basic things that you can achieve by lifting.

Strength. Strength training enhances your ability to lift lots of weight with explosive power—the sort of power Milo needed to lift that bovine barbell. In today's world, strength training is useful if you want to give your legs the power to jump high for a rebound or if you would like to add some forehand power to your tennis game. It can also help you pick up a toddler without throwing your back out or simply make it easier to haul boxes up to the attic.

Endurance. Even if you're exceptionally strong, your muscles need training to maintain their power over long periods of time. Milo was strong, but Bill Rodgers would have run rings around him. Endurance training is a priority, and not only for athletes. Imagine yourself raking all the leaves in your yard next fall and still having energy to do the same for the elderly lady next door.

Size. The emphasis here is on building muscles that look impressive. This is the sort of training that made stars of Sly Stallone's biceps.

Big muscles, by the way, are not necessarily strong muscles. If they were, then bodybuilders would be the strongest lifters—but they're not, Eksten says.

Although we have outlined some specific, highly targeted goals, it is worth noting that most men will go for a combination of these things: larger muscles plus more strength plus more endurance. That's okay, Eksten says, as long as what you're looking for is a solid, all-around conditioning program.

Step 2: Assembling the Blocks

Once you have established what your goals are, you can proceed to structure a workout that will accomplish those goals. While there is always some overlap—lifting for strength, for example, will have at least some effect on your size and endurance—the various techniques really aren't complementary. That's why you have to define your goals up front—to decide if what you're after is to become bigger, stronger, or longer-lasting. Then you can pick the workout that's right for you.

The basic building blocks of a weight-training workout are incredibly simple, consisting of just four things: the amount of weight you lift, how many times you lift it, the number of sets you do, and how much you rest between sets. By making changes in each of these variables, you can achieve virtually any fitness goal, says Thomas R. Baechle, Ed.D., professor and chairman of exercise science at Creighton University in Omaha, Nebraska, and co-author of *Weight Training: Steps to Success.*

Training for strength. When your goal is to get stronger, you need to be lifting weights that tax your muscles to their limits. Dr. Baechle advises lifting between 80 and 100 percent of the amount that you are capable of. He recommends keeping the repetitions low (one to eight) while doing a high number of sets (three to five, or even more).

Since your muscles will be working at their

What Makes Muscles Stronger?

The next time you are in the gym, take a look at the various physiques and note how much weight the men attached to those physiques can lift.

At the bench press, for example, you might see a giant of a man with a barrel chest and biceps the size of your head. He presses about 250 pounds.

Cut to the next guy. He's a tall, lean drink of water, with thin arms and a small chest. Guess what? He also benches 250.

How can two men with such different frames lift the same amount of weight? To a certain extent genetics plays a role. Some men are born to have large physiques, while others are more likely to be lean, says Frank Eksten, strength coordinator in the Department of Athletics and visiting lecturer in kinesiology at Indiana University in Bloomington. What's more, bulk is only one aspect of strength; a more important factor begins in the nervous system.

Obviously, one way to increase the strength of a muscle is to increase the size of the fibers that the muscle consists of. When you subject a muscle to increased tension during lifting, your body releases a protein that increases the thickness of individual muscle fibers and allows them to contract with more force. Further, additional capillaries form to service the muscle's increased need for blood and nutrients, which also make it thicker and larger.

That's one aspect of strength training. The other involves the nervous system. By repeating certain types of lifting movements, you're training not only the muscle but also the nerves that fire the muscle. You are also working the cardiovascular system that supplies the muscle with fuel and removes the waste.

This combination—more and larger muscle fibers working in sync with trained nervous and cardiovascular systems—is what makes muscles strong. It explains how you can be strong without being large.

limits, you're going to need a relatively long period of rest between sets. For most men, resting 2 to 5 minutes will give the muscles plenty of time to recover.

Training for endurance. This involves using relatively light weights (about 70 percent of the maximum that you're capable of) and a high number of repetitions (12 to 20, or more) for two to three sets, says Dr. Baechle. And unlike training just for strength, you want very little rest. He advises resting about 20 to 30 seconds between sets. This not only prepares the muscles for prolonged effort but it also gets your heart and lungs pumping—an essential part of any endurance plan.

Training for size. This requires a middle route between strength and endurance training. Dr. Baechle recommends lifting a moderate amount of weight (70 to 80 percent of maximum capacity) a moderate number of times (8 to 12 repetitions). You'll want to do between three and six sets, with a moderate amount of rest—say, 30 to 90 seconds between sets.

Whatever your fitness goals are, keep in mind that an unbalanced routine is an invitation to injury. Whether you are working for strength, endurance, or size, you don't want to target specific muscle groups to the exclusion of others. For example, many men work hard on the bench to achieve a buff upper body but neglect to work their legs to a similar degree.

Indeed, targeting specific muscles should always be a secondary goal. Instead, do lifts that challenge several muscles at the same time—*compound* exercises like bench presses and leg presses. Gary Hunter, Ph.D., professor of exercise physiology at the University of Alabama at Birmingham, recommends waiting at least 10 weeks after you begin a weight-training program before getting into more targeted lifts. Even after that, he says, you should still maintain a core regimen of basic conditioning exercises for the whole body.

Step 3: Putting It Together

Designing a workout is a little like composing a symphony: Once you have your theme—say, building for strength—you begin writing in what the instruments should play and when. Whichever workout you choose, the following tips will help you get the most from each exercise.

WORK THE BIG MUSCLES FIRST. It takes more energy to work a large muscle than a small one. Just as obvious, you have more energy at the beginning of a workout than at the end. That's why you should begin any workout by targeting the largest muscles and muscle groups, then work downward to the smaller muscles, says Dragomir Cioroslan, head coach of the U.S. Weightlifting Federation and the 1996 U.S. Olympic weightlifting team.

Since the legs are the largest single muscle group in the body, many workouts begin there. Cioroslan often recommends beginning with leg presses. This is a compound exercise that simultaneously works the quadriceps, hamstrings, buttocks, and calves.

From there you can move to a compound exercise for the upper body, like the bench press. Then, when the major muscles have been worked, you can move on to exercises that focus on smaller, specific muscles like biceps, calves, or forearms, says Cioroslan.

STAY CHALLENGED. For workouts to be effective, they should always be moving forward, keeping the muscles stressed and challenged. Wayne Westcott, Ph.D., national strength-training consultant for the YMCA, the American Council on Exercise, and the National Academy of Sports Medicine, recommends the *double-progressive* training system, in which you alternately increase the repetitions and the resistance.

Suppose, for example, you can do eight biceps curls with 50 pounds on the bar. Dr. Westcott advises training until you can do 12 curls with 50 pounds. Then you should increase the resistance to 52.5 pounds. At that weight you may be able to do only 10 repetitions. Train at the heavier weight until you once again can do 12 repetitions. Then increase the resistance to 55 pounds and start again.

GO FROM LESS TO MORE. Gradually increasing the amount of weight you lift from set to set will add intensity to your workout by demanding more effort from the muscles involved. You might start by bench-pressing 50 pounds, for example, then go to 60 pounds for your second set, and 70 pounds for your third.

Whatever the amounts of weight you're using, always go from less to more. Requiring an increasing level of exertion is the most effective way to condition the muscle, Cioroslan says. Gradually building to a peak also gives the muscle a chance to prepare for the greater strains to come.

WORK BACK AND FORTH. Every muscle has its counterpart. The biceps, for example, curl your arms one way, while the triceps pull them back the other way. To keep your workout balanced, it's important to work opposing muscle groups.

"If you train one group and not the opposing group, you run the risk of injury," says Dr. Westcott. "That's the nemesis of all sports-specific training programs: Swimmers get swimmer's shoulder, for example, and runners get runner's knee. If you work the quadriceps on the front of the thigh, make sure you do the hamstrings in back of the thigh. If you do the abdominals, make sure you also do the lower back muscles. If you do biceps, don't forget triceps, and so on."

Another way to keep your workout balanced is the *push-pull* method. The idea is to alternate lifts in which you push the weight away from your body (like triceps extensions or knee extensions) with lifts that pull the weight in (like biceps curls and leg curls). This strategy keeps you from straining the same muscle groups twice in a row and ensures that you will hit the opposing groups evenly, says Dr. Westcott.

Step 4: Avoiding the Plateau

We have explained how important it is to keep your muscles challenged. This is true all the way down to the cellular level. If you keep putting your muscles through the same paces over and over again, eventually the muscle fibers (which are made up of cells) adapt. No longer challenged, they get bored. Progress slows, then stops. You have hit the plateau.

You can expect to hit a plateau somewhere between 12 and 20 weeks after you start lifting, Dr. Hunter says. This first plateau can be especially depressing because, in most cases, the initial progress is so dramatic. But plateauing is a natural response to habitual exercise, and it occurs as readily at three years as at three months.

Some plateaus last a week, others last a month. How long yours lasts depends on what you do about it—if you do anything. Some lifters are perfectly happy staying on a fitness plateau, Eksten says. "I've seen people do the same workout for years," he says. "That's fine: Their goal is to maintain the level of conditioning that they have."

Although there's no way to prevent plateaus entirely, there are ways to minimize the amount of time you spend there. It all boils down to keeping your muscles challenged. The way to do this is to change your workout every five weeks or so, says Dr. Westcott. It doesn't take radical changes either. Tinkering with the basics of your routine—mixing up the exercises, changing the amounts of weights and repetitions, getting more or less rest between sets—is sufficient.

If you usually do bench presses, for example, you may want to switch to an inclined press for a while. While both exercises work the chest, shoulders, and triceps, the slightly different movements involved will activate additional muscle fibers for greater stimulus. Or suppose you have hit a wall doing three sets of each exercise. Try switching to one set while using more weight and maintaining better form, says Dr. Westcott.

When you are trying to beat the plateau, almost any change is good, Dr. Westcott says. Here are a few more strategies you may want to try.

USE THE SAWTOOTH SOLUTION. Also called cycle training or periodization programs, sawtooth training mixes hard stretches of training with planned periods of active rest. Say, for example, you like to do three sets of bench presses with 200 pounds. For a week, drop it down to two sets with 150 pounds—this is the beginning of the active rest phase. A week later, gradually build it back up, going to three sets with 170 pounds for the first workout, 180 pounds for the second, 190 pounds for the third. After that, you are ready to return to where you started and then move on from there to the next higher level.

The rest periods allow the muscles to fully recover from the initial exertion, often with dramatic results. Many lifters will see a surge of progress as they climb out of their self-imposed lull.

On a smaller scale, you can practice the sawtooth pattern within a single week's workout, Dr. Hunter says. For example, on Monday, do three sets of each exercise using the heaviest weights you can lift for six to eight repetitions. On Wednesday, do the same number of sets and repetitions, but cut the weight back to about 70 percent of what you lifted on Monday. Then on Friday, do medium-weight sets, at 75 to 80 percent of your Monday pace. When you return to the gym the following Monday, be prepared for a blastoff.

SLOW TO A CRAWL. Slowing the pace at which you lift can result in substantial gains because it causes muscle fibers to be stressed longer, boosting the intensity of the lift. In one study, Dr. Westcott compared lifters who took 7 seconds per repetition (2 seconds up, 1 second pause, 4 seconds down) to those who took 14 seconds (10 seconds up and 4 seconds down). After two months, the slower-moving group was stronger.

UP THE INTENSITY. A highly effective way to overcome a training plateau is to add what Dr.

Westcott calls "post-fatigue repetitions" to your basic sets. Do a set of any exercise with enough weight so that you can just complete 10 repetitions. Immediately lower the weight 10 to 20 percent and do a few more. Since this demanding technique doesn't allow rest between sets, you don't lose benefits even though you lower the weight.

BUILD A PYRAMID. This torturous technique is another way of tricking your muscles into exerting more effort than they are used to. By lifting heavier and heavier weights in progressive sets, you'll trick the muscle into going beyond the point at which you would ordinarily stop, adding just a little more exertion to each set.

Here's an example. When doing arm curls, start with a pair of dumbbells lighter than you would normally use when doing 10 repetitions. Curl them 5 times. After a short rest, take the next heaviest set of dumbbells and do 5 repetitions. Continue up the rack until you reach a weight that is too heavy to curl 5 times. Then work your way back down through the weights, suggests Dr. Westcott.

Step 5: Making Time

Perhaps the greatest enemy that your muscles face is time. We're not talking aging; we're talking schedule. Simply put, who has time for long workouts? In fact, you don't need a lot of time. Here are a few ways to squeeze the most workout into the shortest possible time.

WORK THE COMPOUNDS. We mentioned earlier that it's a good idea to start a training session by doing compound exercises, which work several large muscle groups at once. Compound exercises are the essence of time efficiency, too. With leg presses, for example, you can work the quadriceps, hamstrings, buttocks, and calves. "In effect," says Dr. Westcott, "you're doing four exercises at once."

SPLIT THE DIFFERENCE. Busy people don't like to stand around doing nothing, yet you're supposed to rest between sets, right? Not necessarily. You can circumvent the rest requirement by alternating upper-body exercises with lower-body workouts. Going from bench presses to leg extensions, for example, lets your chest muscles rest while your legs get a workout.

Experienced lifters sometimes take the split-workout concept to its furthest extreme by eliminating between-set rests entirely. Rather, they quickly move from one set to the next, working different muscle groups without pausing for rest. The technique is called circuit training, and it squeezes the most exercise into the shortest period of time. What's more, it may enhance cardiovascular endurance as well as develop muscular strength.

SPLIT THE WEEK. If your fitness goals are truly ambitious, you may want to expand the split-workout approach to a weekly schedule. For example, dedicate Mondays and Thursdays to lower-body work and Tuesdays and Fridays to upper-body work. Do some abdominal work on all four days, alternating between front abdominals and the side muscles. A split schedule means more trips to the gym (or the basement, if you work out at home), but the trips are shorter. Plus, you don't have to wait the usual 48 hours between workouts, says Dr. Westcott.

REDUCE THE LOAD. Although most lifters complete several sets of each exercise, Dr. Westcott feels that there is no clear evidence that more is necessarily better—at least, not for the average man who is more interested in getting in good general shape than in preparing for the next competition. If time is an issue for you, Dr. Westcott recommends doing no more than two exercises per muscle group and one set per exercise. This will keep your total workout time to 30 minutes.

SCENARIO 1: Losing It Fast

AGE: 38

WEIGHT: 230

HEALTH: He's in good shape generally. Slightly short of breath with minor exertion such as climbing stairs. Blood pressure is healthy, although cholesterol is pushing 210, meaning borderline unhealthy. No significant problems with disease or injury.

EXERCISE ROUTINE: A fair-weather exerciser, he enjoys evening walks of 30 to 45 minutes once or twice a week. During the warm months he gets out to the archery range on weekends; from November to March, he doesn't get out much.

LIFESTYLE: He has a desk job. Is a passionate reader, meaning that he spends an hour or 2 each evening with a book.

WEIGHT GOALS: Wants to lose 50 pounds for his 10th anniversary, two months away.

FITNESS GOALS: No convert to fitness, all he really wants is to lose weight and improve his breathing and endurance so that he can get around comfortably. Would like to lower his cholesterol, but this isn't a high priority.

Most of us can remember a time in our lives when someone pulled us aside to tell us that we were biting off considerably more than we could chew. This gentleman is about to be told that he is biting off *less* than he should chew.

There is no question that he needs to lose weight. There is also no question that he needs to get a lot more active if he is going to lose any weight at all. But trying to lose 50 pounds in two months is a bad idea. "He is in need of a serious attitude adjustment," says John Duncan, Ph.D., professor of clinical research at Texas Woman's University in Denton. "Trying for fast, unrealistic results is one of the great American misconceptions about conditioning."

What's needed here is a shift from short-term to long-term thinking. "It's not about going on a crash diet for two months," says Marjorie Albohm, a certified athletic trainer and director of sports medi-

cine at Kendrick Memorial Hospital in Mooresville, Indiana. "It's about changing your life."

The human body simply isn't designed to lose large amounts of weight quickly. For most men, losing half a pound to a pound a week is about right, says Dr. Duncan. Upcoming anniversary or not, the only way this guy will be successful is to do two things: lower the number of calories consumed each day and get serious about exercise. "Archery is a wonderful sport, but it won't do much for your cardiovascular capacity," says Eric Durak, an exercise physiologist at Medical Health and Fitness in Santa Barbara, California.

This man needs to begin his exercise campaign slowly but determinedly, says Durak. The idea is to do enough to see some improvement (which will keep him going) but not so much as to overdo it (which will cause him to give up). The initial focus should be aerobic conditioning. Given his apparent lack of interest in conventional exercise, Dr. Duncan says, he should look for opportunities to integrate exercise into his daily routine: taking stairs instead of the elevator, for example, or parking farther back in the parking lot and walking the rest of the way. "He needs to think active," Dr. Duncan says. "By putting together a lot of little things, he can build up to 30 minutes of activity a day."

For a more direct approach, he can simply increase his walking from one or two days a week to six or seven, at least 15 minutes each morning and 15 minutes each night. While he is walking, Durak adds, he should try to concentrate on breathing as deeply as possible. By learning to improve his intake of oxygen, he will increase his tolerance for exercise.

Since he loves books, he undoubtedly spends a lot of time sitting on his fanny, which means he also needs to gain some flexibility. Durak recommends incorporating some stretching exercises into his daily routine, especially those that will give him some mobility in the shoulder area, which will pay off on the archery range. (For tips on stretching, see the Flexing and Stretching chapter on page 338.)

The Workout

After a week or two of his increased walking regimen, he can embark on a more vigorous workout routine. His first goal should be overall conditioning. To achieve this, Dragomir Cioroslan, head coach of the U.S. Weightlifting Federation and the 1996 U.S. Olympic weightlifting team, recommends that he do a roughly equal number of exercises for the upper body, lower body, and the midsection. His second goal should be increased endurance. To help him achieve this, Cioroslan recommends that he do a high number of repetitions in each set and a high number of sets for each exercise.

A third goal of this workout is strengthening his self-confidence. He needs, Cioroslan says, to regain a sense of control over his body, to remember what it is like to move with ease and assurance. Getting into shape cuts fatty deposits from the mind as well as from the arteries and the belly.

He should schedule three workouts a week. To start with, rest between sets should be about 1 minute. At that pace each workout should take 45 minutes to 1 hour to complete. "Committing himself to a healthier lifestyle and to a fitness program would be the best anniversary gift that he could give his wife and himself," Cioroslan says. "He has to find the willpower to stay with it."

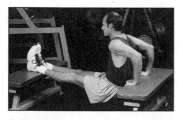

1. Step-ups (page 322) help strengthen several important muscle groups in the upper legs, specifically, the quadriceps (front thigh), hamstrings (back thigh), and gluteal (butt) muscles. Building these muscles will help improve mobility. Try for 15 repetitions with each leg per set.

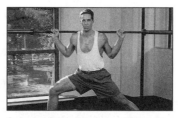

2. Lateral lunges (page 236) will accomplish two objectives: They will strengthen and condition the inner thigh muscles and improve the flexibility of the tendons and ligaments in the hip area. Do 8 to 12 repetitions with each leg per set.

3. Parallel dips (page 272) target two important muscle groups: the triceps (back of upper arm) and the latissimus dorsi (mid and lower back). Torso mobility and upper-body strength will be enhanced. Do 8 to 12 repetitions per set.

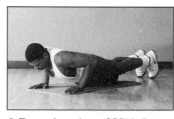

4. The **push-up** (page 286) is the classic exercise for strengthening the arms and shoulders, which will help improve overall conditioning and mobility. Try for 8 to 12 repetitions per set.

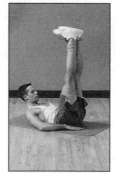

5. Straight-leg raises (page 202) directly target the lower abdominals. This will tone the gut and help improve mobility by enhancing overall stability. Do 15 to 20 repetitions per set.

6. Double-leg scoops (page 215) will challenge the abdominal muscles a bit more than straight-leg raises will. A higher degree of difficulty will help build more midbody muscle tone. Try for 15 to 20 repetitions per set.

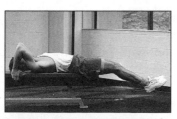

7. Crunches (page 198) are the foundation of virtually any abdominal conditioning routine. They isolate the upper abdominals and help protect the lower back. Work up to 20 repetitions per set.

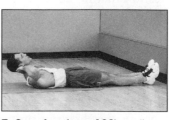

SCENARIO 2: Keeping Up with Time

AGE: 35

WEIGHT: 185

HEALTH: He smokes lightly but has no serious health problems.

EXERCISE ROUTINE: Without fail he plays indoor soccer three nights a week. Periodically lifts weights when friends invite him to the club.

LIFESTYLE: He works freelance construction, mainly as a carpenter. Spends weekends working in the yard or in the garage. Lunch is usually takeout. He has a few beers after work on most days.

WEIGHT GOALS: Wants to lose 20 pounds in 20 weeks (on a bet).

FITNESS GOALS: His arms and legs are already strong, although he has noticed that he can't swing a hammer like he used to. He would also like to develop more leg power for soccer.

Here, we have a man who seems to take reasonably good care of himself and who probably takes his health pretty much for granted. Still, he is 35 now, which means small pleasures are beginning to result in a bit of wear and tear around the edges. It is a good time to think about changing some bad habits. They will be easier to shake now than they will be at 50.

Since he is already in decent shape, losing 20 pounds in 20 weeks may be a reasonable bet, says Marjorie Albohm, a certified athletic trainer and director of sports medicine at Kendrick Memorial Hospital in Mooresville, Indiana. The bet is as good a way as any to kick-start a fitness program—nothing like a little money at stake to provide motivation. But fitness goals should always be long term, she adds, rather than focusing on the next five weeks.

Further, while weight lifting is good, it has to be done regularly to get results. "Soccer is an excellent aerobic activity," she says, "but just lifting weights occasionally isn't going to do much besides providing some social interaction with his friends."

Not surprisingly, all the experts we talked to zeroed in on this man's cigarette habit. "There's no place for smoking in a healthy person's life, period," says Dragomir Cioroslan, head coach of the U.S. Weightlifting Federation and the 1996 U.S. Olympic weightlifting team. They also noted the after-work beers—more for the calories consumed than the alcohol. "Drinking several beers a day is not really compatible with a goal of losing weight," says John Duncan, Ph.D., professor of clinical research at Texas Woman's University in Denton.

Even though being overweight doesn't appear to be this man's problem, he should still keep an eye on his diet, Cioroslan says. "He's probably working pretty hard, physically. But I'd guess right now that he's probably getting too many calories from beer. That's not nutritionally adequate for someone with his energy expenditure."

The Workout

Cioroslan designed this training program to complement and enhance this man's weekly soccer games while at the same time building strength in his hammering arm. The primary goals of the first three exercises are to increase speed, agility, and endurance in the legs. The step-ups are there purely to increase leg strength. The arm exercises will all serve to make this man the meanest man with a hammer since John Henry.

The workout should be done twice a week, 45 to 50 minutes each time. Cioroslan recommends that he rest 1 to 2 minutes between sets, except for the step-ups. For those, he should rest 3 minutes between sets. The longer rest period is recommended for exercises that are geared toward developing pure strength, whereas shorter rests help build endurance.

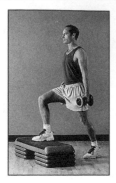

1. Doing **step-ups** while holding dumbbells (page 322) is excellent for strengthening the quadriceps (front thigh) muscles. Not only do they build strength and staying power in the legs but they also bring other muscles into play as you try to maintain your balance. Do 20 repetitions per leg per set.

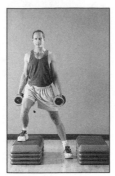

2. **Lateral step-ups** (page 237) are still another way to add strength and coordination to the legs. This exercise particularly targets the inner and outer thighs, hip flexors (front hip), and hamstrings (back thigh), all of which come into play when running side to side on the soccer field. Do 20 repetitions with each leg per set.

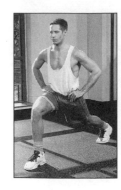

3. The **alternating leg lunge** (page 235) is another power-building exercise for a soccer player's most important body parts—the legs. This exercise works the muscles slightly differently than lateral lunges do. Do 20 to 25 repetitions with each leg per set.

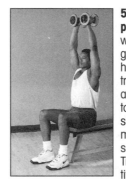

4. **Lateral lunges** (page 236) are perfect for developing the leg muscles necessary for both speed and agility. Do 15 to 20 repetitions with each leg per set.

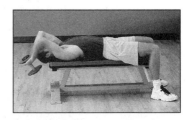

5. **Dumbbell military presses** (page 294) work the three muscle groups involved in hammer wielding: the triceps (back of upper arm), the anterior deltoid (front of the shoulder), and the medium deltoid (outside of the shoulder). Try for six to eight repetitions per set.

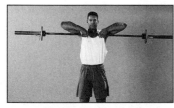

6. The **upright row** (page 296) is a demanding exercise that develops strength in the forearms and the chest as well as the shoulders. Try for 8 to 10 repetitions per set.

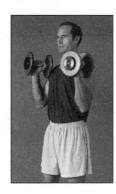

7. As the name suggests, **hammer curls** (page 262) target the muscles used when driving a nail. Specifically, they work the biceps (front of upper arm) and the brachialis (outside of upper arm) muscles. Try for 8 to 12 repetitions.

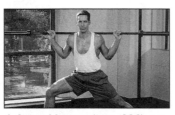

8. **Lying triceps extensions** (page 267) bring the same muscles into play that swinging a hammer does. This exercise will help build the triceps (back of upper arm), adding strength and power. Do 8 to 12 repetitions per set.

SCENARIO **3**: Physical Renewal

AGE: 50

WEIGHT: 220

HEALTH: His blood pressure has reached the point of moderate hypertension and is rising. He is frequently tired, probably because of early-stage diabetes, which doctors say is related to being overweight.

EXERCISE ROUTINE: Doesn't do sports or exercise.

LIFESTYLE: A pharmaceutical representative, he spends 8 hours a day in the car. Cooking is a hobby, so he spends many hours on his feet in the evening. Meets one night a week with fellow gourmets for dinner and drinks.

WEIGHT GOALS: His doctor has advised losing 30 pounds in the next year.

FITNESS GOALS: Hopes to achieve some degree of overall fitness. Would like to get blood pressure and diabetes under control and build up the muscles he uses for standing so that he can work in the kitchen without fatigue.

This man has apparently adopted the same attitude toward his body that New York City once took toward its subways, streets, and parks, which is deferred maintenance. The results in New York are pretty obvious and pretty painful; this man is wise in trying to avoid a similar fate.

His goal of losing 30 pounds in a year is reasonable. In fact, he can probably do it without giving up those weekly feeds with his gourmet friends. Dragomir Cioroslan, head coach of the U.S. Weightlifting Federation and the 1996 U.S. Olympic weightlifting team, does suggest that the group sit down for its feast no later than 7:30 P.M., since calories consumed later in the day don't have as much opportunity to get burned off as those consumed earlier. This man should also limit the Chardonnay to a glass or two at most; fine wine may be the nectar of the gods, but the gods don't have to worry about losing weight.

His next priority, obviously, is to get his body moving again. *Ease* is the operative word here. A

50-year-old man who is overweight with hypertension and diabetes needs to face up to the fact that a heart attack is not out of the question, says Frank Eksten, strength coordinator in the Department of Athletics and visiting lecturer in kinesiology at Indiana University in Bloomington. (Which is why he should check with his doctor before plunging into an exercise program.)

Eksten suggests that he begin by taking simple walks, either outside or on a treadmill, beginning with 15 minutes and working up to ½ hour a day. He can walk as little as two days a week at first, but he should aim for six days a week, Eksten says.

Walking does more than improve cardiovascular fitness. It is also a good way to develop flexibility. Adding 5 minutes of stretching at the end of his walks will help him limber up even more. "That might make him feel a little better about moving," Eksten says. "It will also help him avoid any injuries."

Finally, he should add some strength training to his aerobic regimen as soon as comfortably possible, mainly because of all the time he spends behind a steering wheel. Chip Harrison, strength and conditioning coach at Pennsylvania State University in University Park, notes that a vigorous weight-training workout will substantially elevate his metabolic rate and keep it there for up to 36 hours—far longer than an aerobic workout. The prolonged burn consumes additional calories, even at rest. Strength training also builds muscle, which requires more calories for the body to maintain than fat does. This man can savor the thought of burning fat cells off his waistline even while he is stuck in traffic on the expressway.

The Workout

Given that he is starting from almost zero, this man's workout comes in two phases. The first is an easy-going program involving no weights to help him get started; the second is tougher and will bring him further along. Both workouts, says Cioroslan, are designed to be fun and encouraging.

Phase One of the workout, which should be started along with the walks, will take 20 to 25 minutes and will be repeated twice a week.

In order to concentrate on form, Cioroslan recommends that he complete all the sets of one exercise before moving on to the next. The workouts should be kept 48 to 72 hours apart (Tuesdays and Fridays, for example) so as to give his out-of-shape muscles time to recover. Allow 2 to 3 minutes' rest between sets.

Phase Two of the conditioning plan continues on the two-day-a-week schedule. These workouts are more intense, with exercises divided about equally between the midsection and upper and lower body, says Cioroslan. Some of the exercises require barbells or dumbbells, so he will want to join a gym or buy equipment to keep at home. He will be resting 2 to 3 minutes between sets, meaning that these workouts will take 50 minutes to 1 hour. Once Phase Two has been mastered, he may choose to expand his workouts to include Phase One, adding an additional one to two days per week of exercise.

PHASE ONE

This workout is an essential starting place for someone who is seriously out of shape. Most of the exercises don't require weights, yet the workout puts the body through a wide range of motions.

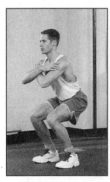

1. The **freehand squat** (page 317) is a basic leg exercise that works the muscles of the upper leg and butt and helps build basic mobility. Do 15 to 20 repetitions per set.

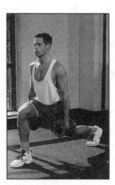

2. Stationary lunges (page 234) are excellent for increasing hip flexibility and for building strength in the inner thigh muscles and butt. Do 8 to 10 repetitions per set.

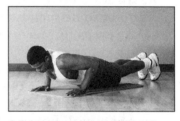

3. The **push-up** (page 286) is the most basic exercise that you can get for strengthening the arms, shoulders, and chest. Try for 5 to 10 repetitions per set.

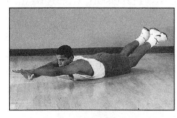

4. Leg and upper-body raises (page 230) work a variety of muscles on the back part of the body, from the hamstrings (back thigh) to the gluteals (butt) and the muscles of the upper and lower back. Try for 8 to 10 repetitions per set.

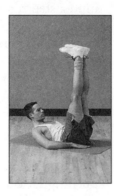

5. Straight-leg raises (page 202) gently tone the midsection by working the lower abdominal muscles and the hip flexor (front hip) muscles. Do 10 repetitions per set.

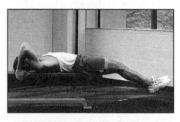

6. Double-leg scoops (page 215) address the lower abdominals and hips in addition to strengthening the lower back. Do 10 repetitions per set.

PHASE TWO

This part of the workout introduces weights and focuses on compound lifts, where several joints and large muscle groups are worked at once. With compound exercises, he can work his entire body in a fairly short time. After three or four weeks of this routine, he should begin to mix and vary the exercises. At any point he feels that he is ready, he should gradually increase the amount of weight lifted or the number of repetitions in order to continue challenging his muscles.

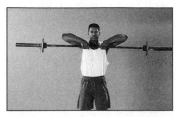

1. The **upright row** (page 296) is a great exercise for the forearm muscles, the biceps (front of upper arm), and the shoulders. It doesn't do the upper back any harm either. Try for 10 to 12 repetitions per set.

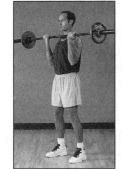

2. Barbell curls (page 257) focus squarely on the biceps (front of upper arm) and can easily be done at home. Try for 8 to 12 repetitions per set.

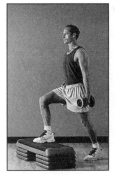

3. Step-ups (page 322) hit two major muscle groups: the quadriceps (front thigh) and the gluteal (butt) muscles. Cardiovascular conditioning is also improved. Do 10 repetitions per leg per set.

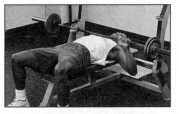

4. The **bench press** (page 277) is another classic exercise that strengthens the entire upper body. Do 6 to 10 repetitions per set.

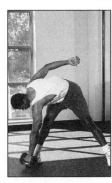

5. Toe touches (page 231) condition the body overall, addressing everything from the hamstrings (back thigh) to the lower back. Do 8 to 10 repetitions per side per set.

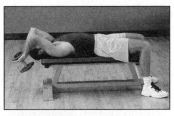

6. Lying triceps extensions (page 267) home in on the biceps muscle's opposite number, the triceps (back of upper arm). Do 8 to 10 repetitions per set.

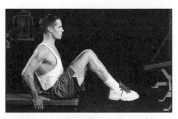

7. Rowing crunches (page 206) primarily hit the upper abdominal muscles as well as the obliques (side) and lower abdominals. Try for 15 to 20 repetitions per set.

SCENARIO 4: Tough to Tougher

AGE: 26

WEIGHT: 170

HEALTH: No problems at all.

EXERCISE ROUTINE: He plays basketball daily, lifts free weights at the gym four days a week, and works out periodically with dumbbells at home. Also swims and runs.

LIFESTYLE: As a doorman at a popular club, he spends evenings and nights on his feet—on display and watching the crowd.

WEIGHT GOALS: Would like to stay about the same or maybe gain a few pounds.

FITNESS GOALS: He is already lean and well-built from his regular lifting and sports. Since, however, a large part of his job is "crowd control," he would like to add more muscle and definition to his midsection.

Apparently, this man is moving too fast to see how fit he already is. Basketball, free weights, swimming, running, a full-time job that requires long periods of standing. And he wants to do more?

"He has to be really careful that he isn't being too intense," says Marjorie Albohm, a certified athletic trainer and director of sports medicine at Kendrick Memorial Hospital in Mooresville, Indiana. "At 26 he can get away with it, but if he keeps on this way, he may run into injury problems or psychological burnout." Indeed, athletes who push too hard may experience overuse syndrome, in which repeated stress on certain parts of the body causes them to break down, says Albohm. Tennis elbow and swimmer's shoulder are classic examples.

Harvey Newton, a certified strength and conditioning specialist and the executive director of the National Strength and Conditioning Association in Colorado Springs, Colorado, adds another possibility: This man may be cheating himself of potential benefits by not giving his muscles sufficient time to recover between workouts.

According to Dragomir Cioroslan, head coach of the U.S. Weightlifting Federation and the 1996 U.S. Olympic weightlifting team, the first thing that he should do is take an honest look at his schedule and think about whether he might need to cut back. He should be getting 7 to 8 hours of sleep a night, and he certainly should wait 48 hours after any intense weight-room sessions before lifting again.

The most obvious way someone in such good condition could make his midsection look even better would be to lose body fat and build more muscle. He is already lean, but if he cuts back on the cheeseburgers that he is probably eating at work, he could get even leaner. That would help the muscles he already has stand out in sharper relief.

At the same time he needs to get the maximum muscle-building advantage from his current training by making sure that he is getting enough protein. Cioroslan recommends that 20 to 25 percent of his daily calories should come from protein. One way that many bodybuilders reach that goal is by using protein powders sold in health food stores. A healthier way would simply be to add a little more high-quality protein foods to his diet, such as lean meat, fish, or low-fat dairy foods, says Peter W. R. Lemon, Ph.D., director of the Applied Physiology Research Laboratory at Kent State University in Kent in Ohio.

Considering his high level of physical activity, one thing this man should be alert to is dehydration and vitamin depletion. He should be drinking at least 8 to 10 glasses of water a day, Cioroslan says. Taking a daily multivitamin/mineral supplement would also be a good idea, he adds.

The Workout

Since this man has the luxury of being able to fine-tune a body that's already in excellent shape, Cioroslan designed a workout focusing on abdominal exercises that call for heavy resistance—as much weight as he can handle and still do a high number of repetitions. The intense, prolonged effort will burn fat and further define the underlying muscles.

Since this man is already risking overtraining, he should only include this workout in his regular weightlifting sessions twice a week.

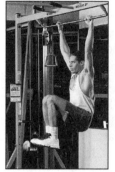

1. Hanging knee raises (page 205) give the lower abdominal muscles a tough workout, and the upper and side abdominals will feel the intensity, too. A strong man should be able to do 20 repetitions per set.

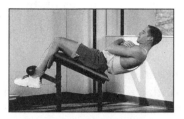

2. Roman chair sit-ups (page 204) are great for hitting all of the abdominal muscles. Begin by doing 20 to 30 repetitions per set, eventually working up to 40 repetitions per set.

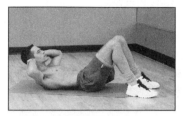

3. The **curl-up** (page 199) is a more-advanced version of the standard crunch. It hits the upper, lower, and side abdominals and will give a gut a harder, more-balanced look. Try for 20 to 25 repetitions per set.

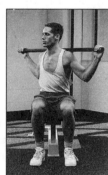

4. Seated twists (page 210) work the oblique (side) abdominal muscles, which will help trim the waist as much as possible, helping to create the ultimate "six-pack" look. Try for 25 to 30 repetitions per set.

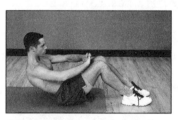

5. Negative sit-ups (page 214) are superb for building endurance as well as strength. Try for 20 repetitions per set.

SCENARIO 5: Mixed Messages

AGE: 30

WEIGHT: 150

HEALTH: He has a little bursitis in each shoulder. Left leg is slightly weak from a ligament injury that occurred 10 years before; this normally isn't a problem, it but can cause slight soreness with extreme exertion.

EXERCISE ROUTINE: Runs 2 to 5 miles in the morning, four or five days a week. Coaches kids' soccer on weekends, which adds a few more miles of stop-and-go running.

LIFESTYLE: He works as a security guard. As a single parent with two children, ages 7 and 9, he spends most of his free time at home.

WEIGHT GOALS: He has always been self-conscious about being thin and would like to increase weight to 165 to 170.

FITNESS GOALS: Eventually, he would like to run a marathon, so his plan is to increase strength and endurance in his legs and perhaps to reduce discomfort in his left leg. He also hopes to get a more buff look by adding a few inches to shoulders, arms, and legs.

Have you ever noticed how many of the things you really want to do in life directly contradict other things you really want to do? Do you pursue your career or your love life? Watch a Michael Jordan special on ESPN or the latest Jim Carrey flick on HBO? Stay lean and run a marathon or put on bulk and slow yourself down?

"A lot of his goals are at odds with each other," says Frank Eksten, strength coordinator in the Department of Athletics and visiting lecturer in kinesiology at Indiana University in Bloomington. "Running a marathon is great, but putting 15 extra pounds of weight on his upper body isn't going to make it any easier. You don't see a lot of bulky marathon runners."

Eksten also points out that training for a marathon isn't going to help him put on the 15 extra pounds that he is hoping to gain. It may, on the other hand, aggravate his leg injury, simply by putting miles of extra stress on an already weak joint. By the same token, if he is really interested in buffing up his shoulders and arms, he has to be careful about aggravating his bursitis.

The bottom line is that he needs to make some choices. "He needs to focus on which of his goals he wants to make his primary goals," Eksten says. "If he tries to do it all, he'll be working against himself."

The first thing he should deal with is the injured leg; this is the weak link that could sabotage all his other goals, says Dragomir Cioroslan, head coach of the U.S. Weightlifting Federation and the 1996 U.S. Olympic weightlifting team. By unconsciously favoring the injured leg, he undoubtedly weakens it further, gradually upsetting his body's natural balance and creating the potential for other injuries.

In addition, he should be especially careful with any stretching exercises involving the knee, Eksten says.

When he gets serious about building up his upper body—perhaps after he takes a year to get the marathon out of his system—he should focus on the bursitis. The conditioning workout given below should help alleviate the pain in his shoulders by strengthening the muscles, ligaments, and tendons and improving blood circulation.

There is nothing exotic involved in putting on 20 pounds. Some of that weight will come from the muscle mass added by a simple weightlifting regimen, but a lot of it will come from the old-fashioned way: eating.

"The main problem I've run into with people trying to put on weight is that they think they need more protein, when, in fact, their protein intake is okay and what they really need is just more calories," says Ann C. Grandjean, Ed.D., assistant professor in the Sports Medicine Program at the University of Nebraska Medical Center and director of the International Center for Sports Nutrition, both in Omaha. The main thing with gaining weight, though, is to be patient. Adding 20 pounds to a lean frame could easily take a year or more.

The Workout

The workout described below, which was designed by Cioroslan, addresses this man's two main objectives. The first four exercises will help to increase his knee and leg strength, while the remaining exercises will help to build up his arms and shoulders.

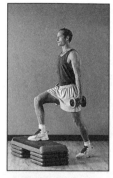

1. Step-ups with dumbbells (page 322) provide a vigorous workout for the quadriceps (front thigh) and gluteal (butt) muscles. This exercise also helps improve knee stability. Do 15 repetitions per leg.

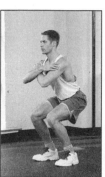

2. Freehand squats (page 317) build leg strength, critical for runners, in the quadriceps (front thigh), hamstrings (back thigh), and gluteals (butt). Strong leg muscles not only boost speed but also help prevent injuries. Do 15 to 25 repetitions per set.

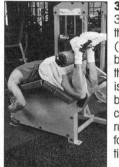

3. Leg curls (page 320) help strengthen the hamstrings (back thigh) and the biceps femoris (back thigh). This exercise is important because both of these muscles are prone to running injuries. Try for 12 to 15 repetitions per set.

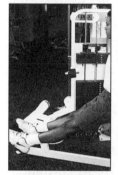

4. Toe presses (page 326) work the calf muscles in the lower leg. This is important for runners because the calf muscles propel the runner forward and absorb a lot of the impact as each stride comes down. Do 15 to 20 repetitions per set.

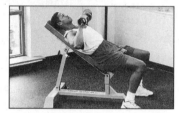

5. Inclined dumbbell presses (page 280) get a lot done at once. They work the upper part of the chest and the front part of the shoulder, while also hitting the triceps (back of upper arm). Do 8 to 12 repetitions per set.

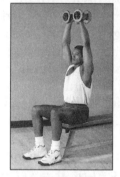

6. The dumbbell military press (page 294) is a classic upper-body strengthening tool, adding bulk and strength to both the arms and the shoulders. Do 8 to 12 repetitions per set.

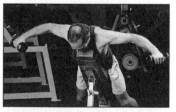

7. Lying lateral raises (page 301) work muscles in the upper back and add strength and stability to the entire shoulder. Doing this exercise will help keep the torso balanced. Try for 10 to 12 repetitions per set.

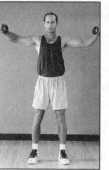

8. Standing lateral raises (page 298) are excellent for building strength and muscle mass in the shoulders. Try to do 8 to 12 repetitions per set.

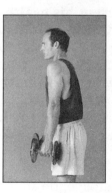

9. Shoulder rotations (page 305) pump blood into the entire shoulder joint, including the tendons, ligaments, and muscles. More blood means that more oxygen and nutrients reach the area, helping to prevent soreness. Do 12 to 20 repetitions per set.

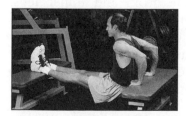

10. Parallel dips (page 272) work all three heads of the triceps (back of upper arm) muscle while maintaining tension in the latissimus dorsi (mid and lower back). Do 8 to 10 repetitions per set.

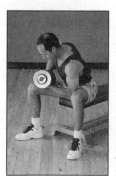

11. Concentration curls (page 264) provide an excellent workout for the biceps (front of upper arm). Because they bring few other muscles into play, the exercise is intensely focused, and you may want to start with lighter weights. Do 12 to 15 repetitions per set.

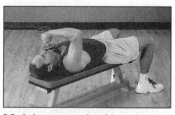

12. Lying cross-shoulder triceps extensions (page 268) help complete an arm workout by adding strength and size to the triceps (back of upper arm), which oppose the biceps. Do 8 to 12 repetitions per set.

SCENARIO 6: From Ground Zero

AGE: 42

WEIGHT: 350

HEALTH: He has been overweight, sometimes severely, for more than 25 years. Is taking medication for high blood pressure and arthritis, both of which resulted from obesity. Has difficulty walking even short distances. His wife usually gets the mail, and he tries not to go up or down stairs more than once or twice a day.

EXERCISE ROUTINE: He played football back in junior high until his weight became a problem. Used to enjoy yard work but now has trouble getting close to the ground. In the last few years has become almost totally sedentary and housebound.

LIFESTYLE: A tenured journalism professor, he has recently cut back on classes because of poor health. Sleeps about 10 hours a day and naps for an hour every afternoon. He rarely has sex due to lack of energy as well as mobility.

WEIGHT GOALS: It is critical that he lose weight to prevent his health from deteriorating further. His doctor has advised getting his weight down at least to 250. Eventually he hopes to reach 200, but after a lifetime of being overweight, his confidence is low.

FITNESS GOALS: Would like to get medical problems under control and improve overall mobility so he can be reasonably active, in bed and out.

This man has a tough job ahead of him. He's so out of shape that he has to get into better condition just to begin getting into shape. He has a lot of work to do, but his condition is certainly not hopeless.

Obviously, he needs to be working with a doctor before starting any exercise plan, says John Duncan, Ph.D., professor of clinical research at Texas Woman's University in Denton. Besides getting his doctor to sign off on any program he undertakes—a must for someone with high blood pressure—he should enlist the services of both a trainer and a nutritionist if he can afford to.

Paradoxically, having so much to accomplish makes his fitness strategy extremely simple. It consists of two parts: losing weight and gaining mobility. Dragomir Cioroslan, head coach of the U.S. Weightlifting Federation and the 1996 U.S Olympic weightlifting team, puts mobility first. "He can't lose weight if he can't move," Cioroslan says.

Perhaps the most difficult challenge will be getting him to move in the first place. Chip Harrison, strength and conditioning coach at Pennsylvania State University in University Park, suggests that an aquatic exercise regimen would be ideal. With a minimum of resistance, he could get back in the habit of using his body.

A second, complementary goal to strive for is sleeping no more than 8 hours a night. Obviously, it doesn't take as many calories to sleep as it does to stay awake and move.

The Workout

Each day should begin with a 10- to 20-minute walk, Cioroslan says. Eventually, he can add some light stretching exercises while he walks: raising his arms over his head, for example, or twisting his torso to the right and left. He can also roll his head or bend down once or twice to pick up a pebble or twig along the way. The frequency of these stretches should be increased until they become a routine that can be repeated four or five times during each walk.

Eventually, he should try walking backward 25 to 30 steps, which will help improve balance and flexibility. When he can do this comfortably, he can add light lunges to the mix to begin building flexibility in the muscles of the groin and upper legs. Cioroslan recommends doing 5 to 10 lunges, using each leg, every morning.

When he can do lunges comfortably, he may want to try lateral lunges (5 to 10 each side) to help develop coordination and agility. The point is to help him reacquaint his body with something that it has largely forgotten: movement, says Cioroslan.

Finally, he should begin doing stationary stretching exercises at the end of each walk, says Cioroslan. These will loosen muscles, ligaments, and tendons that are tight and stiff from lack of use. They will also help increase his agility.

Once he can move comfortably, it's time to move to the more rigorous phase of the workout. This four-day-a-week plan gets progressively more intense as the week goes on. These are meant to be afternoon workouts in order to complement the daily walks, which should be continued.

The first two exercises focus on the lower body, which will increase mobility. Additional exercises address the abdominals, a key area for someone carrying 350 pounds.

MONDAY

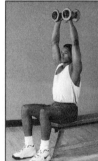

1. Freehand squats (page 317) provide a solid workout without putting too much stress on a body that is out of shape. This exercise works the quadriceps (front thigh), hamstring (back thigh), and gluteal (butt) muscles. Do 15 to 20 repetitions per set.

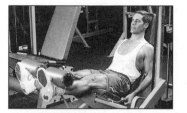

2. Leg extensions (page 319) using very light weight give an intensive workout to the quadriceps (front thigh) as well as the tendons and ligaments around the knee joint. This will further enhance mobility and flexibility. Do 15 to 20 repetitions per set.

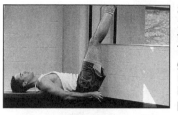

3. Leg raises (page 207) focus stress on the lower abdominals. This exercise will help give strength and flexibility to the midbody. Do 8 to 10 repetitions per set.

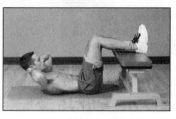

4. Doing **crunches** (page 200) with the legs supported on a bench or sofa will help add strength to the gut while providing good support for the lower back. Try for 15 to 20 repetitions per set.

This lifting workout is a well-rounded routine that starts with exercises for the chest and arms, then moves down to the hips and legs.

TUESDAY

1. The **dumbbell military press** (page 294) is a good compound lift that works the chest, shoulder, trapezius (upper back and neck), and triceps (back of upper arm) muscles. For building upper-body strength, it is among the best exercises that you can do. Try for 10 to 12 repetitions per set.

2. Standing lateral raises (page 298) focus on the shoulders, giving them the strength and flexibility needed to complete the workouts still to come. Try for 10 to 12 repetitions per set.

3. Alternating biceps curls (page 261) are a great way to develop upper-body strength. More specifically, they target the biceps (front of upper arm) and brachialis (outside of upper arm). Do 15 repetitions per arm.

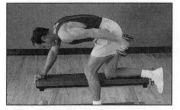

4. Dumbbell kickbacks (page 271) help keep the upper body in balance by working the often-neglected muscles. They hit not only the triceps (back of upper arm), but the shoulders as well. Do 10 repetitions with each arm per set.

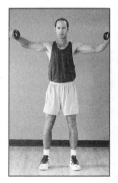
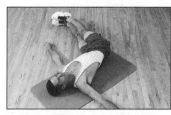

5. Doing **hip rolls** (page 218) is essential for a sedentary body. This exercise helps build flexibility in the hip joint, while strengthening the oblique (side) muscles. Do 10 repetitions on each side per set.

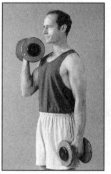
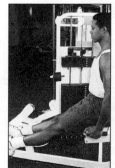

6. Toe presses (page 326) lend strength and flexibility to the calves as well as to the tendons and ligaments in the ankles. This is important for preventing injuries from running or walking, particularly for anyone who is out of shape. Do 20 to 25 repetitions per set.

The following workout will further improve his flexibility and balance, and add muscle mass.

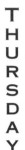

1. Stationary lunges with dumbbells (page 234) provide a rigorous workout to all the upper leg muscles. Begin with a 25-pound dumbbell in each hand, increasing the weight as the exercise gets easier. Do five to eight repetitions per leg per set.

2. The **inclined dumbbell press** (page 280) is a superb exercise that hits the chest, shoulders, and upper arms. It can dramatically improve upper-body strength. Do 8 to 10 repetitions per set.

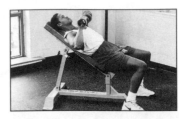

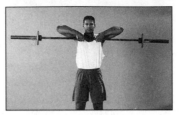

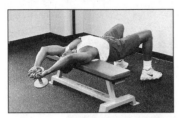

3. Bent-arm pullovers (page 284) work the triceps (back of upper arm), shoulders, and upper chest. It's one of the best exercises for building upper-body strength and flexibility. Do 8 to 10 repetitions per set.

4. A compound exercise, **upright rows** (page 296) work the trapezius (upper back and neck), shoulders, forearms, and upper arms. Start with the barbell empty, adding weight as it gets easier. Do 8 to 10 repetitions per set.

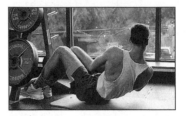

5. Oblique trunk rotations (page 209) home in on the oblique (side) muscles, developing all-important flexibility in the midsection. That's a part of the body that does a lot of twisting and turning in the course of an average day, not to mention during a workout. Do 20 to 25 repetitions per set.

On Fridays he will end the week with his most challenging workout yet, targeting the midsection, back, and legs. Cioroslan continues to stress increased mobility in order to build a firm foundation for further training.

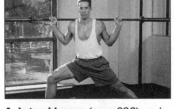

2. Good mornings (page 222) are recommended for working the lower back and legs. Anyone who is severely overweight is likely to be weak in both areas. Do 8 to 10 repetitions per set.

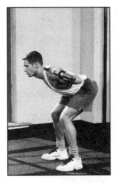

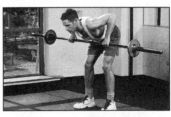

1. Lateral lunges (page 236) work the quadriceps (front thigh) and inner thigh muscles. This exercise is helpful both for strengthening the legs and increasing hip flexibility—key elements in building mobility. Try for four to six repetitions per side per set.

3. Wide-grip rows (page 220) work several major muscle groups, including the shoulders, upper arms, forearms, and latissimus dorsi (mid and lower back) muscles. Start with a moderate weight—perhaps 50 pounds—and increase gradually. Do 8 to 10 repetitions per set.

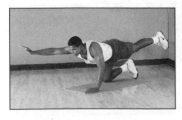

4. Opposite arm and leg raises (page 229) are designed to strengthen the lower back muscles as well as the upper legs and the hips. It is an excellent way to gain overall body stability. Do 15 repetitions per side per set.

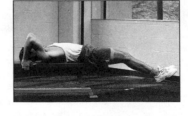

5. Double-leg scoops (page 215) help strengthen and condition the lower back, the lower abdominals, and the oblique (side) muscles. While this exercise can be done on the floor, doing it on a bench adds a substantial degree of difficulty. Try for 15 to 20 repetitions per set.

SCENARIO **7**: Getting Past the Pain

AGE: 39

WEIGHT: 165

HEALTH: He has always been athletic but with age has begun having minor joint stiffness in the neck, knees, back, and shoulders. This has made it impossible to feel truly strong when doing exercise or playing sports.

EXERCISE ROUTINE: Plays basketball at lunch once or twice a week. Attends judo classes three nights a week as he works toward a brown belt.

LIFESTYLE: A school teacher and single man, he has plenty of extra time and would be willing to devote an extra hour or 2 a week to exercise.

WEIGHT GOALS: Would like to maintain current weight.

FITNESS GOALS: To develop extra flexibility to reduce joint pain and expand his potential moves in the martial arts. Would also like to develop more speed and endurance, but without adding bulky muscle.

There is a basic principle in the world of conditioning called the principle of specificity.

"You have to train specifically for the outcome you want," says Ben F. Hurley, Ph.D., director of the Exercise Science Laboratory in the College of Health and Human Performance at the University of Maryland in College Park. "This person has a very specific set of goals related to the activities that he is involved in. What he needs to do is work not only the muscle groups involved in those activities but also the specific motions the muscles are called on to make when he participates in those activities."

He can afford to concentrate on such specific goals because he is in pretty good shape to begin with. This is the type of man that Dragomir Cioroslan, head coach of the U.S. Weightlifting Federation and the 1996 U.S. Olympic weightlifting team, loves to see walking into his gym. The clearer the objective, the clearer the path toward results,

and the easier it is to measure those results.

The joint stiffness may indicate a need for some work on flexibility, and he may benefit from a stretching regimen. Todd Edelson, a physical therapist in Montclair, New Jersey, and a former national weightlifting champion, says a lot of men make the mistake of thinking of stretching as a nuisance—a time-consuming activity that keeps them from getting right into the sports they enjoy playing. "Stretching at the age of 39 is considered a way of preventing injury, not of enhancing performance," he says, "and most men are more interested in performance. Indirectly, though, stretching is a performance-enhancing activity because if you injure yourself, you can't train, and that detracts from performance."

This man needs to spend 15 minutes stretching before each workout, including his basketball games, and 5 minutes stretching after, Edelson says. Since stretching cold muscles can injure them, he needs to warm up first with 5 to 10 minutes of light aerobic activity, such as riding a stationary bike, skipping rope, or jogging in place.

Cioroslan points out that weight training, by strengthening and invigorating the muscles, tendons, and ligaments that surround the joints, can help reduce stiffness, too. That will be one of the benefits of the workouts he's designed to address his other goals: developing speed and endurance.

The Workout

Having specific objectives doesn't necessarily mean that those objectives are in perfect agreement with one another. It's possible to train successfully for both speed and endurance, although not necessarily at the same time. For that reason, Cioroslan has designed two different workouts, one for each objective. He should perform each workout once a week, with a day or more between them. A third workout combining some of the exercises from each could also be added.

SPEED WORKOUT

The basic technique for developing speed is to lift a moderate amount of weight very fast. It's simple: You teach muscles to move quickly by moving them quickly. Cioroslan defines moderate weight as an amount that requires only about 50 to 55 percent of the lifter's maximum effort to lift the required number of repetitions. Since speed is the goal—rather than endurance over a sustained period of time—this man can take a leisurely 2 to 3 minutes to rest between sets, says Cioroslan. That will give his muscles plenty of time to recover and prepare themselves for the burst of explosive energy required in the next set.

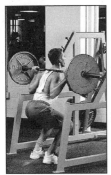

1. Doing **squats** with the barbell behind your neck (page 313) teaches the legs to move more quickly. And by working the tendons and ligaments around the knee, it will help relieve pain there. Do as many repetitions as possible in 10 seconds.

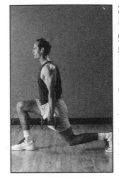

2. Walking lunges (page 321) are a great way to develop strength and flexibility in the lower body and legs. Doing this exercise often will improve reaction speed in particular. Do a minimum of 10 repetitions with each leg, moving as fast as possible.

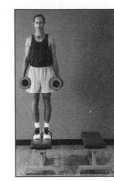

3. Bench lateral step-ups (page 323) also focus on leg strength and agility. It's a great exercise for boosting maneuverability on the court. Do a minimum of 10 for each side, moving as quickly as possible.

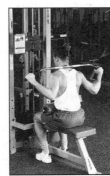

4. Lat pull-downs (page 219) are a great way to strengthen the latissimus dorsi (mid and lower back) muscles, which are essential in the martial arts for throwing an opponent. Try for 15 to 20 repetitions per set.

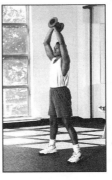

5. Dumbbell swings (page 227) work the hamstrings (back thigh), gluteal (butt), and erector spinae (lower back) muscles. These muscles come into play almost every time when lifting, bending, or running. Do 15 to 20 repetitions per set.

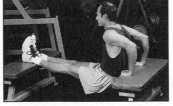

6. Parallel dips (page 272) are another way to target upper-body strength. They work the triceps (back of upper arm) and upper back and stabilize the shoulder joint, which will help relieve soreness. Do 15 to 20 repetitions per set.

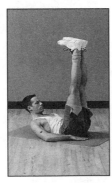

7. Straight-leg raises (page 202) are demanding to the abs and require holding the head up while lifting and lowering the legs. They are great for building strength and endurance in the abs, which is essential for the martial arts. Do 10 to 15 repetitions per set.

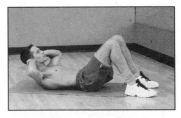

8. Curl-ups (page 199) are an advanced version of the classic abdominal crunch. They focus on the upper abdominals in particular. Do 25 to 30 repetitions per set.

ENDURANCE WORKOUT

The basic principle behind endurance training is to lift a slightly heavier weight load—about 65 to 70 percent of maximum capacity—as many times as possible, explains Cioroslan. Rest between sets should be about half what it was in the speed workout, only 1 to 2 minutes. The same goes for the time between exercises. The idea is to get the muscles used to responding to stress with a minimum of rest over a long period of time. A pretty basic concept, but it works.

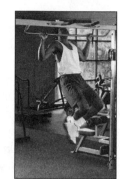

1. Chin-ups (page 225) are simple yet demanding. This classic exercise builds strength in the upper back and biceps (front of upper arm). Do 10 to 15 repetitions per set.

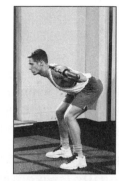

2. Good mornings (page 222) work both the lower back and the middle back, helping improve stability and performance in basketball and martial arts, among many other activities. Do 6 to 12 repetitions per set.

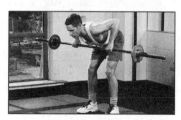

3. The **wide-grip row** (page 220) builds strength and endurance in the back, shoulders, forearms, and upper arms in addition to stretching the hamstrings (back thigh) and gluteals (butt). It also improves blood flow to the shoulders, which will help relieve soreness. Do 15 to 20 repetitions per set.

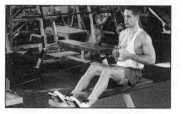

4. Seated rows (page 223) strengthen the muscles on both sides of the upper back and the biceps (front of upper arm). In addition, the movement provides good practice for grabbing and throwing opponents in judo. Do 20 to 30 repetitions per set.

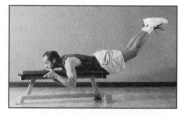

5. Reverse leg extensions (page 241) work three major muscle groups that are key to supporting the lower back: the hamstrings (back thigh), the gluteal (butt), and the erector spinae (lower back) muscles. All are important when it comes to movements like jumping, running, and lifting. Do 25 to 30 repetitions per set.

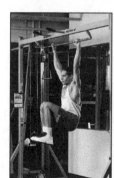

6. Hanging knee raises (page 205) are excellent for building strength and endurance in the lower abdominal muscles and in the hips. Do 10 to 15 repetitions per set.

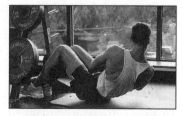

7. Doing a high number of **oblique trunk rotations** (page 209) will add endurance and improve conditioning in the oblique (side) abdominal muscles. Basketball, the martial arts, and other sports typically involve a lot of twisting and turning, movements that depend on the obliques. Do 40 to 50 repetitions per set.

SCENARIO 8: Developing a Healthy Back

AGE: 45

WEIGHT: 190

HEALTH: He had back surgery when he was in his early thirties, followed by a second operation 10 years later. His back is essentially recovered, although sciatic-nerve pain occasionally flares when doing vigorous lifting, bending, or running.

EXERCISE ROUTINE: Plays 18 holes of golf on weekends and occasionally (two or three times a month) plays a round of tennis. Works out regularly at the company gym, spending most of the time doing aerobics, with just a little lifting to tone chest and biceps.

LIFESTYLE: He is an insurance executive who works long hours. Most of his day is spent behind a desk, although he probably walks 2 to 3 miles a day checking on employees on the various floors.

WEIGHT GOALS: After the first surgery, he started developing a gut and never lost it. Would like to lose 20 to 30 pounds or at least 4 inches (from a 38 to a 34) from the waist.

FITNESS GOALS: He definitely would like to strengthen and stabilize his back for added strength and mobility. Reduce and firm up the midsection for added back support.

This man has a desk job, a back problem, a potbelly, and stress. How unusual.

In fact, this is probably one of the most common profiles in the industrialized world. On any given day, it is estimated that between 15 and 20 percent of American adults are suffering from back problems. A goodly proportion of those aching millions have desk jobs, and a lot them are overweight. And, hey, if you don't believe we have a problem with stress in this country, take a look at how people are behaving on the highways.

Actually, this man is coping with his back problem a lot better than most. "He should be proud of himself that he's had two surgeries and he's still engaged in that much physical activity," says Ted Wernimont, director of rehabilitation at the Spine Center at the University of Iowa in Iowa City. "He proves that you don't have to let back problems control your life."

Indeed, staying active is probably why he has minimized his back flare-ups as much as he has, says Wernimont. Staying in good physical condition is one of the best preventive measures known for avoiding back pain; research shows that staying in bed with a backache beyond four days generally makes it worse, not better. His busy lifestyle also suggests that he has a take-charge attitude, one that simply won't tolerate being slowed down by back pain.

So, he is already doing a lot of things right. That's not to say that there isn't room for improvement.

Remember the old football line about the best offense being a good defense? This man needs to think about that. He's not doing enough to defend himself against recurring back pain, even though he has been fairly lucky so far. "The first thing I would do is put this guy on a preventive program," says Todd Edelson, a physical therapist in Montclair, New Jersey, and a former national weightlifting champion.

He spends so much time sitting with his lower back flexed that he needs to balance that with movements that will extend or stretch his lower back, Edelson explains. At least once an hour, he should get up and walk around. He should push his chest out, pull his shoulders back, and, most important, he should maintain a natural curve in his lower back. While he is standing, he can put his hands on his lower back and buttocks and lean backward from his waist, Edelson suggests.

Such a program would make him more flexible, which would reduce the risk of injuries while playing golf or tennis and help counter the effects of sitting behind a desk most of the day.

He also may be in denial when it comes to stress. "He needs to recognize that a stress problem exists, first of all, and then take steps to deal with it," says Wernimont. "We know for certain that stress and pain go together."

The Workout

The first thing that he should do, says Dragomir Cioroslan, head coach of the U.S. Weightlifting Federation and the 1996 U.S. Olympic weightlifting team, is keep up his aerobics routine at the company gym. The following workout will supplement his aerobic workouts by targeting his midsection.

Exercises that combine a high number of repetitions with resistance, as these do, will help build muscle while simultaneously reducing fat. Cioroslan has also included four exercises at the beginning of the workout to help him maintain the tone he likes in his chest and biceps.

Since the goal of these workouts is building muscle (rather than endurance), he can rest for 2 to 3 minutes between sets. While he is resting, he should focus on relaxing his muscles as much as possible and taking slow, deep breaths, says Cioroslan. Teaching himself to take a meditative approach to training will pay dividends outside as well as inside the gym. His history of back trouble means that he needs to take special care to warm up slowly and thoroughly.

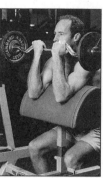

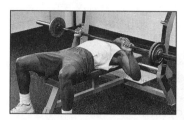

1. Bench presses (page 277) keep the upper body toned by working the chest, shoulder, and arm muscles. Maintaining upper-body strength provides the balanced conditioning necessary to avoid lower back problems. Do 8 to 12 repetitions per set.

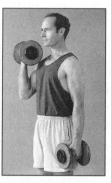

2. Preacher curls (page 258) provide an extremely rigorous workout, specifically targeting the biceps (front of upper arm). Do 8 to 12 repetitions per set.

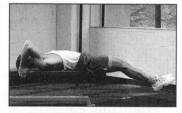

3. Alternating biceps curls (page 261) isolate the biceps (front of upper arm). By keeping the stress focused, they are a great way to add size and strength. Do 10 to 15 repetitions with each arm per set.

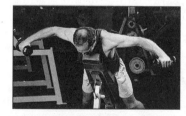

4. Lying lateral raises (page 301) target the shoulder muscles. Keeping the shoulders strong will aid in lifting, which further helps protect the lower back. Try for 8 to 10 repetitions per set.

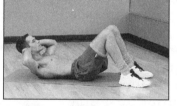

5. Curl-ups (page 199) are slightly more challenging than the standard crunch, effectively working the upper and middle abdominals as well as the hip flexor (front hip) muscles. Working the midbody is perhaps the best way to help prevent lower back problems. Try for 15 to 20 repetitions.

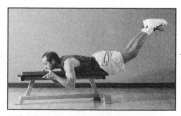

6. Double-leg scoops (page 215), which are more difficult than curl-ups, also work the lower abdominals and hip flexor (front hip) muscles. Do 15 to 20 repetitions per set.

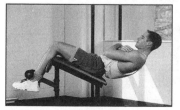

7. Roman chair sit-ups (page 204) add another level of intensity to abdominal workouts. This exercise targets the middle and upper abdominals. Do 20 repetitions per set.

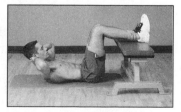

8. Raised-leg crunches (page 200) are a superb exercise for working the abdominals. Again, the goal is to reduce strain on the back by strengthening the front. Do 20 to 25 repetitions per set.

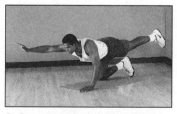

9. Opposite arm and leg raises (page 229) increase the strength of the back muscles as well as those of the trunk, butt, and upper legs. It's a relatively easy exercise that becomes more challenging when the number of reps is increased. Try for 15 to 20 repetitions per set.

10. Reverse leg extensions (page 241) strengthen and stabilize the hamstrings (back thigh), gluteal (butt), and lower back muscles. Strengthening these muscles will help keep the lower back stable and pain-free. Do 15 to 20 repetitions per set.

SCENARIO 9: Driving Concerns

AGE: 32

WEIGHT: 200

HEALTH: A smoker, he has a cough that's getting heavier, and he often gets colds. Otherwise, he is in good shape.

EXERCISE ROUTINE: For most of the past year, he has worked out three times a week. His workouts consist primarily of lifting free weights, concentrating on the chest and arms.

LIFESTYLE: He was recently laid off from his job as a taxi driver. Since he worked the night shift for years, his "morning" doesn't start until afternoon, and he doesn't get to sleep until about 4:00 A.M.

WEIGHT GOALS: He has put on about 15 pounds since getting laid off. Would like to lose the extra padding and get down to 180 to 185.

FITNESS GOALS: Can't afford to join a gym, so he needs a workout program that can be done at home. He would like to toughen up his arms and chest in addition to losing weight.

On just about anyone's list of the world's unhealthiest jobs, cab driver would probably make the cut. Especially a cab driver on the night shift who smokes about two packs a day. But despite having two strikes against him, this guy isn't too much the worse for wear. He is more worried about his pocketbook than his health. In today's job market, who can blame him?

Obviously, he has to quit smoking. There's simply no way to get into shape and still maintain a two-pack-a-day habit, says John Duncan, Ph.D., professor of clinical research at Texas Woman's University in Denton. Once he has kicked the habit, he can get serious about tackling an all-over fitness plan.

Sitting behind a steering wheel 8 hours a day doesn't do much for anyone's flexibility, which is why Todd Edelson, a physical therapist in Montclair, New Jersey, strongly suggests that he start a stretching program to get his unused joints moving again.

Jogging or some other aerobic activity would be an excellent idea, Edelson adds. Since this man is out of shape to begin with, he recommends that he start with a 20-minute walk each day, aiming to gradually get his heart pumping at about 60 percent of his capacity. At that rate he should be able to feel the exertion but not be so out of breath that he can't talk. Ex–cab drivers—or anyone with a sedentary job and a history of smoking who is starting an exercise program—need to treat their hearts very gently for a while, says Edelson.

Eventually, of course, he will need to increase his aerobic time if he hopes to lose some weight. Ben F. Hurley, Ph.D., director of the Exercise Science Laboratory in the College of Health and Human Performance at the University of Maryland in College Park, says that he should gradually increase his walk time, going from a minimum of 20 minutes up to, say, 45 minutes' worth of exercise.

The Workout

Since this man wants to lose 15 pounds (and his smoking habit), aerobic conditioning has to be his first priority. That certainly fits his budget constraints, since you don't have to pay a membership fee to walk or jog around the block.

Adding strength to his arms and chest in addition to the weight loss should be simple enough, especially since he has been doing some upper-body work already, says Dragomir Cioroslan, head coach of the U.S. Weightlifting Federation and the 1996 U.S. Olympic weightlifting team. He doesn't even have to join a gym, Cioroslan adds. All he really needs is a chin-up bar that can be wedged into a door frame, a couple of sturdy chairs, and a pair of 15-pound dumbbells. If his finances are too pinched to accommodate the dumbbells, he can substitute a couple of volumes of an encyclopedia or any other hefty but equally balanced objects.

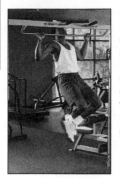

1. Chin-ups (page 225) put the focus on the muscle opposite the triceps, the biceps (front of upper arm). This is a difficult exercise, so start with a low number of repetitions and build gradually. Try for 6 to 10 repetitions.

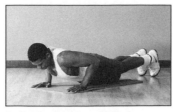

2. Push-ups (page 286) are perhaps the simplest exercise for building the arms and chest, and one of the most effective. Doing up to 40 per set will develop upper-body toughness.

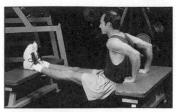

3. Parallel dips (page 272) are difficult but effective, working the triceps (back of upper arm) and keeping the latissimus dorsi (mid and lower back) muscles under constant tension. Start with 8 to 10 repetitions per set, gradually working up to 25 per set.

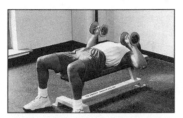

4. Dumbbell bench presses (page 278) work both the triceps (back of upper arm) and the upper chest. Do 15 to 20 repetitions per set.

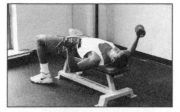

5. Dumbbell flies (page 282) address the chest muscles, specifically the pectoralis major and pectoralis minor. It's an excellent exercise for building chest size and strength. Do 15 to 20 repetitions per set.

6. Alternating biceps curls (page 261) are like a laser beam, focusing the stress totally and intensely on the biceps (front of upper arm). Try for 15 repetitions per set with each arm.

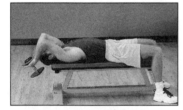

7. Lying triceps extensions (page 267) are probably the single most effective exercise for the triceps (back of upper arm) muscles. Doing these regularly will quickly build strength and mass in the upper arm. Try to do 10 to 15 repetitions per set.

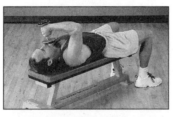

8. Performing **lying cross-shoulder triceps extensions** (page 268) will hit the muscle from a different angle than working both arms at the same time, as when doing lying triceps extensions. Doing these two exercises back-to-back will help prevent training plateaus. Try for 10 to 15 repetitions per set.

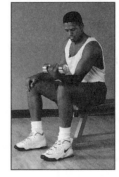

9. Forearm curls (page 273) do a great job hitting the inner and outer sides of the forearms. Do 15 to 20 repetitions per set.

PART VI

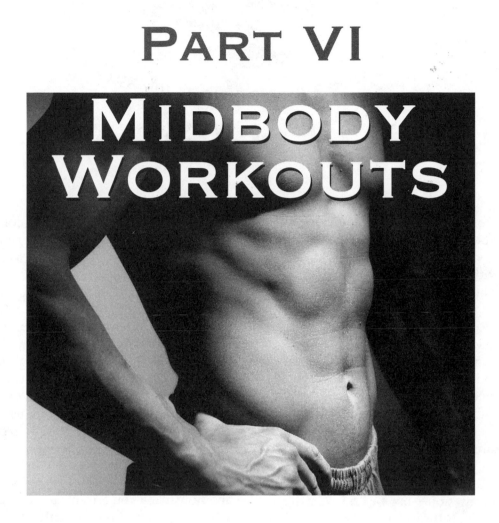

MIDBODY
WORKOUTS

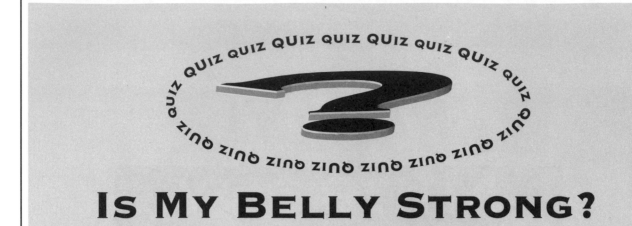

IS MY BELLY STRONG?

Harry Houdini, the great escape artist, was very proud of his abdominal muscles and regularly bragged about their ability to withstand direct hits without damage. One day in 1926, he made that boast once too often.

According to a *Jerusalem Post* report, while Houdini was recovering from a broken ankle, a student decided to test his claim of abdominal strength—immediately and without warning. The blow is thought to have ruptured his appendix. Houdini died soon after on Halloween.

Clearly, it may have been the surprise of the punch rather than any lack of conditioning that laid Houdini low. He knew perfectly well how strong his abs were—it was his business to know. Most of us, of course, don't have Houdini's professional motivation—but we do have flabby reflections in the bathroom mirror to remind us that our midsections could use some work.

How much distance is there between the great Houdini's abs and yours? Take this quiz to find out.

1. How many sit-ups can I do?

This is a trick question. You probably shouldn't be doing sit-ups at all. They can be bad for your back and neck. They don't do that much for your belly either. "There are far too many people doing sit-ups like they did in high school," says Harvey Newton, a certified strength and conditioning specialist and the executive director of the National Strength and Conditioning Association in Colorado Springs, Colorado.

The point here is that if you're doing a lot of sit-ups, you're not doing a lot of crunches, which means that your belly isn't as strong as it could be.

"When you raise your torso with a sit-up, you're exercising your abdominal muscles, but much of the movement is accomplished by the use of the hip flexors," Newton says. While the hip flexors are important for things like walking and doing the twist, they're not the muscles you're going to be showing off at the beach. Crunches, on the other hand, are usually more effective because they put less strain on the back while fully isolating the abdominal muscles.

2. How many crunches can I do?

Since crunches are *the* exercise for working the abs, how many you are able to do in a minute is a good measure of the muscular endurance of your abs.

If you're between 26 and 35 years old and can do more than 45 crunches a minute, you're in excellent shape, says Wayne Westcott, Ph.D., national strength-training consultant for the YMCA, the American Council on Exercise, and the National Academy of Sports Medicine.

In the 36-to-45 age group, anything more than 40 per minute is very good indeed, Dr. Westcott says. If you're between the ages of 46 and 55, you should be able to do more than 35 crunches a minute. Anyone over 56 who can do more than 30 crunches per minute is in stellar shape. Less than 15 is a sign that you're resting on your laurels.

3. How is my back?

Almost every man will experience lower back pain at some point in his life. There are a lot of suspected reasons for that: Having weak abs is one of them. "If your abdominals and lower back muscles are in good shape, you not only decrease the risk of developing lower back pain but you also increase the time it takes you to recover if you do develop pain there," says Gary Hunter, Ph.D., professor of exercise physiology at the University of Alabama at Birmingham.

4. Have I had a hernia?

As with lower back pain, weak abdominal muscles can predispose you to developing an abdominal hernia, in which your insides protrude through a tear in the abdominal wall. Once you've had a hernia, you'll never want another. Keeping your gut in shape is a good way to help ensure that your insides stay where they should.

5. How many leg raises can I do?

There is a simple test for determining abdominal strength—particularly strength in the upper abdominal muscles, says Dragomir Cioroslan, head coach of the U.S. Weightlifting Federation and the 1996 U.S. Olympic weightlifting team.

Lie on your back on a bench, gripping the corners of the bench near your hips. Keep your legs straight and parallel to the floor. Slowly raise your legs to a 45-degree angle. Pause for a moment, then slowly lower them until they are parallel to the floor again. "If you can do that 10 to 12 times, your upper abdominals are in moderately good shape," Cioroslan says. "To be in really good shape, you should be able to do 20 of these or more."

6. How many leg lifts can I do?

Here's another one of Cioroslan's favorites, which measures the strength of the lower abs.

Put two sturdy, well-balanced chairs back-to-back, shoulder-width apart, and lift yourself off the ground with one hand on each chair, arms locked. Keeping your legs straight, slowly raise them in front of you until they are parallel to the

ground, then return. "If you can raise and lower your legs between 8 and 10 times, your lower abdominals are in pretty good shape. If you can raise and lower your legs 15 to 20 times, they're in very good shape," Cioroslan says.

7. Can I pass Doug's Test?

This four-part test of belly strength comes from Doug Lentz, a certified strength and conditioning specialist and the Pennsylvania state director of the National Strength and Conditioning Association. In all four parts you start by lying on your back on a mat with your knees up against your chest, keeping your back flat—no arching allowed.

- Lower one leg slowly to the floor, keeping it slightly bent, until the heel touches the mat. Then bring it back to your chest, and repeat with the other leg. If you can't do this 10 times with each leg without too much trouble, your belly needs work. But if you can do three sets of 10 repetitions, then you can move on to the next part.

- Lower one leg slowly to the floor, keeping it slightly bent. Stop before the heel touches the mat and slowly straighten the leg until it's parallel to (and above) the floor. Hold for a second, then bend the leg and bring your knee back to your chest. If you can do three sets of 10 repetitions, your gut is in good shape.

- This part is identical to the first one, except you're lowering both legs to the floor at the same time, keeping them slightly bent, until your heels touch the mat. Then bring your knees back to your chest. Again, if you can do three sets of 10 repetitions, you're in great shape. Now try part four.

- This part is identical to the second one, except you're lowering both legs to the mat, stopping before the heels touch the mat, and then straightening both legs until they're parallel to the mat. Hold for a second, then bend the legs and bring your knees back to your chest. If you can do three sets of 10 repetitions without arching your back, your abs are in excellent shape.

CRUNCHES AND SIT-UPS
THE BEST EXERCISE IS OFTEN THE SIMPLEST

Granted, all men are different, but there are a few desires—having lots of money, say, or the love of a beautiful woman—that many of us have in common. Next on almost any man's wish list is a treasure more elusive than liquidity and love combined: the six-pack.

We're not talking about beer. We're talking about the dream gut—a midsection in such incredible condition that it looks like beer cans lined side by side beneath your skin.

"That six-pack look is largely a function of two things," says Frank Eksten, strength coordinator in the Department of Athletics and visiting lecturer in kinesiology at Indiana University in Bloomington, "abdominal conditioning and the amount of body fat you have. You have to get your proportion of body fat pretty low to get that look. The older you are, the more difficult that gets because we tend to retain fat as we get older. Also, some people will find it harder than others to get there because of their genetic makeup. But anything's possible. It depends on how hard you're willing to work for it."

The Fat Has to Go

If you're going to achieve that washboard look, you have to lose the extra weight that you're carrying there. But don't kid yourself. It's not enough to lose only the weight around your middle. Why? Because you can't do it. When you exercise, fat is burned globally, not locally. That's why spot reducing—trying to lose weight in one part of your body by intensely working that part—doesn't work. If it did, everybody who chews gum would have a slim face.

"We see people doing all kinds of contortions thinking that they can spot-reduce, and that's just not possible," says Harvey Newton, a certified strength and conditioning specialist and the executive director of the National Strength and Conditioning Association in Colorado Springs, Colorado. "You'll build your ab muscles, but you won't take away the fat."

This isn't to say that you shouldn't be working the abdominal muscles. You should. The abs are designed to contain your organs like a woven basket. The tighter those muscles are wrapped, the more efficiently they keep your insides from bulging out, says Willibald Nagler, M.D., physiatrist-in-chief at New York Hospital–Cornell Medical Center in New York City.

Yet the "corset effect" caused by tight abs only reins in visceral fat, the fat that lies between your muscles and the organs beneath. It doesn't do much for holding in subcutaneous fat, the fat that lies above the muscles and beneath the skin.

There's only one way to burn belly fat. You have to burn more calories than you take in. The two most effective ways of accomplishing this are diet—eating less fat and more fruits, vegetables, beans, and whole grains—and aerobic exercise.

At the same time, however, you should be working your abs. The stronger you make them, the more conspicuous they will become. And once you start stripping away fat from your midsection, their size and shape will become gratifyingly apparent.

Requiem for the Sit-Up

If you're like most men of a certain age, you have probably done your share of sit-ups. Coaches used to like them. They were painful, so presumably they did some good. They were also exhausting, making them an excellent choice for crowd control.

There are two problems with sit-ups. First, they're extremely hard on the neck and back. Second, they work the hip flexor muscles as much as they do the abdominals. In other words, when your goal is to build a hard gut with maximum efficiency, sit-ups don't cut it.

Better by far is the crunch. Crunches are to belly exercises what the guitar is to rock 'n' roll. It's *the* exercise for building a hard gut; everything else is complementary. Unlike sit-ups, crunches take dead aim at the rectus abdominis, the main abdominal muscle that covers the front of the stomach area. More specifically, crunches work the three sections that make up this large muscle, creating the ridges that define the six-pack. A few crunches done properly, some experts say, are worth many more sit-ups. Here's how to do them right.

FOCUS ON FORM. It's as easy to do a sloppy crunch as it is a sloppy sit-up—and with similarly diluted effects. To get the most work from each crunch, you have to maintain perfect form. (To see crunches in action, turn to straight-leg crunches on page 198.) The main point is this: Your shoulder blades should never come more than 4 to 6 inches off the floor. Anything more than that de-

Less Bang for the Buck

You can't spend an hour channel surfing without encountering commercials hawking an endless variety of abdominal machines like the Abworks and AB Sculptor. It's only a matter of time before Fred Flintstone comes on urging us to buy the Abba Dabba Do.

Each of these gadgets is promised to give you the washboard abs of your dreams, and, boy, are people buying. Last year, an estimated 2.75 million ab machines were sold in the United States, racking up about $145 million in sales, according to the New York Times.

Are they worth the money?

Not really, says Marjorie Albohm, a certified athletic trainer and director of sports medicine at Kendrick Memorial Hospital in Mooresville, Indiana. "The ads are really persuasive," she says. "They make people think that exercise will be easier with these machines, which isn't true."

The machines aren't entirely without value, she adds. For example, some guide your body through the same motions that you would use when doing an abdominal crunch. "A lot of people don't know what the correct movements are," she says. "But you can figure the crunch out for yourself without spending a hundred dollars."

creases the benefits. And don't arch your lower back, since that takes strain off your midsection, says Eksten.

BREATHE EASY. Crunches exert a lot of pressure on your midsection—not only on the muscles but also inside your torso. Holding your breath while crunching puts extra pressure on the abdomen, which can lead to hernias, says Dr. Nagler. To be safe and to maintain more control, be sure to breathe in on the way down and exhale on the way up, he says.

STAY IN CONTROL. Jerking yourself upward makes crunches easier. It also makes them less effective. The less you rely on momentum, the more stress you put on the abdominal muscles. Raise your shoulders smoothly and slowly. Try for 10 seconds going up and 10 seconds coming down, says Eksten. Experts say "try" because crunches are tough, and doing them slowly creates a major burn. Enjoy it. That burn is what tells you that your abdominals are getting fit.

EASE INTO THEM. Crunches are hard work. Trying to do too many will make you sore, not fit. Marjorie Albohm, a certified athletic trainer and director of sports medicine at Kendrick Memorial Hospital in Mooresville, Indiana, recommends starting with three sets of 10 crunches, resting 15 to 30 seconds between sets. When you can do this for three workouts in a row, gradually increase the number.

UP THE ANTE. Like any muscle group, the abs need to be consistently challenged in order to improve. Adding more crunches isn't always the answer. "If your goal is toning your midsection, at some point—more than 50 crunches, for example—you reach a point of diminishing returns," Albohm says. "You need to make each crunch harder rather than doing more."

One way to make crunches more intense is to hold a weight plate or dumbbell on your chest. Albohm recommends starting with a 3-pound dumbbell and building gradually from there. Or you can do crunches on an inclined board, in which case gravity, rather than weights, provides the resistance.

Oblique Observations

While you have to work the abs to bring your gut into relief, you don't want to neglect the oblique (love handle) muscles, which run along each side of your torso.

Once again, while there are a number of specific exercises (including crunches) for working these muscles, you also need a generalized approach. "Losing fat from your sides isn't different from losing fat anywhere else," says Wayne Westcott, Ph.D., national strength-training consultant for the YMCA, the American Council on Exercise, and the National Academy of Sports Medicine. "What you need is an aerobic workout that will burn off fat and some strength exercises to tone and shape the muscles that lie underneath."

One point to consider is that when you work a muscle—any muscle—it gets larger, not smaller. If you're seriously working your obliques, don't be surprised when your waist gets larger. Of course, it will be a thicker waist in better condition, and that's good. What you really want to lose is the fat, and working the obliques will help.

WHAT TO BE CAREFUL OF
ABS ARE TOUGH, NOT INVINCIBLE

Abdominal workouts are as safe and simple as it's possible to get. That said, they aren't entirely without risk. Even if you don't strain your gut, you can injure other parts of your body. In addition, since the abs consist of six separate muscles, it's important to hit each of these muscles equally. Otherwise, you won't get the strength—or the washboard look—you're trying for.

To get a well-balanced workout without getting hurt, here is what experts advise.

WATCH YOUR BACK. The lower back is definitely the weak link of the midbody. Even if you're doing crunches instead of the old-fashioned (and back-wrenching) sit-ups, your lower back still is vulnerable, particularly in the early stages.

"Beginners who don't have abdominal strength will typically use their backs when they're trying to do crunches," says Marjorie Albohm, a certified athletic trainer and director of sports medicine at Kendrick Memorial Hospital in Mooresville, Indiana. Using your back not only makes crunches less effective but it also puts strain where you want it least. This is doubly true when you're doing harder crunch variations, such as using an inclined board or holding a dumbbell on your chest.

The key, Albohm says, is never to let your back arch. "By keeping a flat back during your abdominal workouts, you stabilize the back muscles," she says.

The next time you're doing crunches, put your feet up on a couch. That will solidly push your lower back down flat—exactly the position you want it to be in. Then in the future, whether you're doing crunches on the floor or on an inclined board, use that feeling as a frame of reference, Albohm suggests.

MIX THEM UP. Even though the crunch is a superb abdominal exercise, it mostly works the upper abdominal region. "You need to do variations on the crunch that involve other parts of the midsection," Albohm says.

To hit the lower abdominal muscles, for example, you should be doing hanging knee raises (see page 205) as well as basic crunches. To work the oblique (side) muscles, twisting crunches (see page 208) are the way to go.

A variety of crunches does more than provide a well-rounded workout. It also works the abdominal muscles from many different angles, which helps prevent plateaus, those frustrating stretches of time when your workout progress essentially stops.

ALLOW FOR REST. You may have heard that abdominal muscles don't need time to recover the way other muscles do. Indeed, some trainers advise cramming several strenuous ab workouts into a single day. Don't buy it.

"The abdominals need as much recovery time as any other muscle," says Mike Stone, Ph.D., professor of exercise science at Appalachian State University in Boone, North Carolina.

Straight-Leg Crunches

RATING: MODERATELY DIFFICULT

The crunch has eclipsed the sit-up as the most widely recommended exercise for the abs. The reason: Crunches put less strain on your back than sit-ups, and at the same time they do a good job of isolating the upper and lower abdominal muscles.

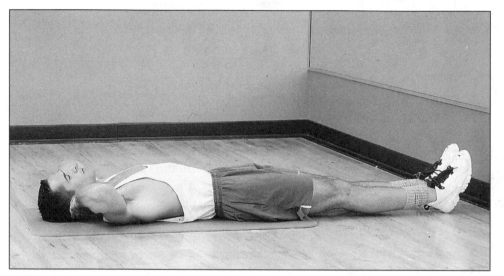

Lie flat on your back, legs extended, knees unlocked. Cup your hands behind your ears, elbows out.

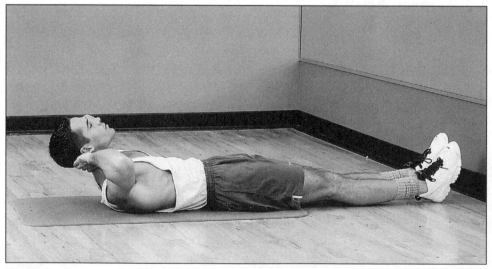

Keeping your lower back in contact with the floor, raise your upper torso a couple of inches off the ground. Look up as you lift your head, neck, and shoulders off the floor. Hold for a second, then lower to the starting position. Immediately begin your next crunch without relaxing in between.

DO IT BETTER

- Avoid pulling your head with your hands, since this can cause injury to the neck or upper back.
- Exhale completely as you crunch. This will help the abdominal muscles contract fully.
- Do your crunches on a mat or carpeted area to lend comfort to your spine and lower back.
- Keep your knees unlocked to prevent unnecessary stress on the knee joints and ligaments.
- To decrease difficulty, cross your hands over your chest.
- To gain additional burn, hold the contraction for 2 to 4 seconds before returning to the starting position.

Curl-Ups

RATING: MODERATELY DIFFICULT

Slightly more difficult than a crunch but safer than a sit-up, the curl-up involves curling your torso into your body (as opposed to a crunch, in which you're pushing your upper body straight up). You may find this bent-knee version easier than the straight-leg variety, since bringing your knees up naturally pulls your lower back to the floor. Your abdominal muscles—the upper, lower, and oblique (side)—all play a part in the curling motion.

DO IT BETTER

• Keep your knees in line with your feet to reduce unnecessary strain on the quadriceps and inner thighs.
• Contract the oblique abdominal muscles as you get closer to the top. The obliques allow you to curl your torso into your knees instead of merely raising your upper body off the floor.
• Avoid pulling your head with your hands, since this can cause injury to the neck or upper back.
• Keep your lower back pressed to the floor to decrease the risk of muscle strain.
• To decrease difficulty, cross your hands over your chest.
• Another way to increase difficulty is to hold each curl-up at the top for a count of two.

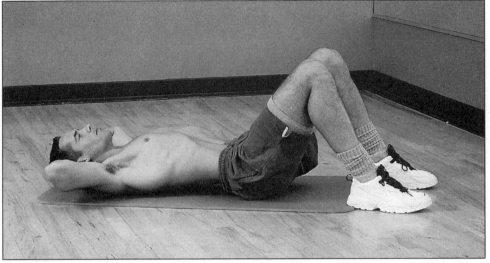

Lie flat on your back with your hands cupped behind your ears, elbows out. Bend your knees at about a 45-degree angle. Place your feet shoulder-width apart and about 6 inches from your butt.

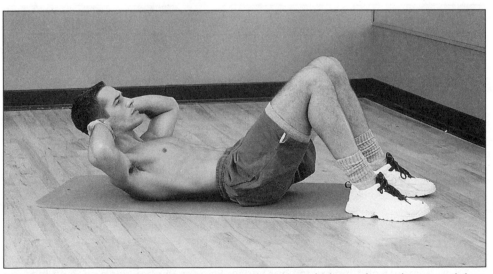

Keeping your lower body stable, curl your upper torso in toward your knees, raising your shoulder blades as high off the ground as you can get them. Move your torso all the way up in a count of two. Concentrate on the contraction of the abdominal muscles. Then count to two again as you return to the starting position. Finish your set without resting between repetitions.

Raised-Leg Crunches

RATING: MODERATELY DIFFICULT

A sensational set of abs is sometimes called a six-pack because there are six distinguishable abdominal muscles. Getting a six-pack begins with the upper abs, which are usually the first to develop fully. This exercise isolates the upper abs—the top four abdominal muscles.

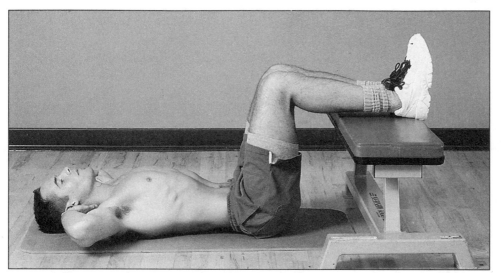

Lie on your back with your knees bent and your feet up on a bench or chair. Your thighs should be perpendicular to the floor and your hands cupped behind your ears, elbows out.

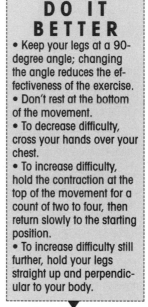

DO IT BETTER

• Keep your legs at a 90-degree angle; changing the angle reduces the effectiveness of the exercise.
• Don't rest at the bottom of the movement.
• To decrease difficulty, cross your hands over your chest.
• To increase difficulty, hold the contraction at the top of the movement for a count of two to four, then return slowly to the starting position.
• To increase difficulty still further, hold your legs straight up and perpendicular to your body.

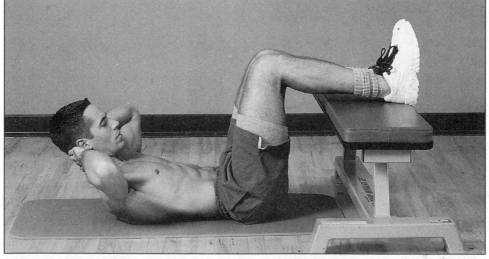

Pull your torso up and in toward your knees, lifting your shoulder blades off the floor for a second. Then lower to the starting position and repeat the movement.

Side Crunches
RATING: MODERATELY DIFFICULT

Also known as oblique crunches, side crunches work the external and internal obliques, muscles that run along the sides of the upper and lower abdominal muscles. Strong obliques do more than make you look good; they can also add power to your golf swing.

DO IT BETTER

• To increase difficulty, hold each crunch at the top for a count of two.
• Concentrate on tensing the oblique muscles throughout the entire movement, up and down, to increase the effects of the exercise.
• Avoid pulling your head with your hands, which could cause injury to the neck or upper back.
• For a very difficult oblique workout, do this exercise on an inclined sit-up board.

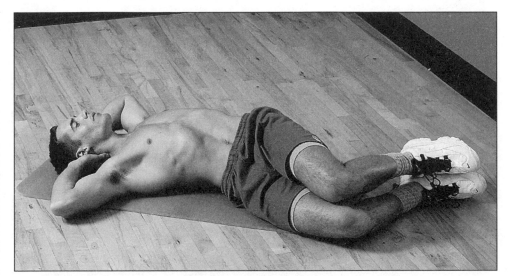

Lie flat on your back with your hands cupped behind your ears, elbows out. With your knees bent at a 45-degree angle, let your legs fall as far as they can to your right side. Your upper body should remain flat on the floor.

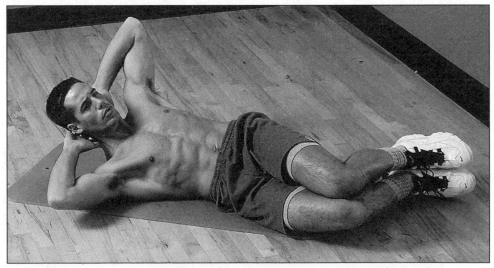

Trying to keep your shoulders parallel to the floor, lift your upper body until the shoulder blades clear the ground. Hold the crunch for a second, then lower to the starting position. Complete one set on your right side, then switch to the left.

Straight-Leg Raises

RATING: DIFFICULT

By raising your legs you are contracting, or shortening, the abdominal muscles and producing muscle tension. Lowering the legs creates an eccentric action—that is, it allows the muscles to lengthen while still remaining tense. To vigorously work the lower abs, which originate in the pelvic area, it's important to maintain the tension throughout the exercise.

Lie on your back on the floor with your hands under your hips, palms down. Press your lower back to the floor. Hold your head up, bringing your chin into your chest, with your shoulder blades off the floor. Extend your legs, knees unlocked and feet flexed, keeping your heels about an inch off the floor.

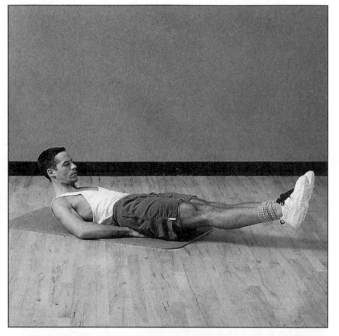

DO IT BETTER

• Keeping your lower back pressed to the floor will reduce the risk of injury to this area of your body.
• Keep your knees slightly bent to prevent injury to the ligaments and joints.
• Do not allow your feet to touch the floor until the end of the set.
• To decrease difficulty, raise each leg separately instead of both legs together.
• To increase difficulty, do this exercise on an inclined board.
• To further increase difficulty, do this exercise holding a basketball or medicine ball between your feet.

Raise your legs until they are perpendicular to your body—or at least as perpendicular as you can get them. Lower them slowly, to a count of two, keeping control of the downward motion. Repeat for your next rep.

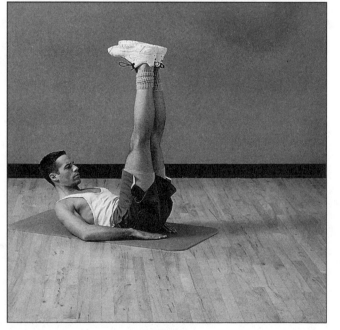

Hip Raises

RATING: VERY DIFFICULT

For runners particularly, hip raises are ideal because they will help increase your range of motion, promoting a longer stride. This exercise works the lower abs, the gluteal (butt) muscles, and the hip flexor (front hip) muscles.

DO IT BETTER

- Make the abs do the work. Kicking with the legs to gain momentum reduces the effectiveness of the exercise.
- Use your hands for balance, not to push your hips up.
- To decrease difficulty, do this exercise with your knees bent, but still keep your feet off the floor.

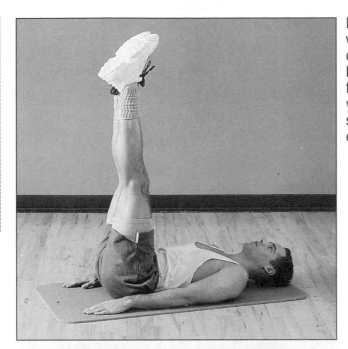

Lie flat on your back with your legs up in the air. Your knees should be unlocked and your toes pointed. Place your hands at your sides with the palms down.

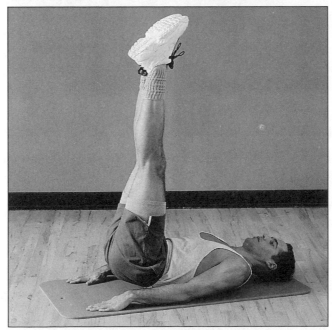

Using your lower abs and shifting your weight toward your shoulders, lift your hips off the floor. Keep your legs in a vertical position throughout the exercise. Hold for a second, then slowly return to the starting position.

Roman Chair Sit-Ups

RATING: DIFFICULT

The Roman chair offers a superb and all-encompassing midbody workout. Roman chair sit-ups are ideal for strengthening and molding the upper, lower, and oblique (side) abdominal muscles as well as the lower back.

Sit on the Roman chair (a slanted sit-up board with feet-support pads will also work). Sit with the tops of your feet secured under the pads with your torso at a 90-degree angle to your thighs. Place your hands across your chest.

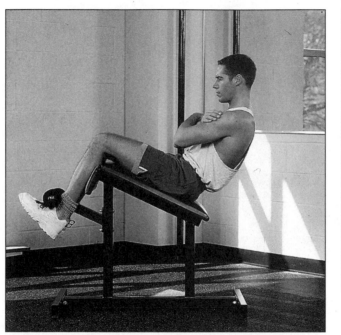

DO IT BETTER

• For maximum effectiveness, do not return all the way to the upward position between repetitions; stopping slightly short will keep the muscles tense and continually working.
• Keep the movement fluid and controlled. Bouncing at the bottom of the movement may cause back injury.
• To prevent injury to the lower back and abdominal area, do not allow your torso to move below the level of your hips.

Keeping your back straight, lower your torso until you feel tension in the abdominal muscles. Raise your body back to the starting position and immediately begin your next rep.

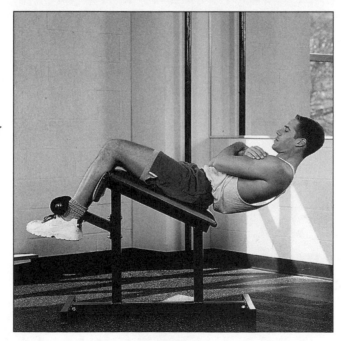

Hanging Knee Raises
RATING: DIFFICULT

This multipurpose exercise strengthens the upper, lower, and oblique (side) abdominal muscles as well as the hip flexor (front hip) muscles. In addition, you get a great stretch for your back and shoulders. You'll need a strong grip—or at least a pair of lifting gloves or a wrist strap—to prolong the hang time.

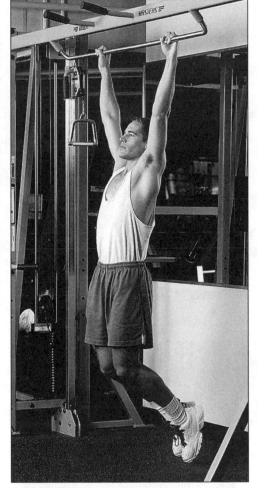

Hang from a bar with your legs extended.

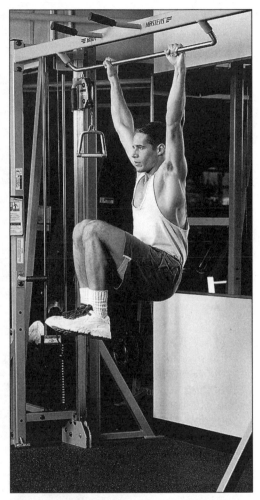

Using your lower abs, bend your knees and raise them as high as you can in a smooth, controlled movement. Your hips will naturally move forward slightly, but don't let the momentum swing your body.

Rowing Crunches

RATING: MODERATELY DIFFICULT

Although the movements used in this exercise are similar to those used in rowing, they have little impact on the back, arms, or legs. This exercise is for the abs only—upper, lower, and oblique (side) muscles.

Sit on a bench with your knees bent and your feet flat on the floor. Grasp the sides of the bench for support and lean back to about a 45-degree angle. Keeping your knees slightly bent, extend your legs and raise them a few inches off the floor.

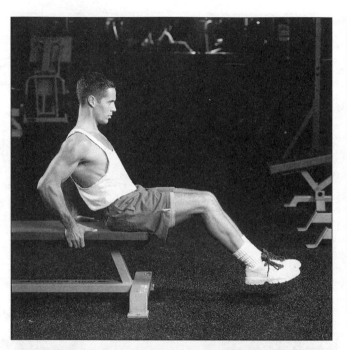

Pull your knees into your chest while bringing your upper body to an upright position. Hold for a second, then simultaneously return your upper body and legs to the starting position.

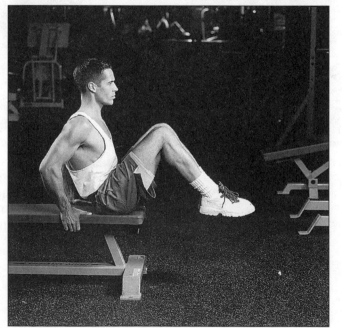

Leg Raises

RATING: MODERATELY DIFFICULT

This intense exercise works the upper, lower, and oblique (side) abdominal muscles. Begin this exercise with your lower back off the bench, slightly arched. As you raise your legs, your lower back presses to the bench.

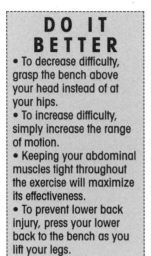

DO IT BETTER

- To decrease difficulty, grasp the bench above your head instead of at your hips.
- To increase difficulty, simply increase the range of motion.
- Keeping your abdominal muscles tight throughout the exercise will maximize its effectiveness.
- To prevent lower back injury, press your lower back to the bench as you lift your legs.

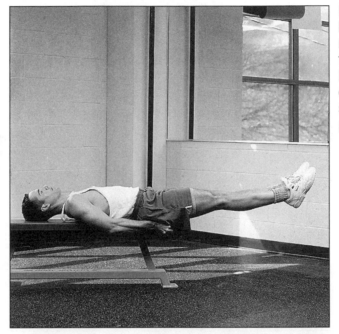

Lie on your back on a bench with your hips near the edge. Grasp the corners of the bench by your hips and extend your legs straight out, toes pointed.

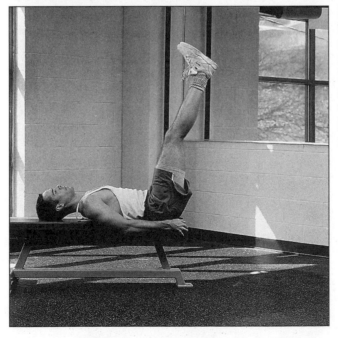

Keep your legs together, knees unlocked, and slowly raise them to vertical. Lower your legs in a controlled motion until your body is completely horizontal. Repeat the motion without resting.

Twisting Crunches
RATING: MODERATELY DIFFICULT

These crunches thoroughly work the oblique (side) abdominal muscles and the upper and lower abs. Done regularly, they may help your waist become smaller, which helps your upper body appear larger.

Lie on your back on the floor with your hands cupped behind your ears, elbows out. Cross your ankles, knees slightly bent, and raise your legs until your thighs are perpendicular to your body.

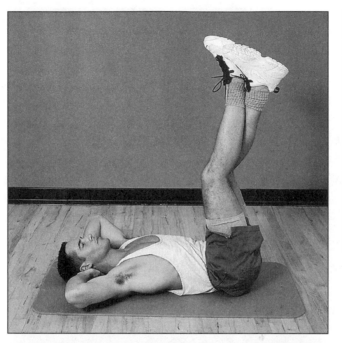

DO IT BETTER
• To maximize muscle burn, hold each contraction for a count of two.
• Avoid pulling your head with your hands, which could cause injury to your neck or upper back.
• To decrease difficulty, cross your hands over your chest. Or do the same motions while keeping your knees bent and your feet flat on the floor, shoulder-width apart.

Bring your left shoulder off the ground as you cross your left elbow over to your right knee. Return to the starting position and duplicate these movements beginning with the right shoulder, crossing your right elbow over to your left knee. Continue to alternate sides until you have completed the set.

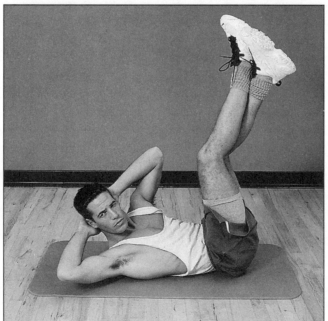

Oblique Trunk Rotations

RATING: DIFFICULT

Many "twisting" sports like golf, basketball, and tennis require intense rotations of the trunk. The muscles involved in twisting movements are the oblique (side) abdominals as well as the upper and lower abs. When doing this exercise, you should feel tension in all these muscles throughout the entire range of motion.

DO IT BETTER

- To reduce stress on your lower back, eliminate the full rotation. From the same starting position, raise your torso up to the right, bring it back to the starting position, then raise to the left for one repetition.
- To increase difficulty, cup your hands behind your ears, elbows out, while doing this exercise.
- To increase difficulty still more, hold a weight plate at the middle of your torso.

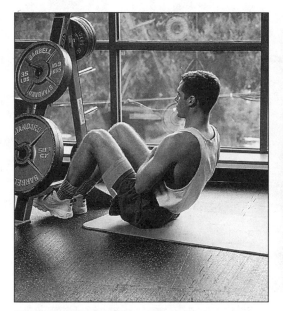

Sit on the floor, hands crossed over your chest and knees bent. Place your feet under a support—the base of a weight machine, for example, or even under your couch—to stabilize your lower body. Hold your torso at a 45-degree angle to the floor.

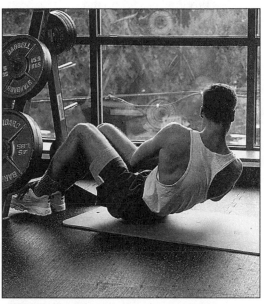

Start by moving your torso to the right, staying to the right as you lower to the back.

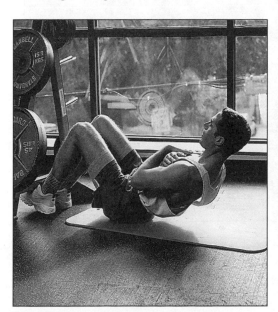

Completing a clockwise rotation, raise your torso on the left side.

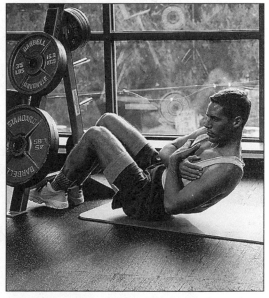

Then repeat the exercise, this time moving down the left side and around to the right.

Seated Twists

RATING: EASY

Fun, safe, and effective, seated twists are among the oldest exercises. They are perfect for hitting the love-handle area—the oblique (side) abdominal muscles.

Grab a stick or light bar about the length of a broomstick. Sit on the end of a bench with your feet slightly apart and flat on the floor. Place the stick or bar behind your head and rest it across your shoulders. Your hands should be as far out toward the ends as you can comfortably reach. Your elbows should remain slightly bent.

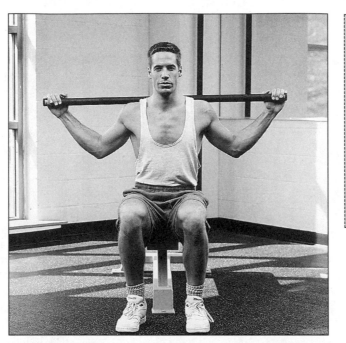

Use your oblique muscles to twist your torso as far to the right as you can while keeping your hips stationary. Repeat the same movement to the left. Continue to rotate right and left, without pausing, until you have completed the set.

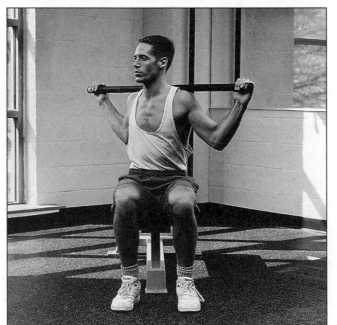

Dumbbell Trunk Twists

RATING: MODERATELY DIFFICULT

Because this exercise works the internal and external obliques (side abdominals), it is often recommended for men who participate in activities that involve trunk rotation, like tennis, canoeing, and golf. And because it keeps the arms at constant tension, it helps work the biceps (front of upper arm) and forearm muscles. In fact, the arm workout is intense; don't be surprised if your arms tire before your abs do.

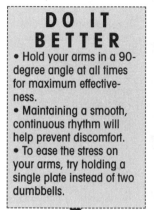

DO IT BETTER

• Hold your arms in a 90-degree angle at all times for maximum effectiveness.
• Maintaining a smooth, continuous rhythm will help prevent discomfort.
• To ease the stress on your arms, try holding a single plate instead of two dumbbells.

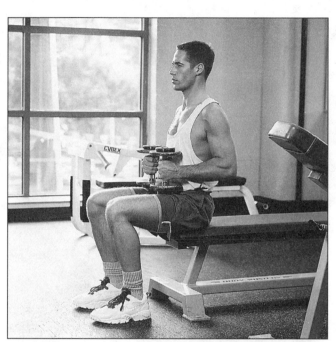

Sit at the edge of a bench with your feet flat on the floor. Keep your chest out and your head aligned with your torso. Hold a dumbbell in each hand, palms facing your body. Bend your arms and bring the weights close to your gut.

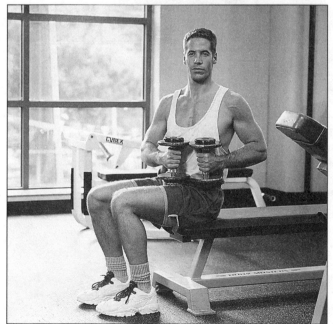

Twist your torso to the left as far as you can comfortably go. When you reach the maximum range of motion, hold for a second, then slowly return to the starting position. Repeat to the right. Continue alternating left and right until your muscles are fatigued.

Cable Crunches

RATING: DIFFICULT

This exercise works all of the abdominal muscles—the upper, lower, and oblique (side). While these crunches can be done using a machine, the method here requires the help of a workout partner.

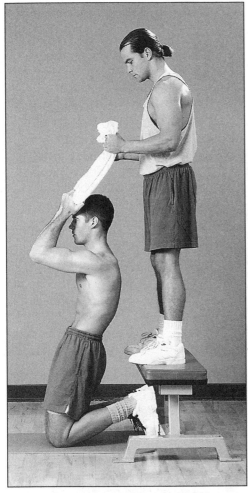

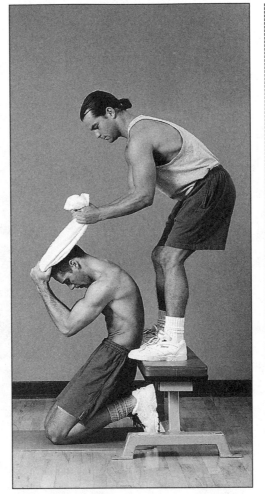

Have your partner stand on a bench or chair, holding a towel with one end in each hand. Kneel on the floor facing away from your partner. Bend your legs at a 45-degree angle. Grab the center of the towel with both hands and hold it at the top of your forehead.

Contract your abs as you curl your torso in and slowly pull on the towel. (Use only your abs, not your upper-body strength.) Curl your body as far in as you can without moving the towel from your forehead or pulling your partner along.

Jumping Flexions and Extensions of the Hips

RATING: DIFFICULT

There are muscles that make it possible for you to bend over and tie your shoes. There are other muscles that make it possible for you to stand back up. Here is an exercise designed specifically to strengthen and develop those muscles: the hip flexors (front hip), hamstrings (back thigh), gluteals (butt), abdominals, and the erector spinae muscles (lower back).

DO IT BETTER

- For maximum effectiveness, fully extend your legs during the backward jump and maintain the alignment of your head and torso.
- Because this exercise employs dynamic force, be sure to stretch beforehand to prevent injury.
- To avoid injury to the toes and ankles, do not raise your legs and feet above shoulder level during the backward jump.
- To increase difficulty, do the exercise without resting at the bent-leg position.

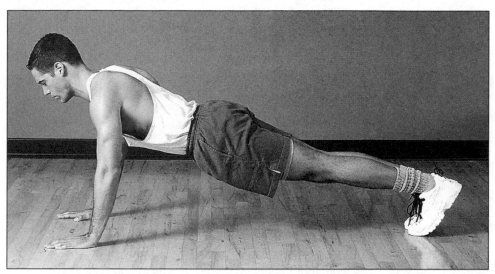

Begin in a push-up starting position. Place your hands slightly more than shoulder-width apart. Your weight should be equally distributed on your hands and toes, and your head should be in line with your torso.

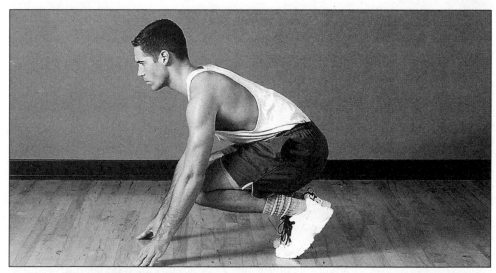

Keeping your hands stationary, jump with your legs, bending your lower body at the hips and knees and bringing your feet up toward your hands. Hold for a second, then repeat, returning to the starting position.

Negative Sit-Ups
RATING: MODERATELY DIFFICULT

For most exercises there is a positive and a negative. The positive is the first half of the exercise (in which the muscles become tense and contract), and the negative is the second half (in which the muscles lengthen but still remain tense). The point of a negative sit-up is to stay within that negative zone until the muscles are fatigued. Unlike traditional sit-ups, this exercise makes the muscles longer as well as bulkier.

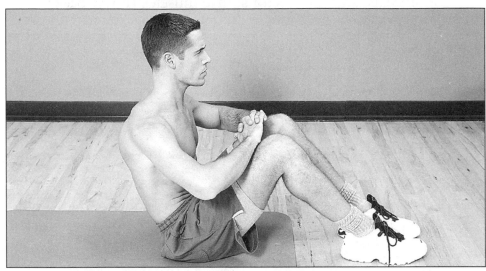

DO IT BETTER

• To put more stress on the lower abs, move your feet farther from your butt.
• Keeping the small of your back rounded as you lower your torso will help prevent lower back injury.
• Raising your torso higher than a 90-degree angle relaxes the abs, reducing the effects of the exercise.
• Lowering your torso below 45 degrees shifts the stress from your abs to the lower back.

Sit on the floor with your knees bent and your feet flat on the floor, shoulder-width apart. Extend your arms with your fingers interlaced, palms facing your knees. Begin with your upper body at slightly less than a 90-degree angle to the floor.

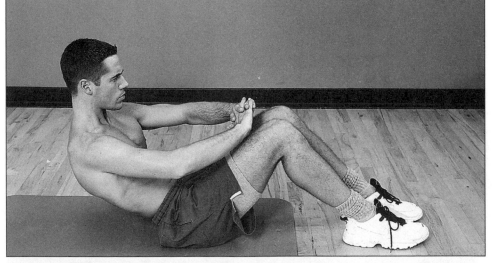

Lower your upper body toward the floor, curling your torso forward and rounding your lower back, keeping the abs contracted. When your body reaches a 45-degree angle to the floor, return to the starting position and begin again.

Double-Leg Scoops

RATING: DIFFICULT

Often used during rehabilitation for lower back injuries, scoops provide great conditioning for the midbody as well. This exercise works the lower abdominals, hip flexors (front hip), and oblique (side) abs. They can be performed at various fitness levels by using a bench or chair or can be done on the floor.

DO IT BETTER

- To do this exercise while sitting (which makes it easier to control), place your hips at the edge of the seat and press your shoulder blades against the back of the chair.
- To reduce strain on the lower back, do this exercise on the floor, with your arms at your sides and palms facedown on the floor.
- To make this exercise most effective, keep your lower back and torso in contact with the bench.
- To increase difficulty, do this exercise while wearing ankle weights.

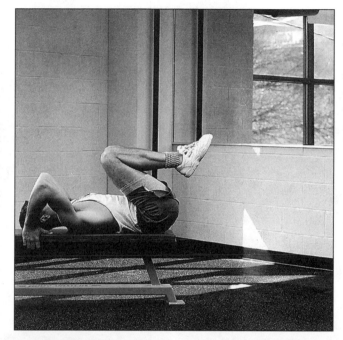

Lie on your back on a bench with your hips at the edge, legs bent at a 90-degree angle. Grasp the bench just above your shoulders. Raise your legs, bringing your knees into your torso.

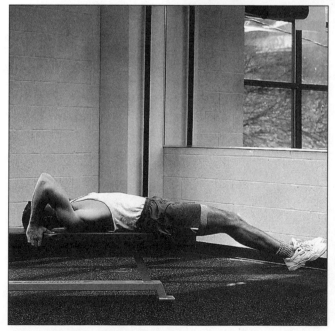

Slowly extend the legs in a downward scooping movement until they are fully extended.

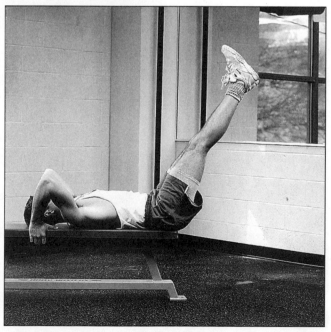

Immediately raise your legs as high as you comfortably can while keeping them extended. Bend your legs and bring your knees back into your torso as you complete a circular motion.

Straight-Leg Rotations

RATING: MODERATELY DIFFICULT

Ideal for Olympic-style weight lifting, pole vaulting, and high jumping, straight-leg rotations help strengthen and develop the hip flexor (front hip) muscles and the oblique (side) abdominals. The muscles worked during this exercise are the same ones used when doing virtually any lifting.

Lie on your back on a bench with your hips at the edge. Grasp the bench above your shoulders. Extend your legs, knees unlocked.

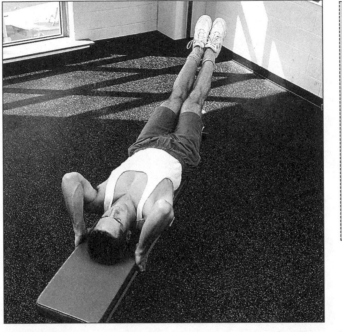

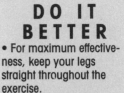

DO IT BETTER
• For maximum effectiveness, keep your legs straight throughout the exercise.
• Keeping the movements smooth and fluid will help prevent injury to the lower back.
• To increase difficulty, do this exercise while wearing ankle weights.
• To increase difficulty even more, do this exercise from a hanging position.

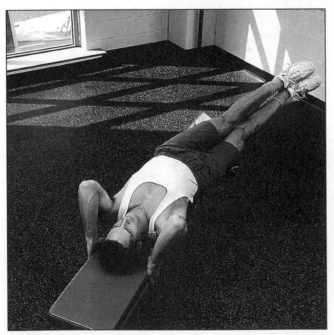

Rotate your legs to the right in a clockwise movement, using your full range of motion.

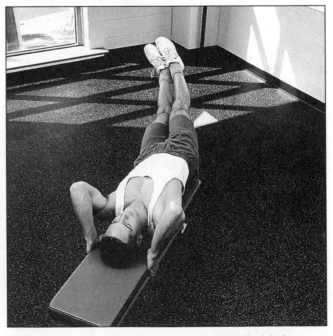

Then repeat the motion, this time to the left side in a counterclockwise motion.

Leg-Overs

RATING: EASY

This exercise works the oblique (side) abdominals, while also giving an excellent stretch to the lower back and hips. You can also use leg-overs as a warm-up or cooldown for any sport.

DO IT BETTER

• Allow your hip to follow through while crossing your leg over. This gives a nice stretch in the hip, which helps prevent injury to the lower back.

• Keep both shoulders on the floor throughout the entire range of motion for maximum effectiveness.

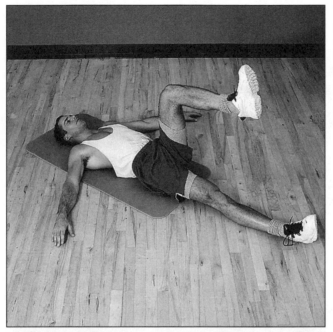

Lie flat on your back, arms out to your sides, palms on the floor. While keeping your right leg straight, bend your left knee at a 90-degree angle.

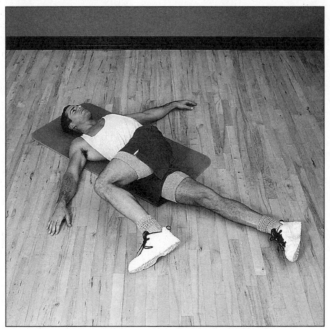

Cross your left knee over your body and lightly touch the floor on the opposite side. Return to the starting position, then repeat. After completing one set, switch to the right leg.

Hip Rolls

RATING: DIFFICULT

If skiing and soccer are your sports of choice, this rotation exercise may be for you. As you roll from side to side, you put stress on the oblique (side) abdominal muscles. At the same time it gives a good stretch to the lower back and hips.

Lie on your back with your arms straight out to your sides, palms facing down. Extend your legs straight in the air. Keep your feet together, knees unlocked.

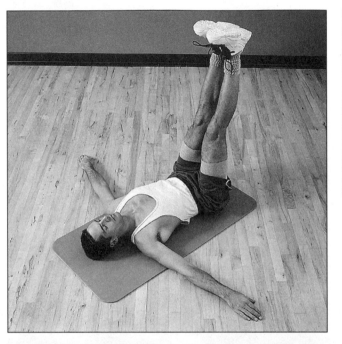

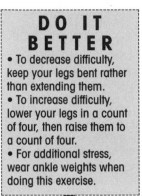

DO IT BETTER
- To decrease difficulty, keep your legs bent rather than extending them.
- To increase difficulty, lower your legs in a count of four, then raise them to a count of four.
- For additional stress, wear ankle weights when doing this exercise.

Slowly lower your legs to the left and touch the floor with the outside leg and foot. Without resting, raise the legs back to the starting position, then lower them on the other side, again touching the floor with the outside leg and foot. Continue alternating from the left to right side until you have completed a set.

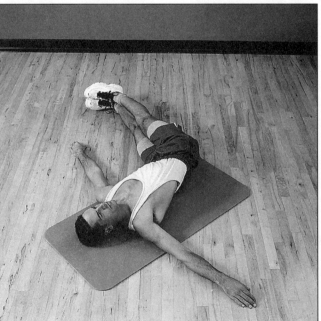

Lat Pull-Downs

RATING: MODERATELY DIFFICULT

When you're looking for a whole-back workout, this exercise is a good place to start. It primarily works the latissimus dorsi (mid and lower back), teres major (below shoulder blade), and the rhomboids (upper back). Because it is done with a machine, the movements are easy to control.

DO IT BETTER

- Concentrate on spreading your lats on the downward pull; don't pinch your shoulder blades together.
- Don't let your upper body move forward as you lower the bar, which could cause back or neck injury.
- The same exercise can be done pulling the bar to the front. Some find this version to be more comfortable and easier to control.

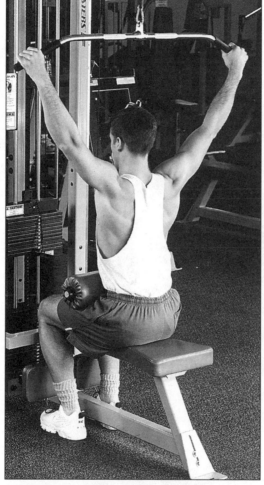

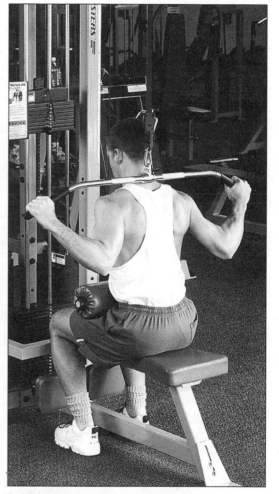

Sit (or kneel if there isn't a seat) at a lat pull-down machine. Grasp the bar overhead, placing your hands shoulder-width (or more) apart. Your palms should face away from your body. Keep your upper body straight and your eyes forward.

Pull the bar behind your head until it reaches the top of your shoulders, keeping your upper body upright throughout the movement. Then return your arms to the starting position and repeat.

Wide-Grip Rows

RATING: DIFFICULT

This is an extremely versatile exercise, working not only the muscles in the back but also the rear deltoid (shoulder) muscles. In addition, the bent-over position provides a terrific stretch for the hamstring (back thigh) and gluteal (butt) muscles. And because this exercise requires that you keep your stomach tight and back flat, your abs and lower back reap the benefits as well.

Stand with your feet shoulder-width apart, knees slightly bent. Bend at the waist until your upper body is straight and parallel to the floor. Grab the barbell, using a wide (more than shoulder-width) grip, palms facing your body.

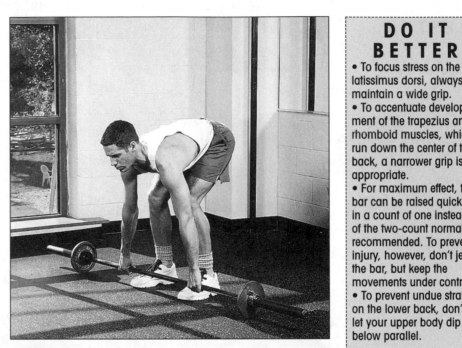

DO IT BETTER

• To focus stress on the latissimus dorsi, always maintain a wide grip.
• To accentuate development of the trapezius and rhomboid muscles, which run down the center of the back, a narrower grip is appropriate.
• For maximum effect, the bar can be raised quickly in a count of one instead of the two-count normally recommended. To prevent injury, however, don't jerk the bar, but keep the movements under control.
• To prevent undue strain on the lower back, don't let your upper body dip below parallel.

Raise the bar in a count of two until it touches your chest. Your elbows should be higher than your back. Slowly lower the barbell to about the middle of your shin, then repeat.

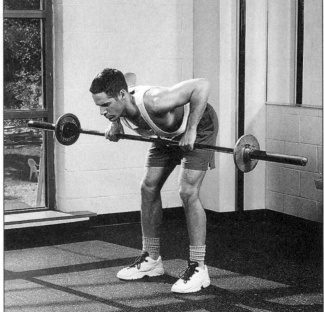

T-Bar Rows

RATING: DIFFICULT

This exercise is recommended for strengthening the back and developing good posture and form, which is particularly important if you participate in sports that put a lot of stress on the lower back, like bowling. It works all the back muscles and the rear deltoid (shoulder) muscles. While most health clubs have a T-bar apparatus, you can do this exercise using a barbell wedged in a corner. Because of the potential for injury, good form is essential. You want to keep your lower back flat or, at most, slightly arched, but never curved.

DO IT BETTER

• Stand on a 6-inch platform with the bar still between your legs. This helps increase the range of motion and optimize development of the back muscles.
• When using a T-bar machine, putting your hands wider than shoulder-width apart will maximize stress on the latissimus dorsi muscles.
• This exercise can be done by grasping the bar with only one hand, without the use of attachments, straps, or ropes. This helps isolate the muscles on each side of the back.

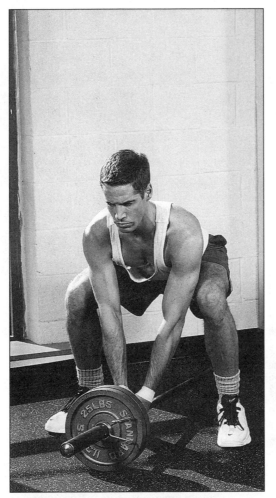

Using an Olympic-size (45-pound) bar, wedge one end in the corner and place a weight plate on the other end. Wrap two wrist straps around the bar just below the weight and encircle your hands around the bar at this point. You could also use lifting gloves or your bare hands. Straddle the bar, keeping your knees slightly bent. Your chin should be up, your chest out, stomach in, shoulders back, and back flat.

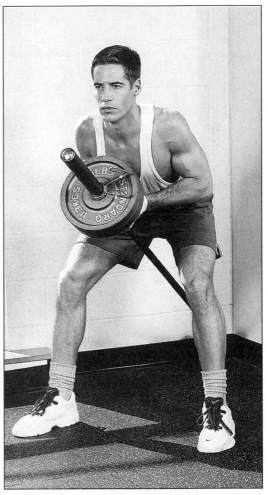

Pull the bar to your chest, slightly arching your back and letting your elbows rise above your chest. Slowly lower the bar to arm's length, then continue with the next repetition.

Good Mornings

RATING: DIFFICULT

Not recommended for beginners, this exercise requires some effort, so you'll need to be alert—and have a strong lower back. This is an extensive midbody workout involving your hamstrings (back thigh), gluteals (butt), abdominals, and all of the back muscles, especially the erector spinae (lower back).

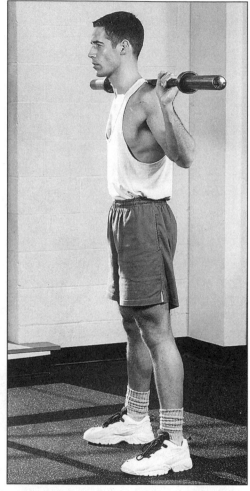

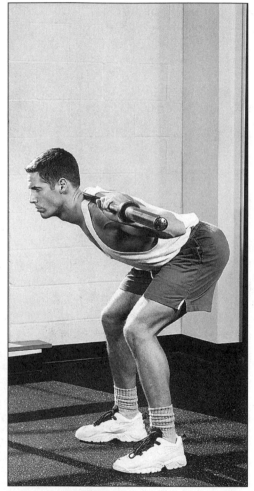

DO IT BETTER

• Contracting your abs throughout the entire range of motion will help keep your body stable.

• Because this exercise is extremely difficult, it's a good idea to start with an empty bar until your form is perfected.

• To increase difficulty, have a friend provide extra resistance by pressing on your upper back as you return to the starting position.

• To do this exercise without weights, hold a towel behind your neck and pull on the ends to create resistance.

Stand with your legs shoulder-width apart, knees unlocked. Hold a barbell across your shoulders, with your hands slightly more than shoulder-width apart, palms facing out. Keep your upper body straight, your shoulders back, and chest out. Lean forward slightly at the waist.

Bend slowly at the waist, keeping your back straight, until your upper body is parallel to the floor. Your eyes should be looking forward, not down. Slowly return to the starting position, then repeat.

Seated Rows

RATING: MODERATELY DIFFICULT

This exercise is perfect for sculpting the entire back, particularly the upper middle back. Seated rows work the latissimus dorsi (mid and lower back), trapezius (upper back and neck), and the rhomboids (upper back) as well as the middle and rear deltoid (shoulder) muscles. It also works the teres minor (outside the shoulder blade), infraspinatus (shoulder blade), and biceps (front of upper arm) muscles.

DO IT BETTER

• Using a wider grip will put more tension on the lats. A narrower grip, by contrast, puts more emphasis on the midback region—the trapezius and rhomboid muscles.

• To isolate each lat separately, fit the machine with a single-arm attachment. Reduce the weight and pull back one arm at a time.

• Keeping your back straight will help maximize stress on the target back muscles.

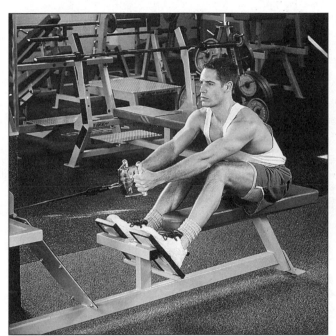

Sit at a pulley row machine. Anchor your feet against the foot pedals, with your knees slightly bent. Keep your back straight as you lean forward, bending at the waist. Grasp the handles with a narrow grip and pull back. Your arms should be fully extended, with your body leaning forward slightly.

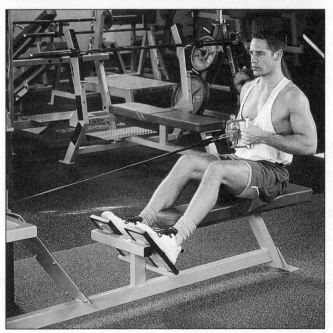

Pull the handles until they touch your chest, bringing your body into an upright position. Your elbows should be pointing behind you, with your knees unlocked. Hold for a second, then return to the starting position.

High Pull Extensions

RATING: DIFFICULT

The demands exerted on your body by this exercise are similar to those of the clean and jerk, the Olympic-style lift. Not only does it build muscle strength and size but it also increases speed and force. It's an extremely versatile exercise, working the hamstring (back thigh) and gluteal (butt) muscles as well as major muscles in the back, shoulders, and arms.

Stand with your feet shoulder-width apart and your knees slightly bent. Squat to pick up the bar, placing your hands slightly more than shoulder-width apart, using an overhand grip. Keep your back flat and your head in line with your back.

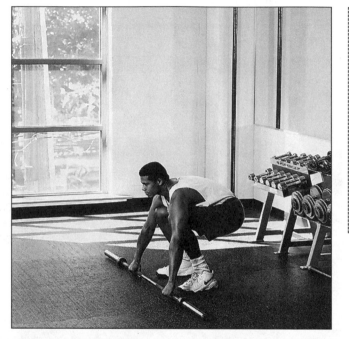

DO IT BETTER
• To decrease difficulty, use just the bar or a light weight.
• For maximum effectiveness, keep the bar close to your body throughout the entire range of motion.
• To increase difficulty, bounce up on your toes at the maximum range of motion. To work the calves, stay up on your toes for a second.

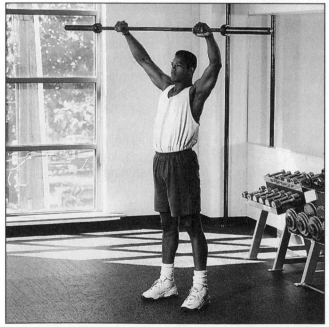

Begin standing as you raise the bar in a vertical movement. Raise the bar above your head, keeping your elbows unlocked. Keep your wrists bent so that the bar and your palms are parallel with the floor.

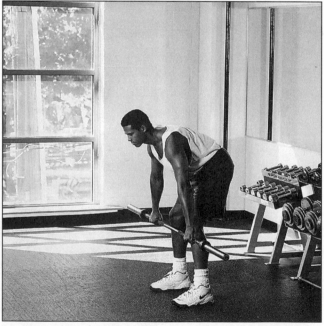

Slowly lower the barbell, keeping it close to your body, to just below knee level, keeping your lower back flat. Repeat the movements. Don't let the bar touch the floor between repetitions.

Chin-Ups

RATING: DIFFICULT

This exercise looks easy, but it requires that you raise your entire body weight. It works all the major upper body and midbody muscles, including those in the back, chest, and arms.

DO IT BETTER

• If you can't do chin-ups on your own, have a friend help lift you up. Then lower yourself slowly, keeping the motion under control.
• To decrease difficulty, do this exercise with your hands closer together.
• To further decrease difficulty, use an underhand grip.
• To increase difficulty, use a wide grip and pull yourself up so that the bar comes behind your neck.

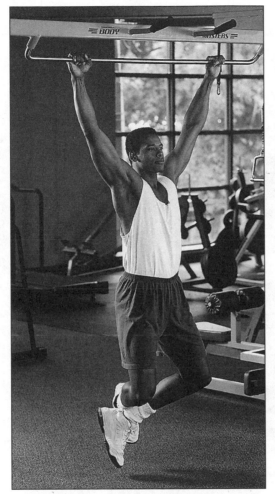

Grasp a chin-up bar, using an overhand grip and placing your hands as far apart as possible. Hang from the bar with your legs slightly bent and your ankles crossed.

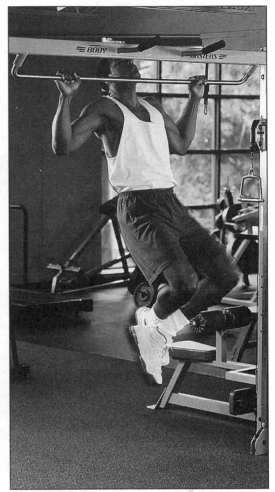

Slowly pull yourself up until your chin is over the bar. Hold for a second, then return to the starting position. Repeat without resting.

One-Arm Dumbbell Rows

RATING: MODERATELY DIFFICULT

Unlike most back exercises, this one is done using one arm at a time. Since your back muscles come in sets of two (one on each side), this exercise makes it possible to isolate and strengthen the weaker side, bringing all the muscles into balance. Although the arm and shoulder muscles come into play, this exercise primarily works the back—specifically, the latissimus dorsi (mid and lower back), rhomboids (upper back), and trapezius (upper back and neck) muscles.

With a dumbbell in your left hand, rest your right knee and right hand in the center of a bench. Place your left foot firmly on the floor, knee slightly bent. Keep your back straight and your eyes facing down. Let your left arm hang down with the elbow unlocked, palm facing the side of your body.

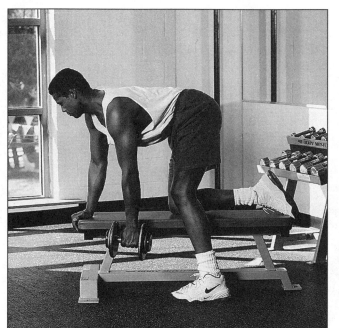

DO IT BETTER

• To decrease difficulty, use a wrist weight instead of a dumbbell.
• You can also do this exercise using a Theraband (available at most sporting goods stores). Step on the middle of the Theraband. Pull the band across the front of your body with the working arm and follow the same steps as when using weights.
• To increase stress on the shoulders, begin with your palm facing the front of your thigh and rotate your palm in toward your torso while you lift.

Pull the dumbbell up and in toward your torso, raising it as high as possible to your chest. Your left elbow should be pointing up toward the ceiling as you lift.

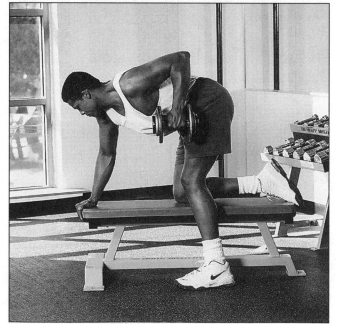

Dumbbell Swings

RATING: MODERATELY DIFFICULT

While most exercises are designed to be done in slow, controlled movements for safety and effectiveness, this one should be done with accelerated effort. The explosive nature of the activity enables you to utilize more fibers within each muscle, while expanding your range of motion. Unlike most back exercises, the dumbbell swing provides a high level of conditioning for the erector spinae (lower back) muscles as well as the hamstring (back thigh), deltoid (shoulder), and gluteal (butt) muscles.

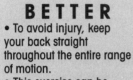

DO IT BETTER

• To avoid injury, keep your back straight throughout the entire range of motion.
• This exercise can be hard on the back, so begin with very light weights and high repetitions.
• To incorporate more leg muscles into the workout, rise up on your toes after reaching the maximum range of motion.

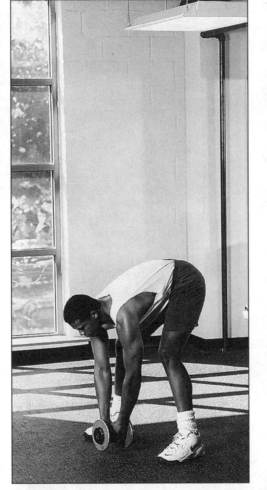

Hold a dumbbell with both hands. Stand with your feet more than shoulder-width apart, knees unlocked. Bend at the waist while holding the dumbbell between your shins, arms fully extended. Keep the weight off the floor.

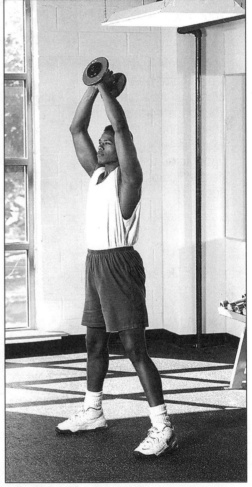

Swing the dumbbell until it's over your head, simultaneously standing upright. Hold the dumbbell over your head for a second, then bend at the waist as you return to the starting position.

Back Extensions

RATING: MODERATELY DIFFICULT

The abdominal and lower back muscles overlap and work together to move your trunk, whether for lifting or twisting. The key to developing strong abdominal muscles lies in developing a sturdy lower back, and vice versa. These extensions are the best lower back exercises you can do. And since the lower back muscles intersect the butt muscles, which in turn overlap the leg muscles, this workout creates tension throughout the midbody.

Get in position on a back extension station. Your ankles should be locked behind the padded bars, with your upper thighs resting on the platform and your hips over the edge. Fold your arms across your chest. Bend at the waist, lowering your upper torso until it's perpendicular to the floor.

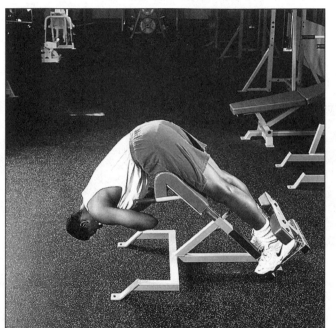

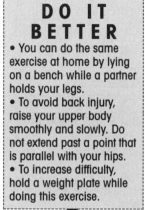

DO IT BETTER

• You can do the same exercise at home by lying on a bench while a partner holds your legs.
• To avoid back injury, raise your upper body smoothly and slowly. Do not extend past a point that is parallel with your hips.
• To increase difficulty, hold a weight plate while doing this exercise.

Keeping your arms folded across your chest, raise your upper body until your back is in line with your lower body. Hold for a second, then return to the starting position.

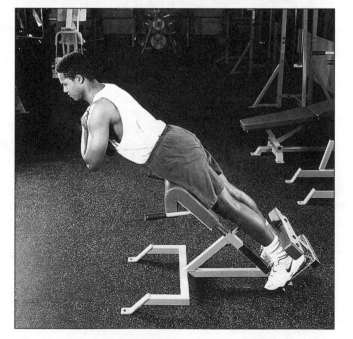

Opposite Arm and Leg Raises

RATING: EASY

Most exercises are not meant to push your body beyond the normal range of motion. Here is an exercise designed to push you slightly past that point, but never to the point of pain. Although there is not any weight involved with this exercise, it will still increase the strength of all of the back muscles and the gluteal (butt) muscles.

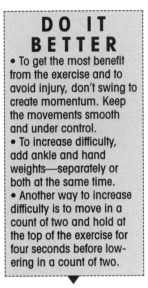

DO IT BETTER

• To get the most benefit from the exercise and to avoid injury, don't swing to create momentum. Keep the movements smooth and under control.

• To increase difficulty, add ankle and hand weights—separately or both at the same time.

• Another way to increase difficulty is to move in a count of two and hold at the top of the exercise for four seconds before lowering in a count of two.

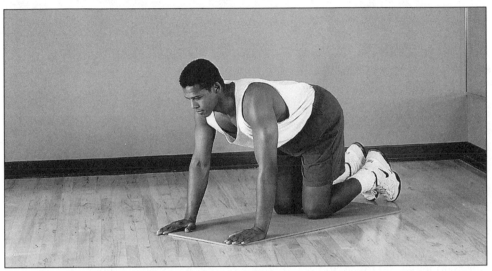

Get down on your hands and knees. Keep your back straight and your head in line with your spine. You should be looking straight ahead, not down.

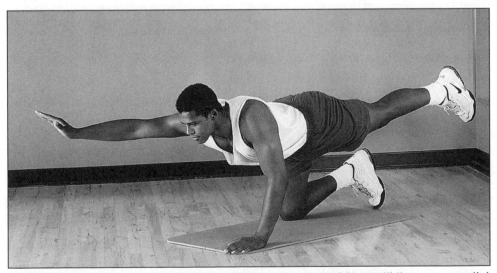

Simultaneously raise and straighten your right arm and left leg until they are parallel to the ground. Hold for 2 seconds, then slowly return to the starting position. Repeat with your left arm and right leg.

Leg and Upper-Body Raises

RATING: MODERATELY DIFFICULT

You know that you're supposed to lift with your legs to prevent back injury. Leg and upper-body raises are designed to target the delicate erector spinae (lower back) muscles, which are at greatest risk for injury when you lift improperly. Try this exercise, which also strengthens and develops the hamstring (back thigh) muscles and the gluteal (butt) muscles. You need all of these muscles to lift anything at all.

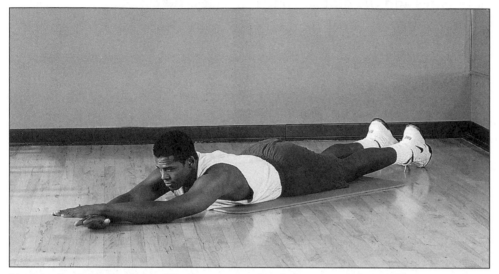

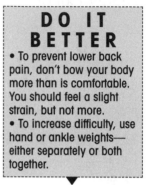

DO IT BETTER
• To prevent lower back pain, don't bow your body more than is comfortable. You should feel a slight strain, but not more.
• To increase difficulty, use hand or ankle weights—either separately or both together.

Lie facedown on the floor with your arms extended over your head. Keep your hands together, palms facing down, knees unlocked, and toes pointed.

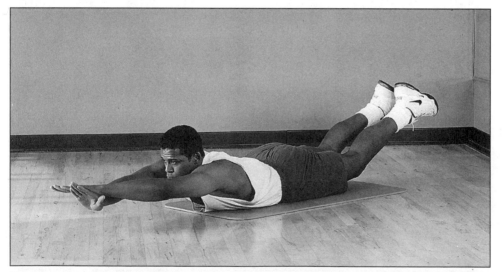

Slowly raise your legs and arms at the same time, raising them as high as comfortably possible. At the maximum range of motion, hold for a second, then slowly return to the starting position.

Toe Touches

RATING: EASY

Long a favorite of calisthenics classes, this exercise, traditionally done without weights, is an excellent way to strengthen the lower back and to some degree the hamstring (back thigh) and gluteal (butt) muscles.

DO IT BETTER

- This exercise can be hard on the lower back, so move slowly and with control.
- To help your body get used to the movements, do the exercise several times without a weight.
- Progressively increase the repetitions before increasing weight. You want to work on increasing flexibility before strength.

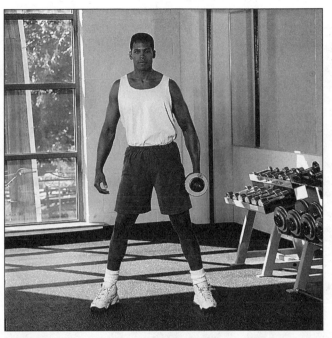

Hold a dumbbell in your left hand, with your feet shoulder-width apart, knees unlocked.

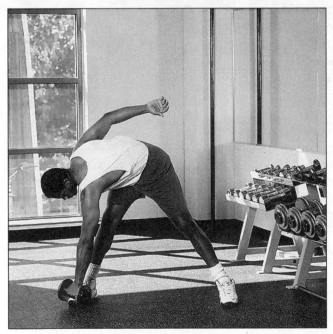

Bending forward and to the right, touch the dumbbell to your right foot. Return to the starting position, then repeat. After several repetitions to the right, switch to the left.

Romanian Dead Lifts

RATING: MODERATELY DIFFICULT

A slight variation on the standard dead lift performed by power lifters is the Romanian dead lift. This exercise strengthens nearly every major muscle in your body—including those in the legs, back, shoulders, and arms—but is less stressful than the traditional dead lift. When doing these dead lifts, you'll want to use less weight because you start by holding the weighted bar, rather than hefting it off the floor.

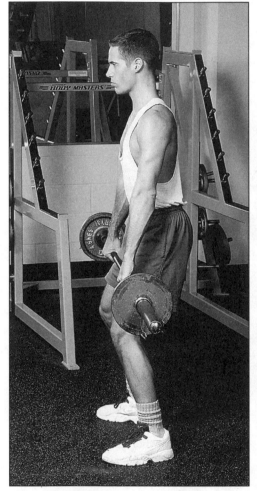

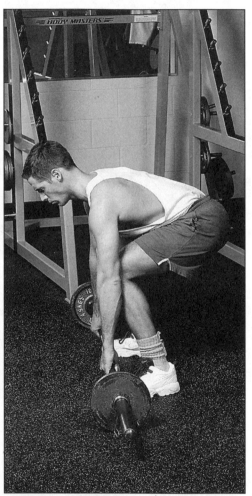

DO IT BETTER

• When starting out, use the bar without adding weights until you're comfortable with the movements.
• This exercise is hard on the lower back, so use lighter weights than you would for traditional dead lifts.
• Maintain a flat back and use slow, controlled movements throughout the entire exercise.
• To decrease difficulty, set the bar down between repetitions.
• To increase difficulty, stand on a 4-inch platform. The extra stretch will benefit the hamstrings and gluteal muscles as well as the erector spinae muscles of the back.

Hold a lightly weighted barbell at midthigh level, with your hands more than shoulder-width apart, palms facing your body. Hold the barbell against your legs with your arms fully extended, shoulders back, and chest out.

Keeping your back flat and your knees slightly bent, bend forward at the hips, keeping the bar close to your thighs. Lower the bar toward the floor, going as far as you comfortably can. Slowly return to the starting position, keeping your back straight throughout the exercise.

Duck Squats

RATING: MODERATELY DIFFICULT

Once you do this exercise, you'll see how it got its name. It primarily works the gluteal (butt) muscles, but also hits the adductor (inner thigh) and quadriceps (front thigh) muscles. These squats are unique because they work these muscles at angles different from any other exercise.

DO IT BETTER

• To protect your knees, don't bounce at the bottom of the movement and don't turn your knees in toward the front of your body.

• To work the calf muscles, rise up on your toes when rising to the starting position. Only try this if you have good balance.

• To decrease difficulty, do the same exercise without holding weights.

• To increase difficulty, hold a dumbbell in each hand at shoulder level. Press them above your head as you squat, then return to shoulder level as you rise.

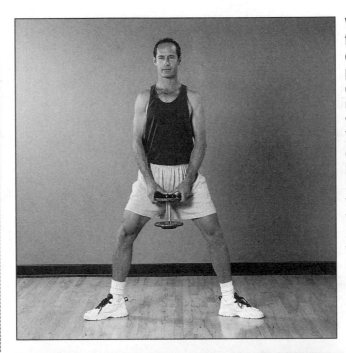

With your feet more than shoulder-width apart and your toes pointing out, hold a dumbbell by the end, using both hands, with your arms extended. Your chest should be out, your shoulders back, abs tight, and back straight. Keep your head in line with your spine and look straight ahead. There will be a slight forward lean to your upper body, which is natural.

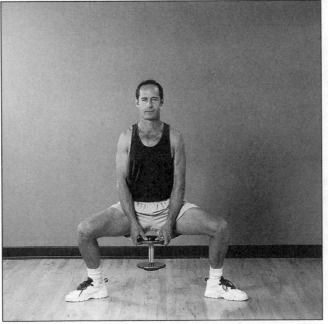

Squat until your thighs are parallel to the ground. Keeping your feet flat on the floor, slowly rise, keeping your hips slightly forward and your abs tight. Do not lock your knees at the top. Continue with the next rep.

Stationary Lunges
RATING: MODERATELY DIFFICULT

This is a superb exercise that works the gluteal (butt) and quadriceps (front thigh) muscles, while putting very little stress on the knees. It also strengthens the hamstring (back thigh) muscles, which help keep your body balanced through the entire range of movement. This exercise is superb for improving speed and flexibility.

Stand with your head in line with your spine, your back straight and your feet shoulder-width apart. Hold a dumbbell in each hand, with your arms hanging down, palms facing your body.

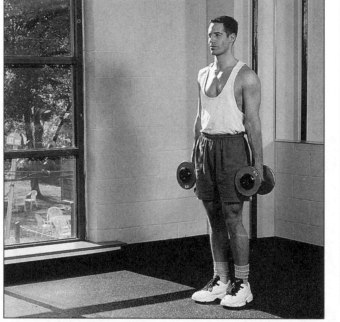

DO IT BETTER
• To strengthen the tendons in the knee and develop the hip flexors, do this exercise with the foot of the working leg turned toward the center of the body.
• This exercise requires good balance, so you may want to start out doing it without using weights.
• To increase difficulty, replace the dumbbells with a barbell placed behind your neck.
• To incorporate more of the gluteal muscle, place the foot of the working leg on a platform at least 6 inches high.

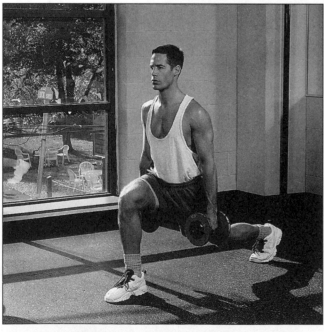

Take a long step forward with your right foot. Bend your leg until your right thigh is parallel to the floor. Your left leg should be extended, knee slightly bent and almost touching the floor.

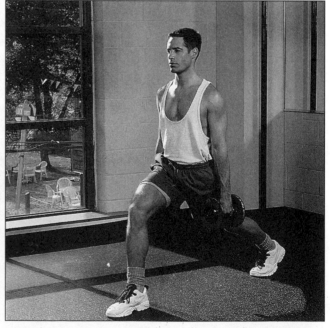

Keep your right foot stationary as you straighten your right leg. Continue bending and straightening the right leg. Switch legs and repeat on the left side.

Alternating Leg Lunges

RATING: MODERATELY DIFFICULT

This is a dynamic, explosive exercise in which no weight needs to be used. It helps build strength and coordination by working the quadriceps (front thigh), hamstring (back thigh), gluteal (butt) muscles, and hip flexor (front hip) muscles. If you play basketball, soccer, or other sports in which agility and speed are important, this exercise is a good choice.

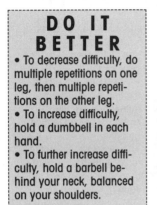

DO IT BETTER

- To decrease difficulty, do multiple repetitions on one leg, then multiple repetitions on the other leg.
- To increase difficulty, hold a dumbbell in each hand.
- To further increase difficulty, hold a barbell behind your neck, balanced on your shoulders.

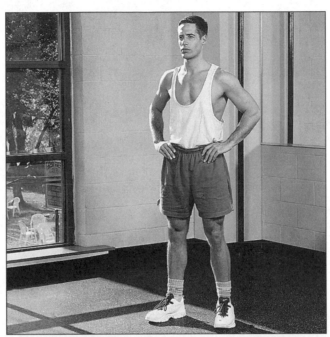

Stand with your feet shoulder-width apart, hands on your hips. Keep your upper body upright and your head in line with your spine.

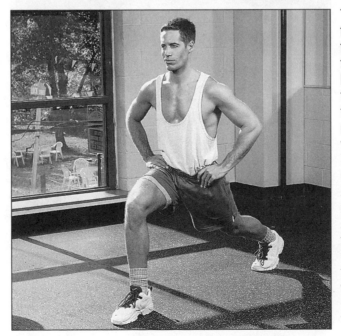

Take a long step forward on your right foot. Firmly plant that foot on the floor and bend your knees until the right thigh is parallel to the floor. Don't let the right knee extend past your right foot. Your left leg should be extended behind you, knee slightly bent, heel raised. Immediately step back with the right foot, pressing your left heel to the ground. Your feet should be shoulder-width apart. Repeat using the left foot; continue alternating.

Lateral Lunges

RATING: MODERATELY DIFFICULT

Many activities—tennis, volleyball, even dancing—require lateral movements. These lunges are recommended for strengthening the adductor (inner thigh) and abductor (outer thigh) muscles as well as the hamstring (back thigh) and gluteal (butt) muscles.

Balance a barbell behind your neck, resting it on your shoulders. Place your hands slightly more than shoulder-width apart. Your feet should be shoulder-width apart with your knees unlocked and the toes pointing out slightly. Keep your chest out, shoulders back, stomach tight, and back straight. Your head should be in line with your spine.

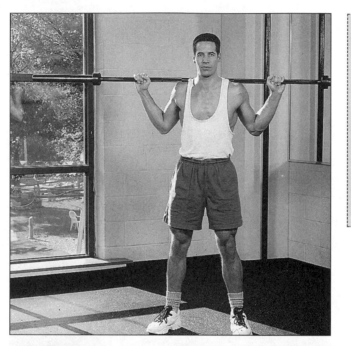

DO IT BETTER
• To protect your knees, don't let them extend past your toes.
• When pushing off the leading leg, push back rather than up, which could cause you to lose balance.
• To decrease difficulty, replace the barbell with dumbbells, one held in each hand.

Step to your right, landing heel to toe, pressing your hips down until your right thigh is parallel to the floor. Your left leg should be extended with the left foot planted firmly on the floor. Your right foot will point to the side while your left foot points forward and your torso faces forward. Hold for a second, then push back with the right leg and return to the starting position. Continue on the right side for one set, then switch to the left.

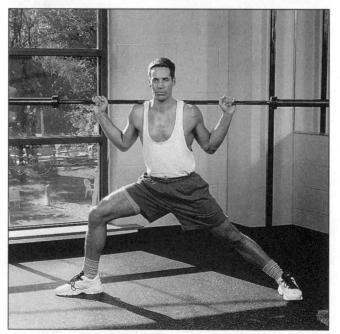

Lateral Step-Ups

RATING: DIFFICULT

Virtually all activities require at least some lateral movements. Lateral movements bring a variety of muscles into play, including the abductor (outer thigh), adductor (inner thigh), hip flexor (front hip), and hamstring (back thigh) muscles. In this exercise, the higher you raise your legs, the more you involve the hips. Try alternating your steps between two wooden blocks, each about a foot high.

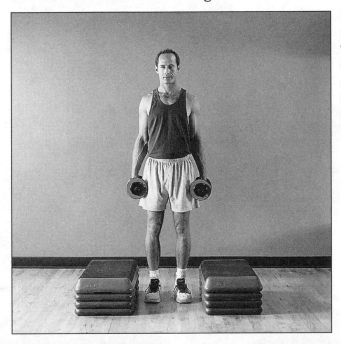

DO IT BETTER

• To increase difficulty, raise the height of the steps.
• For ease and control, try lateral step-ups using only one stack of steps or blocks. Step up to the right and down to the right—moving from one side of the step to the other—as you do the exercise.
• To further increase difficulty, include a one-legged squat at the top of the movement.
• For an aerobic gain, increase the frequency and speed of the step-ups.

Place the steps slightly more than shoulder-width apart. Hold a dumbbell in each hand, arms fully extended down at your sides, palms facing your body.

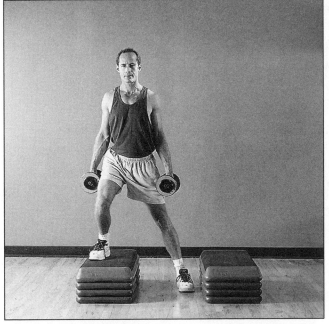

Beginning with the right foot, step up, placing your foot as far to the right on the step as you comfortably can, shifting your weight to the right foot.

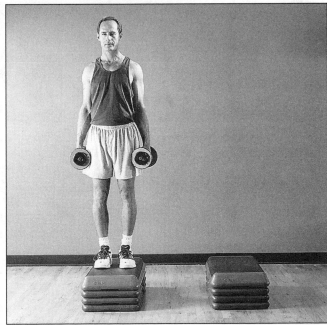

Follow with your left foot, putting it next to the right. Beginning with the left foot, step down, one foot at a time, and return to the starting position. Then repeat the movements, this time leading with your left foot.

Standing Kickbacks

RATING: EASY

This exercise works both the gluteal (butt) and hamstring (back thigh) muscles. It's especially recommended for runners, because damaged hamstrings are a common running injury.

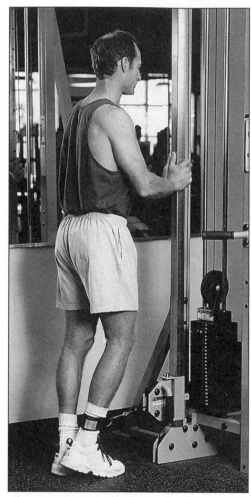 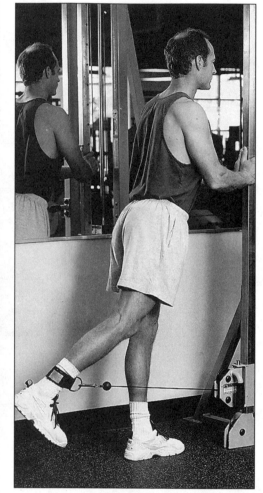

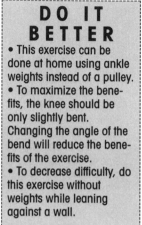

DO IT BETTER
• This exercise can be done at home using ankle weights instead of a pulley.
• To maximize the benefits, the knee should be only slightly bent. Changing the angle of the bend will reduce the benefits of the exercise.
• To decrease difficulty, do this exercise without weights while leaning against a wall.

This can be done using a Theratube (available at sporting goods stores) or a cable pulley machine. Using the cable pulley machine, attach the ankle strap around your right ankle. Stand facing the weight stack. Use your hands for balance by holding on to the equipment at about waist height. Keep your head in line with your spine.

Keep your right knee slightly bent as you move your right leg straight back until you feel tightness in your butt. Do not overextend your leg to the point of discomfort. Bring your right leg back to the starting point. Complete one set, and then work the left leg.

Sprinter's Start Jumps

RATING: MODERATELY DIFFICULT

This is one of the few exercises that increases strength and flexibility in the groin area—particularly in the transversus abdominus, the deepest abdominal muscles that run from the hip to the bottom of the pelvic area. It also works the muscles that enable you to bring your legs together—known collectively as the adductor (inner thigh) muscles.

DO IT BETTER

- Before jumping, use the starting positions to stretch, holding the stretch for 30 seconds on each leg.
- To focus stress on the quadriceps and hamstrings, keep your movements straight—don't allow your legs to go out to the sides.
- Increasing the frequency and intensity of the jumps will incorporate aerobic stress into the workout.

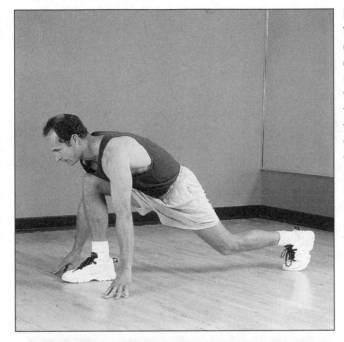

Begin in the race position with your hands down and arms extended. Bend your right leg to the front of your body, keeping the thigh parallel to the floor. Do not extend your right knee past your toes. Extend your left leg behind your body, knee slightly bent. Support the weight of your left leg on your toes and the ball of your left foot.

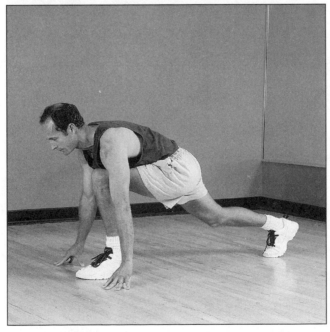

Jump and alternate legs, bringing the left leg forward and extending the right leg back. Allow your weight to rest on both arms, while pushing your hips and legs up at the same time. Hold for a second, then jump again.

Kneeling Leg Kicks

RATING: EASY

This exercise is good for increasing hip flexibility and improving running time. No weights are required, but adding ankle weights will put helpful stress on the hamstring (back thigh) and gluteal (butt) muscles.

Get down on your hands and knees.

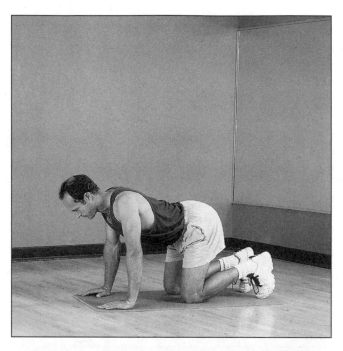

Keeping your right knee slightly bent, raise the right leg until the thigh is parallel to your torso. Hold for a second, then return almost to the starting position. Immediately raise the leg again before it touches the floor. Complete one set with the right leg, then switch to the left.

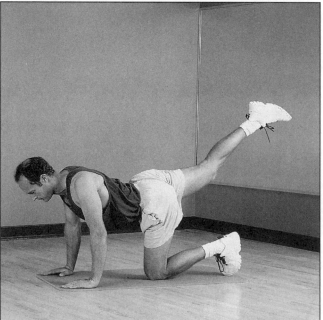

Reverse Leg Extensions

RATING: MODERATELY DIFFICULT

This is one of the best exercises for developing the hamstring (back thigh), gluteal (butt), and erector spinae (lower back) muscles without putting pressure on the lower back. Indeed, it's often used to treat lower back injuries because it strengthens all the extensor muscles that stabilize the area.

DO IT BETTER

• Keeping your toes pointed will help keep the legs straight and increase your range of motion.
• This exercise can be done using a Roman chair. Rest your abdomen on the body support pad and hang on to the foot pads, using an underhand grip.
• To increase difficulty, attach one end of a Theratube to a leg of the bench or table and the other end to your feet. Adding ankle weights will also increase difficulty.
• To make this exercise even harder, at the top of each movement, bend your legs and bring your heels in toward your butt.
• Avoid raising your thighs above a level parallel to the bench, which could cause lower back injury.

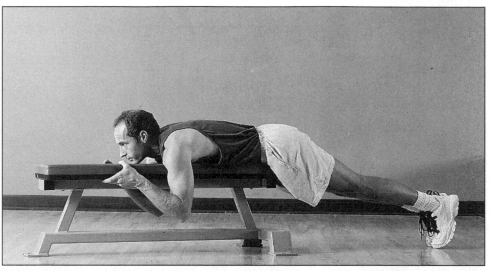

Lie facedown on a bench or table with your hips at the edge, legs together, knees slightly bent and toes touching the floor. Grab the sides of the bench above your head to keep your upper body stable as you move your legs. Hold on firmly to avoid sliding off the bench.

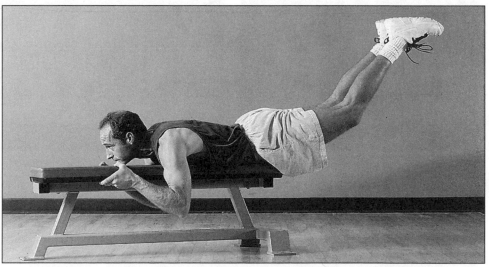

Raise your legs slowly, keeping your feet together, toes pointed, until your thighs are about parallel to your torso. Hold for a second, then slowly lower the legs to the starting position. Do not allow your feet to touch the floor until you have completed one set.

Standing Back Leg Swings

RATING: EASY

Football players have long recognized the value of ballet for increasing agility. This exercise, which is similar to warm-up exercises used in ballet, is recommended for loosening and strengthening the hip flexor (front hip) muscles and the leg extensor (front thigh) muscles as well as the hamstring (back thigh) and gluteal (butt) muscles. It's also used to increase the range of motion in the legs.

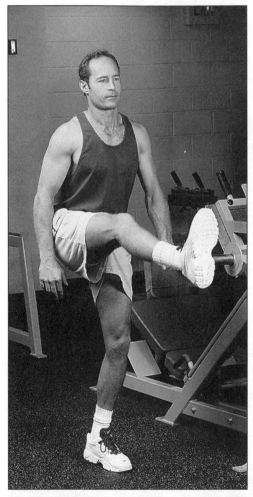

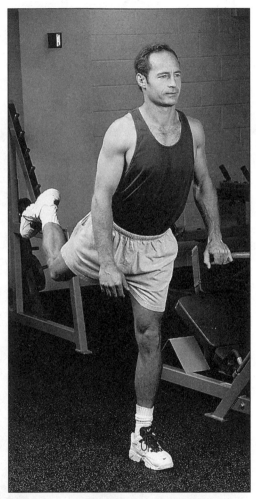

Stand with the left side of your body next to a stationary object, like a ballet warm-up bar or an exercise machine, and hold on with your left hand. Support your weight on your left leg, with the right leg slightly bent. Raise the right leg as high as possible in front of your body. Hold for a second.

Allow the right leg to fall and swing behind your body as far as it will comfortably go. Hold for a second, then swing back to the starting position. Repeat to complete the repetitions in the set, then switch to the other leg.

Kneeling Leg Raises

RATING: EASY

In addition to strengthening the abductor (outer thigh) and gluteal (butt) muscles, this exercise promotes tremendous hip flexibility by working the hip flexor (front hip) muscles. Many athletes use this exercise to loosen muscles in between heavy weightlifting sets. It can also be used as a warm-up before running or jumping.

DO IT BETTER

- To avoid straining your neck, keep your head in line with your spine and your arms perpendicular to the floor.
- To maximize the effects of the exercise, don't rotate your foot outward.
- To bring more muscles into play, point the toes toward the floor. This will help target the gluteal and outer thigh muscles.
- To increase difficulty, add ankle weights when doing this exercise.

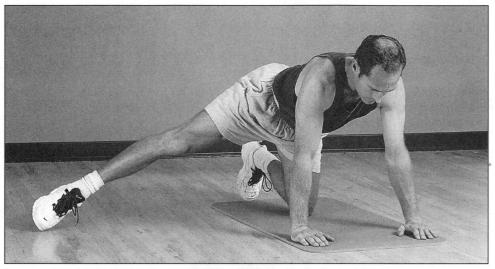

Get down on your hands and knees with your arms fully extended and your back flat. Extend your right leg out to the side so that your knee is facing forward. Your foot, with the toes pointed, should be resting on the floor.

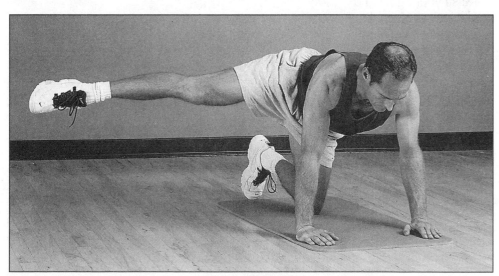

Raise your right leg until it is parallel with the floor—or as close to parallel as you can comfortably get. Hold for a second at the top of the movement, then lower the leg slowly. Before it touches the floor, immediately raise it again. Continue on the same side to finish the set, then switch legs and repeat on the left.

Abductions

Abduction of the thigh means moving your thigh away from your body. This is an important exercise since these muscles are normally neglected and can be slow to strengthen. Leg abductions work two of the three gluteal (butt) muscles and the tensor fascia latae (a band of muscle down the side of the thigh).

Lie on your back with your arms extended at your sides, palms down. Keep your head and lower back flat on the floor. Bend your left leg and plant your left foot firmly on the floor, as close to your butt as is comfortably possible. Extend your right leg, with your foot flexed and toes turned in so that your hip is rotated inward.

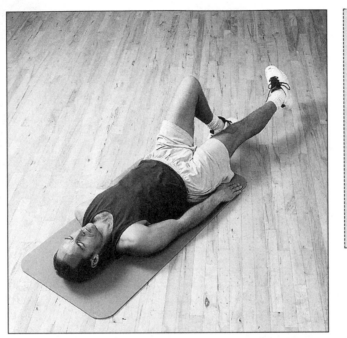

DO IT BETTER

• Keeping your toes turned in throughout the entire range of motion will maximize stress on the target muscles.

• To increase difficulty, loop a Theratube around your ankle and attach the other end to a stationary object, to increase resistance.

• To further increase difficulty, do this exercise using ankle weights.

Raise your right leg a few inches off the floor and pull it away from the center of your body as far as you comfortably can without twisting your torso. Slowly return to the starting position, beginning the next repetition without resting your foot on the floor. After completing a set, repeat using the left leg.

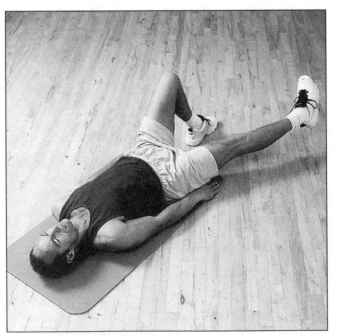

Adductions

RATING: EASY

The groin muscles aren't strengthened by most daily activities and so are prone to injury, particularly when you're running, jumping, or doing heavy lifting. This exercise works the adductor (inner thigh), quadriceps (front thigh), and hip flexor (front hip) muscles.

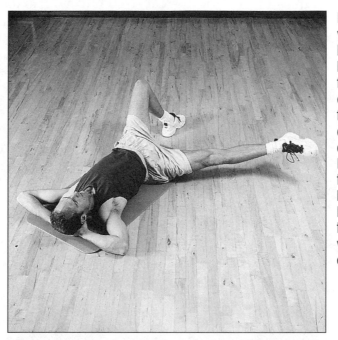

Lie on your back with your hands behind your head. Keep your lower back pressed to the floor. Bend your left leg and plant your left foot firmly on the floor, as close to your butt as is comfortably possible. Extend your right leg to the right side of the body as far as you can. Flex your right foot and turn the toes out so that your thigh is rotated outward.

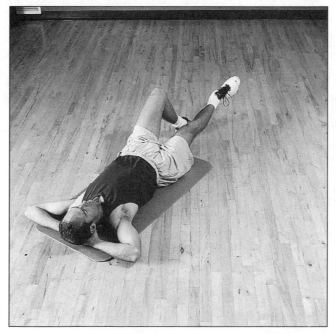

Pull the right leg in toward the center of your body without twisting your torso. Slowly bring the leg back to the starting position, then proceed with the next repetition without resting your foot on the floor. After completing a set, repeat using the left leg.

Sideways Raises

RATING: VERY DIFFICULT

This tough, midbody exercise is emphatically not recommended for beginners. It's a great workout for the abdominal, oblique (side), gluteal (butt), and quadriceps (front thigh) muscles. As you try to stabilize your body on one knee, you'll see that sideways raises are also great for developing balance and coordination. They also improve flexibility in the ankles, knees, and hips and provide a great stretch to your back.

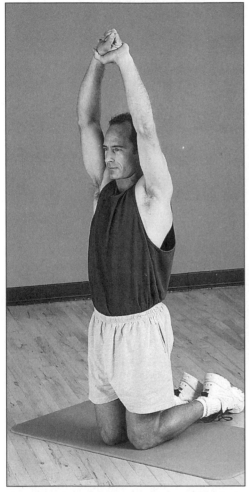

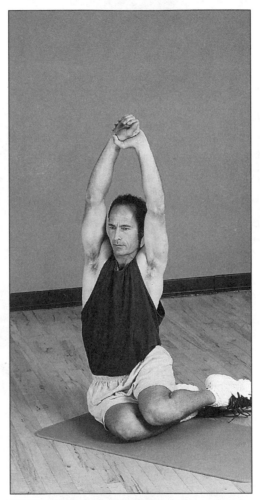

DO IT BETTER
• The exercise is extremely effective, but only when done with control. Do the movements slowly, without rocking or jerking.
• For the workout to be most effective, keep your arms fully extended and your torso straight.
• To increase difficulty, increase the frequency of repetitions. Be sure to move your body through the entire range of motion.

Kneel on a mat with your arms extended above your head, your left hand holding your right wrist. Maintain a straight upper body, keeping your head aligned with your spine.

Sit back on your heels. Lower your buttocks to the right until the right side of your butt and hip touch the floor. Hold for a second, then pull your torso up using your arms, obliques, and quadriceps. Return to the starting position with your torso centered over your hips. Switch hand positions, so that your right hand is holding your left wrist, and repeat to the left side.

Lying Leg Raises
RATING: EASY

In runners and soccer players particularly, hip pain may be caused by a tight iliotibial band—a tendinous band that runs from the ilium (the main hipbone) to the tibia (the shinbone). This is one of the few exercises that will stretch this band. At the same time, it stretches and strengthens the external quadriceps (front thigh), hip flexor (front hip), and oblique (side abdominal) muscles.

DO IT BETTER
• To prevent injury to the neck, don't pull on your head while doing the exercise.
• If you have injured your neck in the past, do this exercise without holding your head up.
• To increase difficulty, wear an ankle weight. Or have a partner press on the side of your shin as you perform the movement.

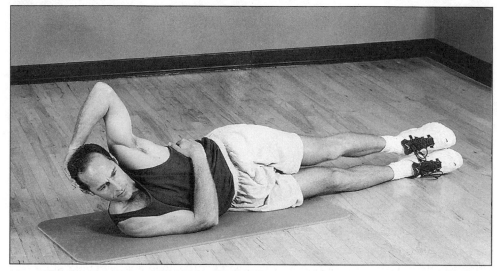

Lie on the floor on your right side, with your legs straight and aligned with your upper body and your toes pointed. Bend your left arm and reach behind your head, gently cupping the right side of your head just behind your right ear. Keep your right arm in front of your body. It should be bent at a 90-degree angle, right hand placed on your left side.

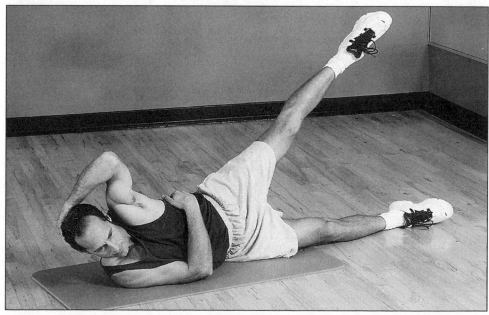

Raise your left leg as high as you comfortably can while using your oblique muscle to hold your head and torso up. Hold for a second at the top, then slowly return to the starting position. Finish a set, then switch sides and repeat.

Lying Leg Kicks

RATING: EASY

This is one of the few leg exercises that can be done comfortably by people with lower back pain. In fact, it is often recommended to help relieve back pain. Because of the position, it puts little stress on the lower back, while still stretching and strengthening the hamstring (back thigh) and gluteal (butt) muscles.

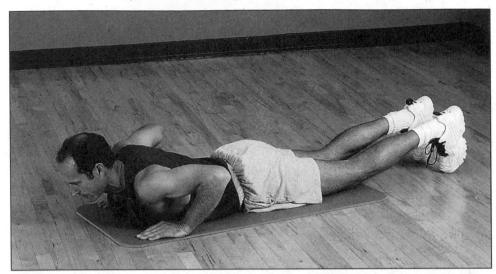

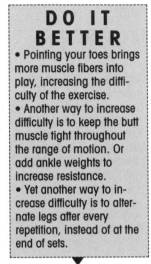

DO IT BETTER

• Pointing your toes brings more muscle fibers into play, increasing the difficulty of the exercise.
• Another way to increase difficulty is to keep the butt muscle tight throughout the range of motion. Or add ankle weights to increase resistance.
• Yet another way to increase difficulty is to alternate legs after every repetition, instead of at the end of sets.

Lie facedown on the floor and support your upper body on your hands, with your elbows bent and close to your body. Your head should be in line with your spine, with your upper chest and shoulders off the floor.

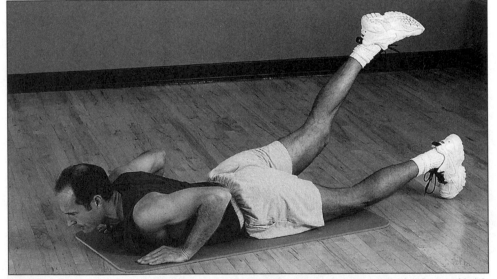

With the knee slightly bent, raise your right leg as far as it will comfortably go. Hold for a second, then slowly return to the starting position. Finish the set, then switch sides and work the other leg.

Midbody Circuit

If you do anything more vigorous than lying in bed all day, then a strong midsection is essential. The following workout was designed by Dragomir Cioroslan, head coach of the U.S. Weightlifting Federation and the 1996 U.S. Olympic weightlifting team, to provide a superb workout for the abdominal and lower back muscles. When doing this workout, be sure to do the exercises in the order given. You always want to start with exercises that involve the greatest number of large muscles and joints, and then finish up with exercises that work single joints and smaller muscle groups.

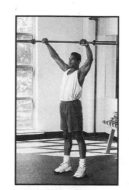

1. High Pull Extensions (page 224)

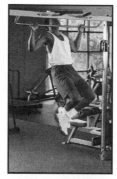

2. Chin-Ups (page 225)

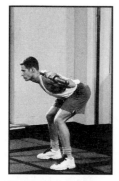

3. Good Mornings (page 222)

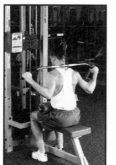

4. Lat Pull-Downs (page 219)

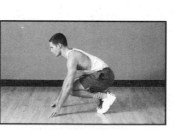

5. Jumping Flexions and Extensions of the Hips (page 213)

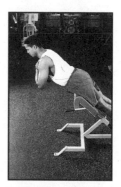

6. Back Extensions (page 228)

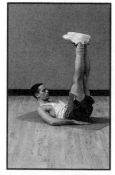

7. Straight-Leg Raises (page 202)

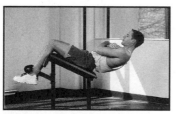

8. Roman Chair Sit-Ups (page 204)

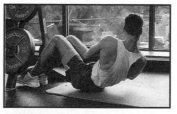

9. Oblique Trunk Rotations (page 209)

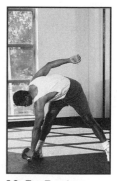

10. Toe Touches (page 231)

PART VII
UPPER-BODY WORKOUTS

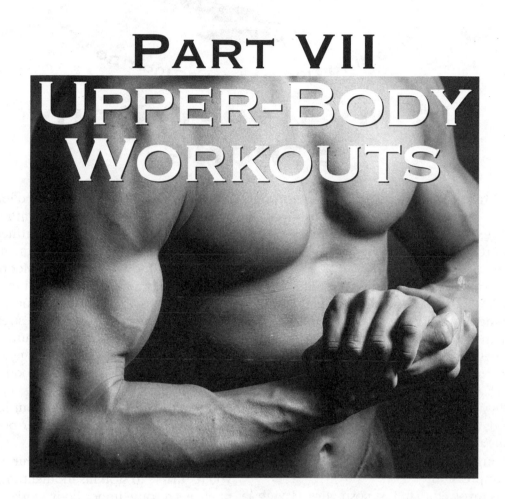

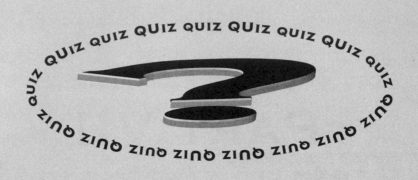

IS MY UPPER BODY STRONG?

Something all Americans have in common, one of those experiences that brings us together as a people, is wondering whether the news anchors on television look as good in person as they do on the screen.

Not a chance. The dirty little secret of TV news is what a lot of the stars look like when they stand up after the newscast is over. Their bottoms are wider than their shoulders, and their legs are about 2 feet shorter than you would expect.

The point here isn't to make fun. After all, these folks are no more or less fit than the rest of us. But they know a lot about what makes people look good, and it's no accident that the camera's view stops above the waist. Having an upper body that's strong and in shape conveys a powerfully positive impression.

More is involved than just cosmetics. Having a strong chest, arms, and shoulders is an immeasurable asset, whether you're hauling garbage cans or changing a tire. Conversely, having too little upper-body strength means that other parts of your body, especially the lower back, take on more work than they're designed to handle.

Is your upper body strong? Take this quiz to find out.

1. You come home from work, and your five-year-old son comes charging downstairs and leaps into your arms. Can you catch him and hoist him up over your head in one smooth motion without doing serious damage to yourself?

"A five-year-old is a pretty good load, especially considering the momentum from his run," says Marjorie Albohm, a certified athletic trainer and director of sports medicine at Kendrick Memorial Hospital in Mooresville, Indiana. "Ideally, you'd want to lift him using your legs, but if he's coming at you quickly and unexpectedly, you may have to rely on strength."

If you can make the lift, hold him aloft for 20 seconds, and set him back down gently with no soreness the next day, you have good upper-body strength.

If you can lift him okay, but your lower back is a bit sore the next day, your upper-body strength is about average.

If your son goes flying over your head because you're unable to stop his momentum, you definitely need some upper-body work.

2. Ever since your nephew joined the wrestling team, he has been acting like a Stallone clone. He thinks he's stronger, faster, and badder than anyone else at school, and now he's coming after you. He wants to bet $10 that he can do one more push-up than you can. You've always had good upper-body strength, and you're pretty sure you can beat the cocky little guy. Should you take the bet?

Push-ups are a great test of strength and muscular endurance, says John Porcari, Ph.D., an exercise physiologist and executive director of the La Crosse Exercise and Health Program at the University of Wisconsin in La Crosse. "If you do a few push-ups and you're breathing hard, that means your muscles are unfit," he says.

There's no question that as men get older, they begin losing upper-body strength. But if you've kept yourself fit, you shouldn't have a problem giving the kid a run for his money. Assuming you're 35 years old, here's the measure.

- **35 or more push-ups: You're in good shape.**
- **16 to 34 push-ups: You're in average shape.**
- **15 push-ups or less: You're in poor shape—and should limit the bet to $1, tops.**

3. You have just bought a house without central air. Now that summer is coming on, it's time to descend to the basement to uncover the air conditioner, haul the monster back upstairs, and heft it into the living-room window. The problem, of course, is that the unit is bulky, and it weighs about 100 pounds. Are you up for the job, or should you call in some friends?

More is involved than just upper-body strength. Just getting the thing off the floor is going to call on the legs, hips, and lower back—pretty much the same muscles needed when doing squats, says Frank Eksten, strength coordinator in the Department of Athletics and visiting lecturer in kinesiology at Indiana University in Bloomington. "You should be able to squat your own body weight," Eksten says. "Maybe not the first time, but it's a goal that can be easily obtained." If you can't even get the thing off the floor, assuming you don't have an injury of some kind, you certainly need some work.

Once you're standing upright with the air conditioner in your arms, you'll need to heft it into the window. This is where you'll certainly need a fair bit of upper-body strength. Most men, says Eksten, should be able to do it without too much trouble. "If you can't do it without getting some help, then you're probably not at a very good level of fitness."

4. Can you make love as long as you would like?

Unlike some of the convoluted positions that you might find in the *Kama Sutra*, the missionary position doesn't demand a lot of upper-body strength. "What's called for here is basically stabilization—using the muscles to prevent fatigue," Albohm says.

If you can go through a full-length sexual encounter in the missionary position without once thinking about your arms, congratulations: Your upper body and your sexual stamina are both in fine condition.

If you find yourself switching positions solely because your arms and shoulders are getting tired, you definitely need some upper-body work.

5. A friend just cut down a dead tree in his yard, and he has offered you free wood for your fireplace if you're willing to come and get it. Can you load a cord of hardwood without spending the next three days in bed?

"Loading wood is tricky because it's so heavy and so monotonous," Albohm says. "That's a setup for injury because the repetitiveness of it lulls you into forgetting to lift with your legs. Unless you have good body strength, that means you're going to compromise your back."

If you can load the wood with no injuries and no soreness the next day, your upper-body strength is good.

If you have average upper-body strength, you'll get the wood to your garage, but for the next few days your back and shoulder muscles will remind you of the extra burden that you have put them through.

If you have poor upper-body strength, you're probably going to throw your back out—and wind up paying the teenager next door to load the wood.

WHY UPPER-BODY STRENGTH MATTERS
SAVING YOUR BODY, KEEPING YOUR LOOKS

When you stand in front of a mirror, what do you see? The first thing that men tend to focus on—sometimes with satisfaction, more often not—is their bellies. After that, the areas of most concern are the biceps, shoulders, and chest. "Beach muscles," one trainer calls them, and in every weight room in America, you can bet those are the body parts that most men are working on.

While vanity fuels much of the attention that we give our upper bodies, there are other reasons for keeping them strong. "We don't think of needing upper-body strength in a lot of things we do, especially if we have desk jobs," says Marjorie Albohm, a certified athletic trainer and director of sports medicine at Kendrick Memorial Hospital in Mooresville, Indiana. "But once we get outside or start doing sports or hobbies, having it contributes immensely. Also, the more efficient we can make our upper bodies, the less energy we will expend. We'll have a greater quality of life."

This last point was confirmed in research conducted by Gary Hunter, Ph.D., professor of exercise physiology at the University of Alabama at Birmingham. In one study, people in their sixties and seventies walked on a treadmill while holding a box of containers filled with water. The amount of water varied; the idea was to make it heavy enough that people were carrying about 40 percent of their maximum capacity—roughly, the same load they would move by carrying a heavy bag of groceries.

These same people then embarked on a strength-training program that included bench presses, overhead presses, and arm curls. After 16 weeks, the amount of effort needed to hold the containers of water was reduced by about half. What's more, their blood pressures and heart rates declined dramatically.

What this study shows is that having a fit upper body allows you to complete everyday tasks with less stress, both on your muscles and on your cardiovascular system. "A younger man might not have any problem lifting a bag of groceries," Dr. Hunter says, "but a 50-pound bag of fertilizer is a different story. If you can do those sorts of jobs more easily, it will reduce wear and tear on your heart."

Preventing Pain

An important benefit of upper-body strength is that it helps you avoid some particularly troublesome injuries. As a trainer and physical therapist, Albohm deals daily with repetitive-stress injuries such as bursitis and tendinitis. Repetitive-stress injuries result from any kind of activity—from word processing to tennis—that subjects muscles, tendons, and ligaments to consistent stress. Joints, especially shoulders, are particularly vulnerable.

Not surprisingly, arms, shoulders, necks, and backs are more resilient and resistant to injury when they're strong and in good condition. "If you have good upper-body strength," Albohm says, "you'll be able to prevent these problems—and that means preventing time lost from your job."

There's no question that keeping your upper body strong can go a long way toward saving your lower back. Back pain is one of the most pervasive health problems in America. Even if you make a conscious effort to lift heavy objects carefully, no one does it correctly every time. Having good upper-body strength will help you weather those lapses because it will compensate for the extra strain that you're putting on your lower back.

Appearances Count

Most of us feel a little guilty when it comes to worrying about our appearance. This may have something to do with our Judeo-Christian heritage—sinful pride, and all that. But in truth, feeling good about how you look can vastly improve your self-confidence, and self-confidence in today's competitive world is nothing to take lightly. "We need to be realistic and acknowledge that a fit appearance is important," Albohm says. "Upper-body strength has a lot to do with that, especially for men."

There are many ways in which a strong upper body can give your self-image a little shot of adrenaline. For starters, research shows that people make a better impression when they stand straight and tall without slouching. Having strong shoulder and upper back muscles makes it easier to maintain that upright bearing, says Dragomir Cioroslan, head coach of the U.S. Weightlifting Federation and the 1996 U.S. Olympic weightlifting team.

For those with a little extra weight around their middles, a strong upper body can provide a valuable optical illusion: When men with well-developed chests and shoulders stand up straight, the stomach seems to shrink.

"Why do you think women like to wear puffy shoulder pads?" says Thomas R. Baechle, Ed.D., professor and chairman of exercise science at

What Women Want

In pursuit of love, men spend untold amounts of time building their biceps, broadening their chests, and strengthening their backs. The general feeling is that a buff upper body, like nectar in a rose, is what attracts the female of the species.

Research suggests, however, that women aren't as interested in the shape of men's bodies as men are in theirs. In his book What She Wants: A Man's Guide to Women, Curtis Pesmen notes that while women may admire a buffed rhomboid from afar, what turns them on up close is more likely to be the look in a man's eyes, the sound of his voice, or the feel of his handshake.

"Women may want mystery and fantasy in their 'stars,'" Pesmen writes, "but they prefer approachability and sensuality in the men they actually take as their lovers."

Women have many different ideas about what makes men attractive, and these ideas often have little to do with bulging pecs. "I pay more attention to the eyes, hands, and butt than the arms and chest," says Petrina Dawson, a lawyer from Mountain Lakes, New Jersey. Wyatt Townley, an editor and poet who lives in the Midwest, lets her eyes drift farther south. "I'm weird," she says, "but I've always been fascinated by the curvature of men's calves."

Pam Black, a business writer in New York City, says that she likes arms and chests well enough, but that massively developed upper bodies are a definite turnoff. "When I see the men at the gym who are the real bodybuilders, I don't find that attractive. It's too pumped up and intimidating."

Creighton University in Omaha, Nebraska, and co-author of *Weight Training: Steps to Success.* "If your shoulders are wider, it makes your stomach look trimmer."

Men's suits are padded in the shoulders, just as women's are, says Warren Christopher, clothing and grooming editor for *Men's Health* magazine. It's not as obvious, usually, but there's enough filler in there to create the illusion of a fuller upper body.

In particular, tailored clothing is designed with proper posture in mind. "It will be easier for you to get a good fit if you're in good condition," Christopher says. "If you are standing tall and have good posture, the jacket will hang correctly."

What to Be Careful Of
Balance Is Essential

A lot of us spend a lot of our workout time focusing on exercises that develop our chests, shoulders, and arms. That's fine up to a point, but all that upper-body work can, if you're not careful, cause some problems.

Chief among those problems are overuse injuries, which include tendinitis, bursitis, and muscle strain. You often won't feel the pain from overuse injuries right away.

What you will keep are the days (or weeks) of soreness. The most vulnerable spots are the big joints: the wrists, elbows, and especially the shoulders. Many trainers will tell you that some of the most common overuse injuries occur in men doing too much upper-body work. In fact, overuse injuries are far more common than acute injuries such as spraining an ankle or dislocating a shoulder.

"Acute injuries do happen in the weight room," adds Frank Eksten, strength coordinator in the Department of Athletics and visiting lecturer in kinesiology at Indiana University in Bloomington. "But they're rare."

Knowing how to avoid serious injuries is self-evident. Not so obvious (because the damage is more subtle) are ways to prevent the micro-tears in muscle fibers caused by overuse. Here are a few tips.

GET THE BLOOD FLOWING. "Sometimes in the gym I see someone walk in and, with no warm-up whatsoever, go over to the bench press, lie down, and start pressing away," says Eksten. "You have to warm up before an exercise."

He recommends doing a two-phase warm-up before working your upper body. First, get your whole system ticking by doing 5 minutes of aerobic exercise: riding a stationary bike, jumping rope, jogging, running in place—whatever will get your heart going and cause you to break a sweat.

Once that's done, warm up the muscles that you'll be working. For example, if you're going to be benching, do a set without adding weight to the bar, or you can do calisthenics that target the specific muscles. For the chest, a set of push-ups is a good starting place.

STAY IN BALANCE. The body is a finely balanced mechanism that can easily be thrown out of kilter by exercising one muscle while neglecting its counterpart. That happens a lot with upper-body work, when men are often thinking more about how good their bodies look than how effectively they are functioning.

"We see a lot of injuries when people overdevelop the quadriceps and neglect the hamstrings," says Eksten. "Or they overwork the chest and neglect the upper back muscles. They get imbalances of opposing muscle groups, which lead to injuries because that changes the biomechanics of the body."

SPREAD IT OUT. Just as you always want to work each muscle's counterpart, it's also good to take care of the rest of your body. For example, if your routine consists of 10 exercises that work the chest and none that hit the legs or back, chances are you're going to start hurting. It's okay (desirable, actually) to concentrate exercises on one particular target area, but only if you're also taking care of overall conditioning.

Barbell Curls

RATING: MODERATELY DIFFICULT

If you want to develop massive, well-defined arms, this exercise is a must. It concentrates energy on the biceps, the large muscle group located mainly in the upper arms.

DO IT BETTER

• Keep the bar under tight control using only your biceps; swinging the bar or using other muscles to assist reduces its effectiveness.

• Standing with your back against a wall will help keep your upper body straight.

• To protect your elbow joints, don't bounce the bar at the bottom of the curl. Keep the motion smooth and fluid.

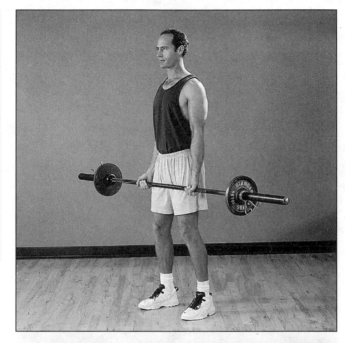

Stand with your feet shoulder-width apart, knees slightly flexed. Hold the barbell with your palms facing up and spaced slightly more than shoulder-width apart. Your arms should be fully extended, with the bar resting lightly on your upper thighs.

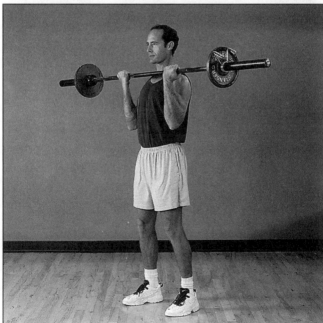

Keeping your upper arms close to your sides, curl the barbell toward your collarbone. Pause for a second at the top of the curl, then lower the bar to the starting position.

Preacher Curls

RATING: DIFFICULT

As with standing curls, this exercise works the biceps (front of upper arm). Because it keeps the upper arms stabilized, however, it provides maximum stress, making each repetition more efficient. And because it's done sitting, it's easier on your back than standing curls.

Sit on the bench with your arms hanging over the platform. Your elbows should be low on the platform, with your armpits almost touching the pad. Hold the curling bar with your palms facing upward and your hands spaced closer than shoulder-width apart.

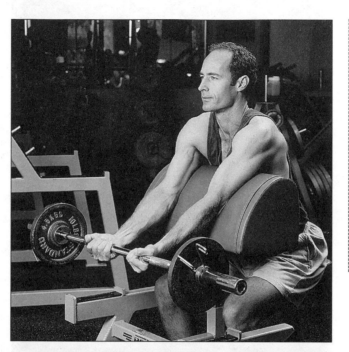

DO IT BETTER
• Keep your elbows and upper arms in contact with the platform throughout the exercise. This prevents the back and shoulders from coming into play, focusing stress on the biceps.
• Keep your wrists straight to prevent unnecessary strain on the joints.
• Don't let your arms overextend at the bottom of the curl, which could cause injury to the elbow joints.

Keeping your upper arms in contact with the pad, curl the bar toward your chin. Hold for a second, then slowly lower to the starting position.

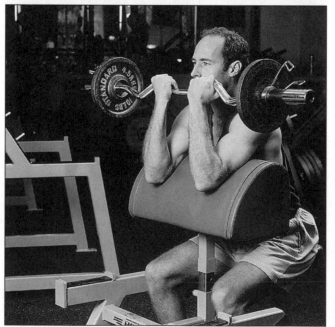

Reverse Grip Biceps Curls

RATING: EASY TO MODERATELY DIFFICULT

This exercise complements standard biceps curls by working the muscles from a slightly different angle. Working muscle groups from different angles gives them more balance, resulting in a more pleasing symmetry. It also makes them stronger and less prone to injury.

DO IT BETTER

• To increase the difficulty of this exercise, use a narrower grip, moving your hands closer together on the bar.
• Another way to increase difficulty is to do this exercise on a preacher bench.
• Don't sway during lifting because the resulting momentum brings other muscles into play, reducing stress on the biceps. Jerking or swaying also increases the risk of injury.

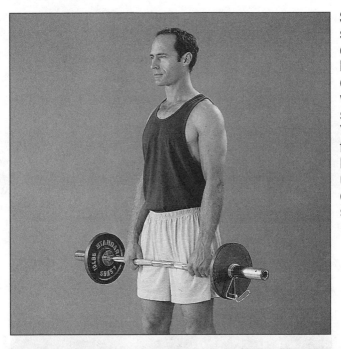

Stand with your feet shoulder-width apart and your knees slightly bent. Hold the barbell in an overhand grip with your hands spaced shoulder-width apart. Your arms should be fully extended with the bar resting against your upper thighs. Keep your elbows close to your sides.

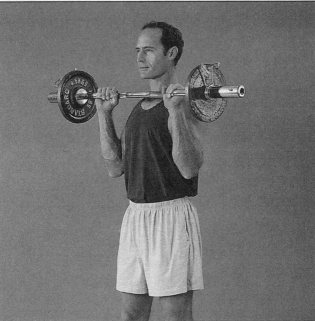

Curl the bar toward your collarbone. Pause at the top for a second, then slowly lower the bar to the starting position.

Cable Curls
RATING: EASY TO MODERATELY DIFFICULT

The biceps consist of three muscle groups: the biceps brachii (front of upper arm), the brachialis (outside of upper arm), and the brachioradialis (upper forearm). This exercise works all three groups. To do this exercise, you need a low pulley on a multi-station weight machine.

Stand facing the pulley with your feet shoulder-width apart and about 1½ feet away from the pulley. Keep your knees flexed and your back straight. Hold the bar using an underhand grip. Your shoulders should lean back slightly.

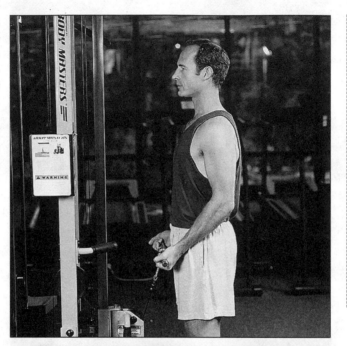

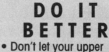

DO IT BETTER
• Don't let your upper arms move away from your body, which will reduce stress on the biceps.
• To maximize your range of motion and increase flexibility, start each curl with your arms fully extended.
• This exercise tends to pull the body forward. Keeping your chest out and your shoulders back will maximize the benefits.
• For added difficulty, attach a loop handle to the cable and perform this exercise one arm at a time.

Keeping your upper arms tight against your body, slowly curl the bar toward your chin. Pause for a second at the top, then slowly lower the bar to the starting position.

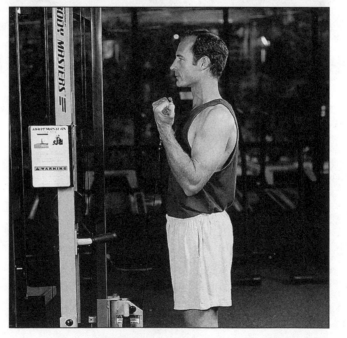

Alternating Biceps Curls
RATING: MODERATELY DIFFICULT

The twisting motion of this curl works not only the biceps (front of upper arm) muscles but also the forearm supinator muscle, increasing overall arm strength and stability. Also, the alternating curls permit you to concentrate on one set of muscles at a time, thus maximizing the workout of each arm.

DO IT BETTER

• To decrease difficulty, this exercise can be performed in a seated position on the edge of a bench. Arm position and lifting technique remain the same.

• To increase difficulty and improve your range of motion, rotate your wrists at the top of the lift, turning them outward to the sides of your body.

• Keeping your upper arms close to your body and your elbows stationary will maximize stress on the target muscles.

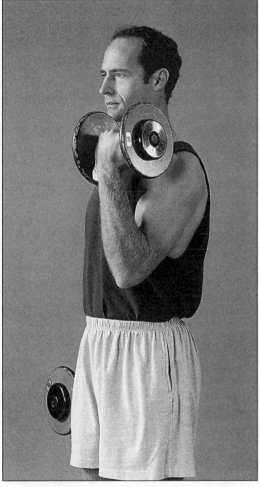

Stand straight with your feet shoulder-width apart and your knees slightly flexed. Hold a dumbbell in each hand with your arms down at your sides and the palms facing in. Slowly curl the left dumbbell up toward your collarbone. As you do the curl, rotate your arm so the palm faces up. Pause for a second at the top of the lift, then slowly lower the weight to the starting position.

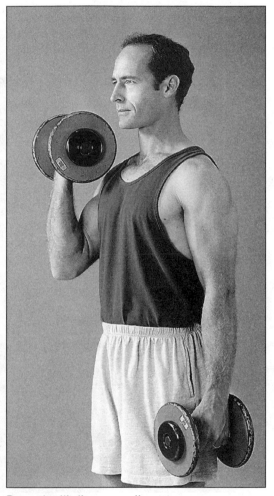

Repeat with the opposite arm.

Hammer Curls

RATING: EASY

If you have ever pounded a nail, you know how to do this exercise. Unlike regular biceps curls, in which the palms turn upward as you lift, there is no twisting movement involved with this exercise. It's particularly good for isolating and building the biceps (front of upper arm) muscles.

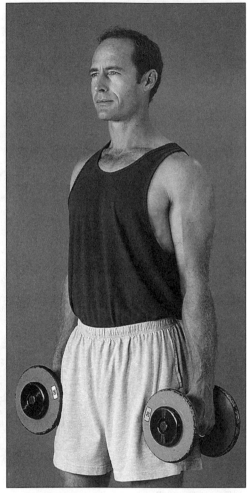

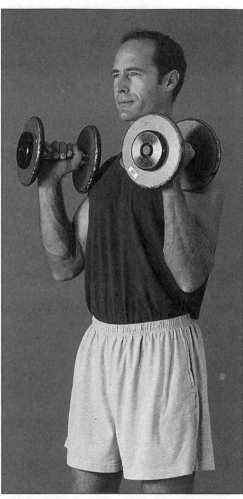

DO IT BETTER

• Maintain strict control during the downswing. Allowing the dumbbells to bounce at the extended position can injure the elbows.

• To decrease the difficulty, do this exercise while sitting.

• Because this exercise utilizes such a simple movement, it is easy to let your mind wander. Don't allow that. Concentrate on what you are doing and squeeze the muscle as you raise your arm. You won't get good results if you just go through the motions.

Stand straight with your feet shoulder-width apart and your knees flexed. Hold a dumbbell in each hand with your arms fully extended down at your sides and the palms facing your thighs.

Keeping your upper arms and elbows stationary, slowly curl the dumbbells until the ends touch your shoulders—don't rotate your wrists. Hold for a second, then slowly lower the dumbbells to the extended position.

Inclined Dumbbell Curls

RATING: MODERATELY DIFFICULT

Don't be fooled by the relaxed position required for this exercise. The reclining position puts a lot of stress on the biceps (front of upper arm) and the supinator muscles near the elbow. And because the bench provides good back support, you're less likely to strain a back muscle than when doing standing curls.

DO IT BETTER

• To increase difficulty and improve your range of motion, rotate your wrists at the top of the lift so that the palms turn outward.

• Keep the weights under constant control; letting your arms swing downward reduces stress on the muscles, making the exercise less effective.

• Keeping your head in contact with the inclined-bench pad will help prevent neck strain.

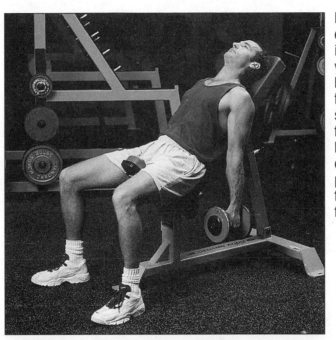

Holding a dumbbell in each hand, sit on the inclined bench, keeping your head and upper body in full contact with the bench. Your feet should be flat on the floor. Let your arms hang down, fully extended and perpendicular to the floor, with your palms facing your body.

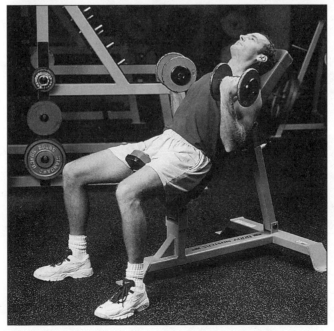

Slowly curl the dumbbells up to your shoulders, keeping your upper arms stationary and your elbows pointed down. Your palms should turn up during the lift until they face your shoulders. Hold for a second at the top, then slowly lower your arms to starting position.

Concentration Curls

RATING: EASY

True to its name, this exercise is very effective at isolating the biceps (front of upper arm) muscles because it allows very little extraneous body movement. Since it works one arm at a time, it maximizes force on the individual muscles.

Sit in a chair or at the end of a weight bench with your feet a little more than shoulder-width apart. Hold a dumbbell in your left hand, palm facing up, with your arm fully extended. Rest your left elbow on your left inner thigh. With your right hand on your right knee, bend forward slightly, keeping your back straight.

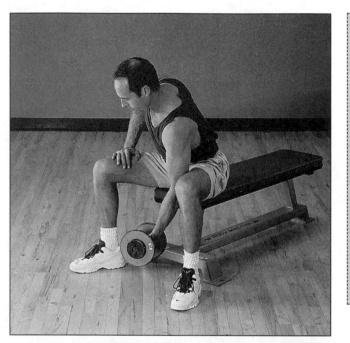

DO IT BETTER

• For better support, brace your elbow and upper arm solidly against your thigh, and lean on your opposite hand.
• To maximize stress on the muscle, don't swing the weight or use your back or shoulders in the lift.
• The leaned-over position required for this exercise makes it easy to slouch—which can cause back and shoulder strain. Keep good posture by concentrating on flattening your lower back and keeping your shoulders down and relaxed.

Curl the dumbbell up toward your shoulder, keeping your upper arm perpendicular to the floor. Hold for a second, then lower the dumbbell to the starting position. Finish the set, then repeat with the other arm.

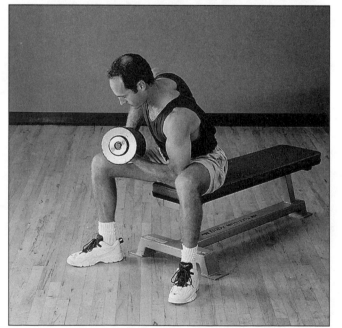

French Curls

RATING: DIFFICULT

This exercise was once known as the nose breaker because the weight was lowered directly over the nose (today, it's lowered toward the top of the head). Even with the change of position, though, this exercise can be dangerous if not done with good control. Use it to develop the three heads of the triceps (back of upper arm) muscles.

DO IT BETTER

• Overhead lifts can be dangerous because a weight could easily slip and hit your face. Begin by using light weights, and preferably a spotter, to prevent accidents.

• Don't arch your back or clench your abdominal muscles when bringing the weight back up.

• If you can't do this exercise without bringing additional muscles into play, use lighter weights so that you can complete the movement using only your arms.

• To increase the overall stability of the elbow joint, substitute light dumbbells for the bar. Using dumbbells requires more coordination, which brings more supporting muscles into play.

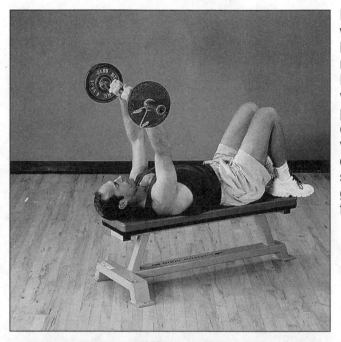

Lie on your back on a weight bench with your knees bent and feet resting on the bench. Hold a curl bar over your chest, with your palms facing up and away from you and your arms fully extended. Your hands should be in a narrow grip position, spaced 4 to 6 inches apart.

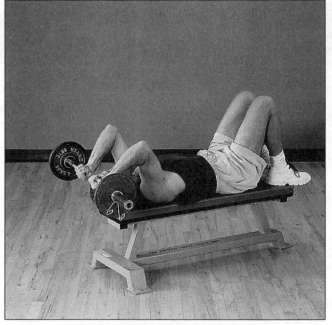

Keeping your upper arms stationary, slowly bend your elbows, lowering the weight toward the top of your head. Then slowly return the bar to the starting position.

Standing Triceps Curls

RATING: MODERATELY DIFFICULT

This exercise employs an unusual grip. Rather than holding the dumbbell by the bar, use both palms to hold it by the end. The two-handed grip provides more control and is safer than the traditional one-handed grip.

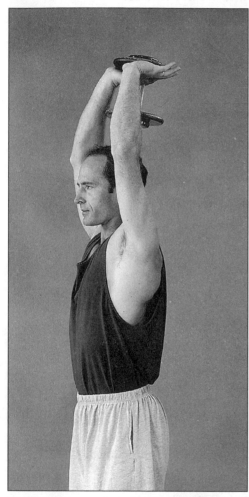

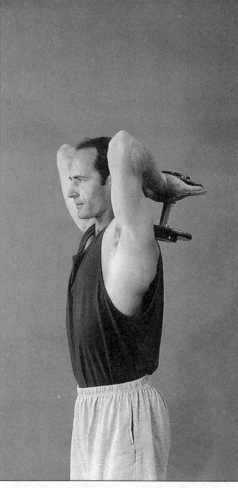

DO IT BETTER
• Doing this exercise while sitting keeps your back more stable and helps reduce the risk of strains.
• Keeping your shoulders down and relaxed while extending your arms will also help prevent strains.
• When using dumbbells with removable plates, make sure the plates are tightly fastened; they can easily slip off when the bar is held in a vertical position.

Stand with your feet shoulder-width apart, your knees slightly bent, and your back straight. Using both hands, hold the dumbbell over your head, with your thumbs around the bar and the weight resting on your palms. The bar should be perpendicular to the ground. Start with your arms fully extended over your head, keeping your shoulders relaxed and your head up.

Keeping your upper arms close to your head, lower the dumbbell behind your head as far as it will go. Hold for a second, then raise to the fully extended position.

Lying Triceps Extensions
RATING: DIFFICULT

This exercise works both the triceps (back of upper arm) and the anconeus, a short, triangular muscle that helps straighten the elbow.

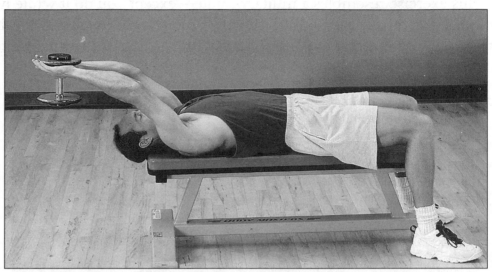

Lie on your back with your head slightly extended over the end of a weight bench, with your feet flat on the floor. Hold a dumbbell with both hands, with your thumb around the bar and the weight resting on your palms. Fully extend your arms at a slightly greater than 45-degree angle, with the weight over the top of your head. Keep the bar perpendicular to the ground.

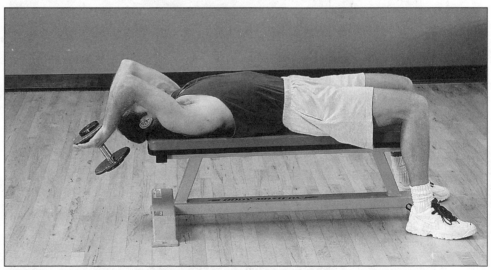

Keeping your upper arms stationary, slowly bend your elbows, lowering the weight until it is behind your head. Hold for a second, then slowly return to the starting position.

Lying Cross-Shoulder Triceps Extensions

RATING: DIFFICULT

This exercise resembles a military salute—except you do it while lying on your back. It looks deceptively easy, but it's actually quite tough. The across-the-body movement is strenuous and difficult to control. Start with a lighter-than-usual weight until you get the hang of it.

Lie on a bench with your head near one end, keeping your knees bent and your feet flat on the floor. Hold a dumbbell in your right hand, with your arm extended straight up from your body and your palm facing your feet.

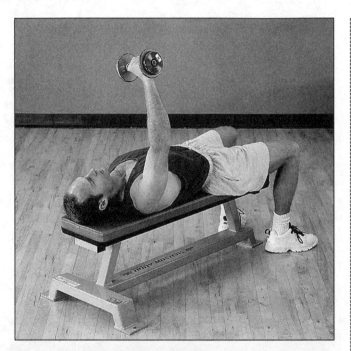

DO IT BETTER

- Overhead lifts can be dangerous if elbows collapse or the weight is dropped, so be sure to use light weight and a spotter, if possible, when first attempting this movement.
- Use a spotter, when possible, whenever using heavy weights. This can prevent injury to your shoulders and/or face.
- To produce a greater stretch in the triceps and a more powerful muscle contraction, you must keep your upper arm and elbow stationary as you do this exercise.
- Completely straighten your arm at the extended phase of the exercise to produce maximum development.

Keeping your upper arm and elbow stationary, slowly lower the dumbbell across your upper chest until the end touches your left shoulder. Slowly extend your arm back to the starting position. Finish the set, then repeat with the other arm.

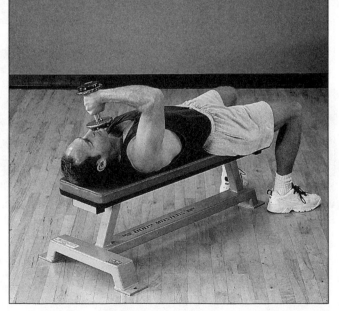

Triceps Push-Downs

RATING: MODERATELY DIFFICULT

Triceps exercises are a great preliminary to a chest workout because these muscles work with the chest when lifting weights on the bench. This is an excellent all-around exercise that works all three heads of the triceps (back of upper arm) muscle. To do this exercise, you need a high pulley cable, which is usually part of a multistation weight machine.

DO IT BETTER

• It's a good idea to regularly change handgrips (or use different handles). By changing the angle at which you work the muscles, you'll develop more balance and power.
• To get the most benefit, push down only with your arms—don't bring the upper body into play.
• To prevent elbow injury, don't forcefully extend your elbows at the bottom of the extension. Straighten your arms slowly to a point where you're comfortable, but not beyond that.

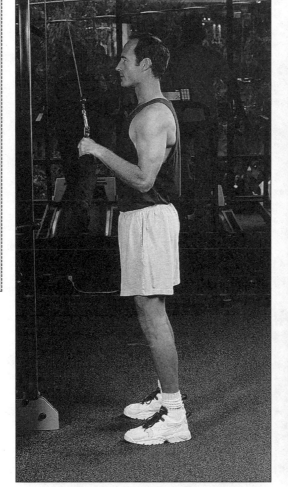

Stand facing the overhead pulley cable, with your legs shoulder-width apart and knees slightly bent. Hold the bar with both hands in a narrow grip, palms facing down. Hold the bar about chest high, keeping your elbows and upper arms close to your body.

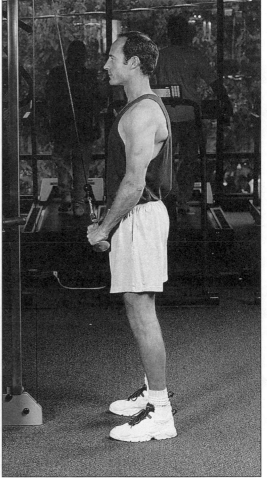

Slowly and smoothly extend your elbows, pressing the bar down as far as you can. Keep your wrists locked and straight. Hold for a second at the fully straightened position, then slowly allow the bar to rise to the starting position.

Triceps Pull-Downs

RATING: EASY TO MODERATELY DIFFICULT

This exercise works the entire triceps, but it's especially good for strengthening the lateral head, which is on the outer back part of your upper arm. This exercise calls for a high pulley, which is found on most multistation weight machines.

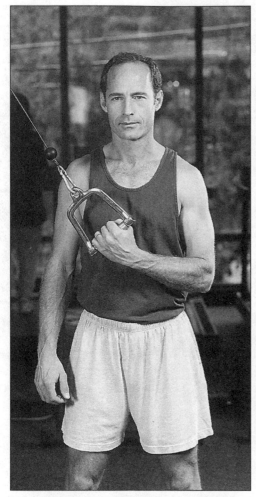

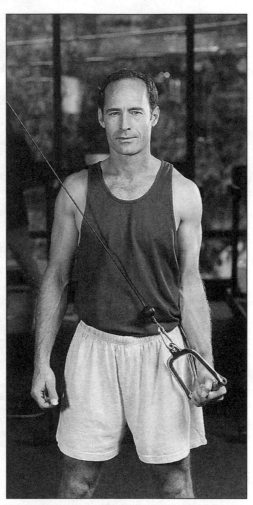

DO IT BETTER

• Resist the temptation to lean into the pull, which allows the stomach or shoulders to assist the lift.

• It's important to fully extend and contract your arm in a slow, controlled manner. If you can't do this movement without jerking or swaying, move to a lighter weight.

Stand sideways in front of the overhead pulley, with your right shoulder closest to the equipment. Your legs should be shoulder-width apart with your knees slightly bent. Grip the pulley handle with your left hand, palm facing you. Keep your upper arm vertical with your elbow bent at about 90 degrees. Step back from the machine and bend forward slightly at the hips, keeping your back straight.

Slowly pull the handle down across your body until your arm is fully extended. Hold for a second, then slowly return to the starting position.

Dumbbell Kickbacks

RATING: MODERATELY DIFFICULT TO DIFFICULT

The term *kickback* is used to suggest a monetary payoff of some sort. It's an appropriate name for this exercise, which is so tough that you may find yourself wanting someone to pay you for doing it. Because this exercise isolates the triceps (back of upper arm) muscles, you don't get much help from the surrounding muscles; it's a challenge to maintain good form and control.

DO IT BETTER

- Keep your shoulders down and relaxed but not hunched; hunching causes the back to curve, putting strain on the shoulders and neck.
- Make sure that the bench supporting your free hand is low enough to keep your back horizontal, which will help prevent injuries.
- If you can't move the weight with complete control, without swinging, go to the next lighter weight.

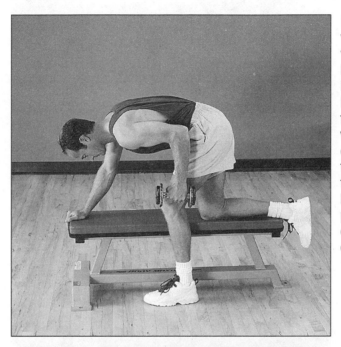

Holding a dumbbell in your left hand, support yourself on an exercise bench with your right knee and your right hand. Keep your left foot on the ground, with your back straight and parallel to the floor. The arm holding the dumbbell should be bent with your elbow pointing toward the ceiling and the weight close to your rib cage.

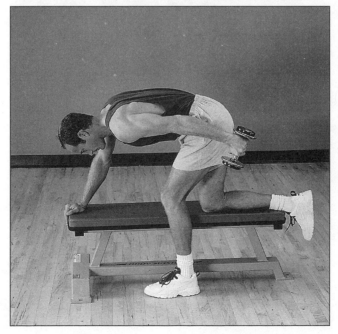

Straighten your left arm and extend the weight behind your body, keeping your upper arm parallel to the ground. You should feel the triceps (back of upper arm) muscles fully contract. Then bend your arm and bring the weight back to the starting position.

Parallel Dips

RATING: DIFFICULT

This tough exercise brings all three heads of the triceps (back of upper arm) muscles into play. You don't need weights, but you will need two exercise benches—or two sturdy chairs.

Place the exercise benches side by side, about 3 to 4 feet apart. With your arms shoulder-width apart and fully extended, hold on to the edge of one bench. Put your heels on the facing bench, suspending your butt slightly forward from your hands.

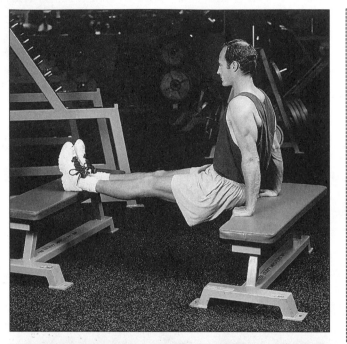

DO IT BETTER
• To increase the difficulty of this movement, put a weight plate across your lap.
• To prevent yourself from slipping, keep about 6 inches of your leg on the bench—don't just put your heels on the edge.
• Keeping your legs straight will help focus the most stress on the triceps.
• To decrease difficulty, allow your heels to rest on the floor instead of on the bench.
• This exercise puts a lot of pressure on the wrists. If you're weak in that area or have had previous injuries, leave this exercise alone.

Slowly bend your arms and lower your body toward the floor. Go as low as you can without touching the floor. Then extend your arms, raising yourself back to the starting position.

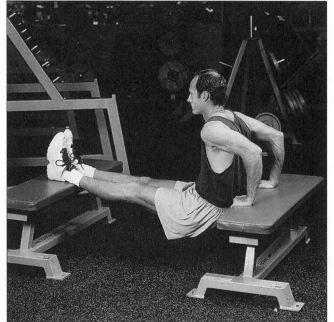

Forearm Curls

RATING: EASY

There's more to developing a tough grip than strengthening the muscles in the hands. You need to work the forearms and wrists as well. This exercise strengthens a series of muscles located in the forearms—the wrist flexors (underside of forearm), hand abductors (inside of forearm), and hand adductors (outside of forearm). Because it strengthens the muscles surrounding the wrists, it also helps prevent injuries.

DO IT BETTER

• Keeping your lifting arm firmly planted against your thigh will focus the most stress on the wrist, making the exercise more effective.
• To work both wrists at once, substitute a barbell for the dumbbells.
• Opening your hands slightly as you lower the weight will help increase your range of motion.

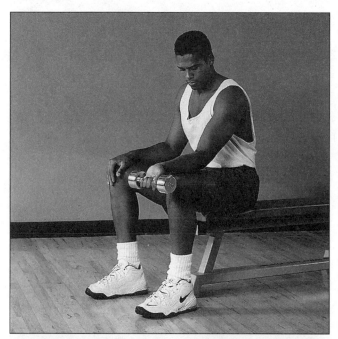

Sit on a weight bench with your legs a little more than hip-width apart. With your palm up, hold a dumbbell in your left hand. Lean your left forearm on your left thigh, with the back of your wrist positioned just slightly over the knee for maximum mobility. Rest your right hand on your right thigh. Keep your body upright, slightly leaning on your left leg for comfort. Allow the left wrist to bend back naturally as the weight pulls it down.

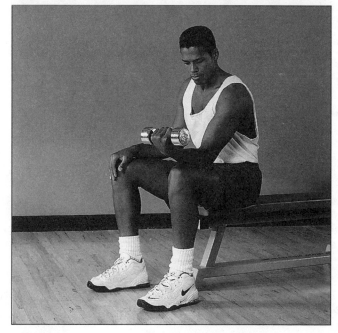

Using the wrist only and keeping the rest of your arm stationary, curl the dumbbell toward your body as far as it will go. Hold for a second, then return to the starting position.

Forearm Extensions

RATING: EASY

When you want a stronger backhand for tennis or racquetball, this exercise can help. Unlike forearm curls, which primarily work the muscles on the inside of the forearm, this exercise works the outer muscles. It's a good idea to do both exercises for developing strength, balance, and flexibility.

Sit on a weight bench with your legs a little more than hip-width apart. Hold a dumbbell in your left hand with your palm down. Lean your left forearm on your left knee, with your wrist positioned just slightly over the knee for maximum mobility. Let your right hand rest on your right thigh. Keep your body upright, slightly leaning on your left leg for comfort. Allow the left wrist to bend naturally as the weight pulls it.

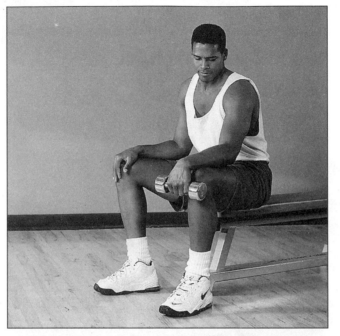

Using the wrist only and keeping the rest of your arm stationary, curl the dumbbell as far as you can. Hold for a second, then return to the starting position.

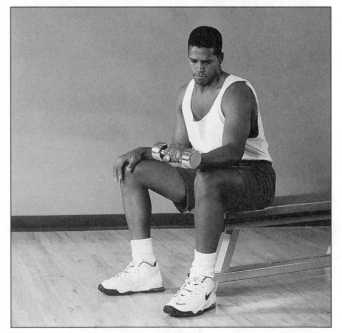

DO IT BETTER

• The muscles worked in this exercise are generally weaker than those on the opposite side of the arm, so you'll want to use a lighter weight than you did for the forearm curl.
• To work both wrists at once, substitute a barbell for the dumbbells.
• To maximize stress on the forearm, keep it on your thigh during the lift.
• As with abdominal and calf muscles, the forearms require regular, long-term workouts to increase in size and strength.

Wrist Rolls

RATING: MODERATELY DIFFICULT TO DIFFICULT

If you're only going to do one wrist exercise, this should be the one. It works muscles in the wrists, fingers, and the outer forearm. To do it, you'll need a wrist roller, which in most gyms is found in the free-weight room. You can also make your own by attaching one end of a 5-foot cord to the middle of a dowel (about 14 inches long), with the other end tied to a weight plate.

DO IT BETTER

• This exercise is surprisingly difficult, so begin by using a light weight.
• Stand against a wall for added support.
• To work the muscles that flex your wrists forward, roll the rod clockwise. Turn it counterclockwise to work the muscles that flex your wrists backward.

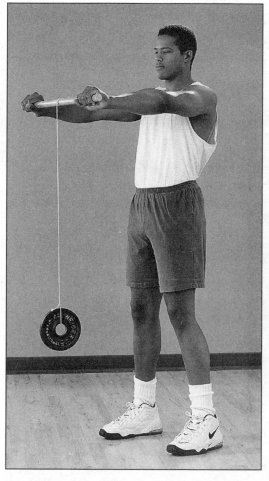

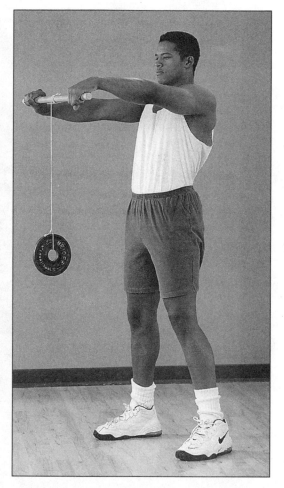

Stand with your feet shoulder-width apart, holding the wrist roller with both hands, arms extended in front of you and parallel to the ground. Grip the roller near the ends, with your palms down. The cord should be completely unwound, with the weight dangling in front of you.

Using your wrists only, slowly roll up the cord, using long, exaggerated twisting movements. Keep your arms up and your body still. When the weight is rolled all the way on the bar, slowly unwind it, letting it return to the starting position.

Grip Strengtheners

RATING: EASY

You need a strong grip not just for lifting weights or playing sports, but also for such things as gardening, playing the piano, and moving furniture. A spring-loaded grip trainer, or gripper, can help. There are two types available: the standard, nonadjusting gripper and the adjustable-resistance type. The adjustable type is best because it allows you to increase the resistance as your strength improves.

Hold the handles between your thumb and fingers. Squeeze the handles together. Slowly release and repeat.

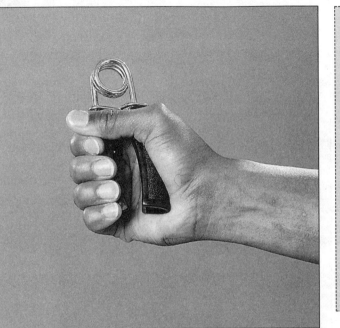

DO IT BETTER

• Squeeze and release the gripper using slow, steady resistance. This will help prevent muscle tears and cramping.
• If you don't have a gripper, a tennis ball will also work.
• To get blood circulating and your hands warmed up, swing your arms several times before gripping.
• Another way to strengthen your grip is with Power Putty. This is a squeezable, claylike putty that comes in different toughnesses for adding (or subtracting) resistance.

Bench Presses

RATING: MODERATELY DIFFICULT

Most men would say that their most important fitness goal, besides trimming their waist, is building a stronger chest. Of all the chest exercises, the bench press is probably the most widely used—and for good reason. It works the pectoralis (chest), deltoids (shoulder), and triceps (back of upper arm) muscles.

DO IT BETTER

- To maximize stress on the chest muscles, keep your elbows pointing out and your chest high.
- Use complete control when lowering the barbell, making sure not to bounce the weight off your chest at the bottom of the lift. Besides cheating on the lift (using momentum makes the lift easier, hence less effective), this can cause back or shoulder strains as well as a bruised chest.
- Avoid arching your back and keep your head on the bench to avoid injury to the neck or back.
- To increase difficulty, use a narrower or wider grip. A narrower grip will work more of your lower and inner pectoralis; a wider grip works more of the upper and outer pecs.

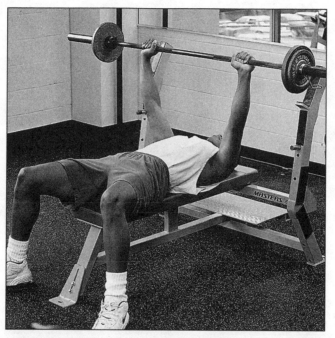

Lie on a weight bench with your head under the barbell rack and your feet flat on the floor. With your arms a bit more than shoulder-width apart, hold the barbell with an overhand grip. Press the barbell off the rack and hold extended at arm's length.

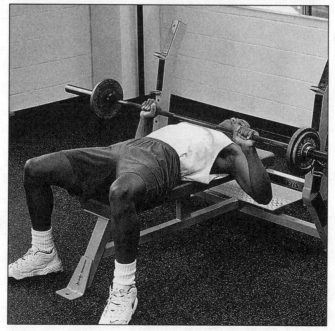

Slowly bend your elbows, lowering the weight to the middle of your chest (about 1 inch below your nipples). Hold for a second, then slowly press the barbell up to the starting position. Hold for a second, then repeat.

Dumbbell Bench Presses

RATING: MODERATELY DIFFICULT

Although the basic movement of this exercise is nearly identical to the bench press, using dumbbells requires your arms to work harder to balance and support the two separate weights. This means the muscles are more fully stressed and developed, and joints become stronger.

Lie flat on a weight bench with a dumbbell in each hand, arms fully extended and perpendicular to the floor. The dumbbells should be almost touching. Your feet should be flat on the floor; your palms should be facing your feet.

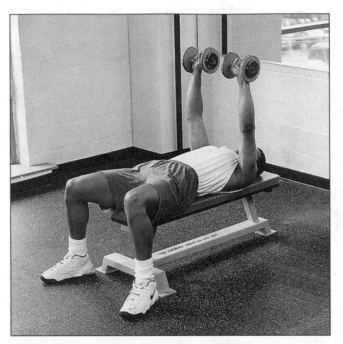

Slowly bend your elbows and lower your arms straight down, until the weights are just above either side of your chest. Pause for a second, then slowly bring your arms back up again. Keep the weights under control, without arching your back or allowing the weights to bounce.

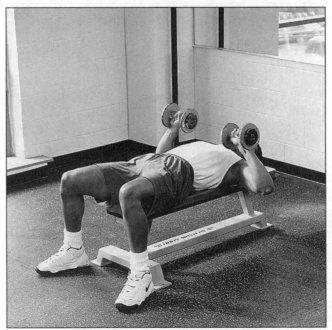

Inclined Bench Presses

RATING: MODERATELY DIFFICULT

This exercise helps build the upper and outer pectoralis (chest) muscles and shoulders. It also works the serratus anterior (located around the upper and outer rib cage)—the so-called boxer's muscle. This muscle is essential for throwing powerful, horizontal punches.

DO IT BETTER

- Wearing a weight belt will provide additional lower back support, helping prevent strains and injuries.
- If you're arching your back to lift the weights, you need to use a lighter weight.
- Keep your hips and head solidly on the bench to prevent neck and back strains.
- To increase difficulty, vary the spacing of your grip. This will stress your muscles from different angles, helping create muscle balance and working the muscles to their fullest capacity.

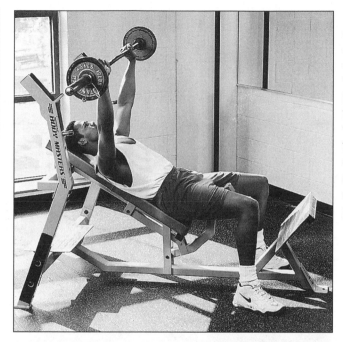

Lie on a 45-degree inclined bench. With your arms shoulder-width apart and palms facing your feet, hold on to the barbell. Keep your back flat on the bench and your feet flat on the floor. Press the weight off the barbell rack and completely extend your arms until they are perpendicular to the floor.

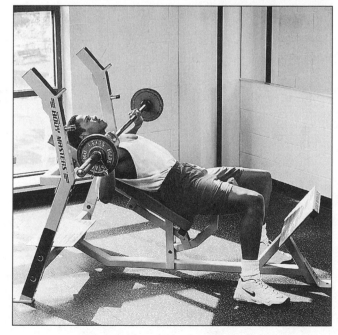

Bend your elbows and slowly lower the barbell to just above your chest, between your shoulders and nipples. Keep your elbows pointing out. Pause for a second, then slowly raise the barbell over your chest again. Use good control and try not to arch your back or bounce the bar off your chest.

Inclined Dumbbell Presses

RATING: MODERATELY DIFFICULT

Another variation of the standard press, this movement works the triceps (back of upper arm) and is especially good for developing the upper pectoralis (chest) muscles. The angle of the inclined bench helps isolate the pecs, putting most of the stress on the upper chest.

Lie on a 45-degree inclined bench with your arms fully extended and perpendicular to the ground. Using an overhand grip, hold a dumbbell in each hand, with your palms facing your feet. Your arms should be shoulder-width apart, your back flat against the bench, and your feet flat on the floor.

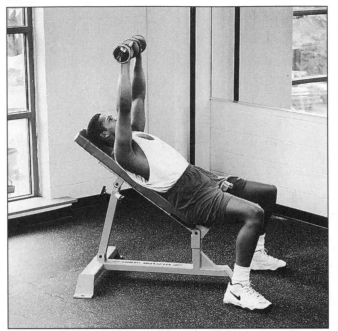

DO IT BETTER

• To support your lower back and prevent injury, it's a good idea to wear a weight belt when doing this exercise.
• This exercise can be dangerous, so always use a spotter when lifting heavy weights.
• To work your pectoralis and deltoids to the fullest, lower your elbows as far as they will go when bringing the weight down.

Slowly lower the weights to your shoulders, keeping your elbows pointing out. Pause for a second, then slowly extend your arms again. Use good control and try not to arch your back or bounce the dumbbells off your chest at the bottom of the lift.

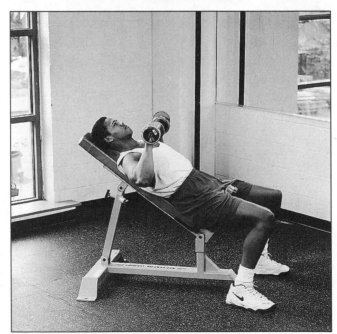

Declined Bench Presses

RATING: DIFFICULT

Changing body position—by lying on a straight, declined, or inclined bench—stresses muscle groups at different angles, leading to good muscle balance. The declined bench causes most of the muscular stress to be exerted on your lower pectoralis (chest) muscles. Because your body is inverted, this is the most difficult—and potentially dangerous—of all the bench presses. Use lighter-than-usual weights and be sure to have a spotter ready to help out.

DO IT BETTER

• Keep your back, head, and shoulders in contact with the bench throughout the exercise to provide maximum support.
• To prevent back strain, avoid bouncing the bar off your chest.
• Periodically changing the spacing of your hands will work the muscles from different angles, helping create more muscle balance and working the muscles to their fullest capacity.

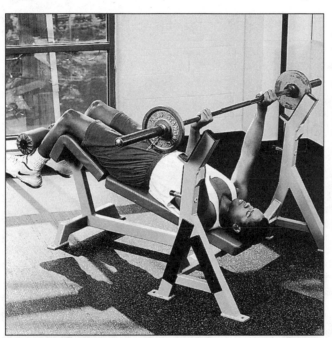

Lie on a declined bench with your head under the barbell rack and your knees over the far end of the bench. Hook your feet under the support pads. With your arms shoulder-width apart, hold the bar using an overhand grip, palms facing your feet. Lift the bar off the rack and hold it straight over your chest.

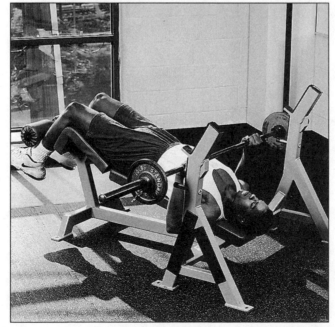

Slowly bend your elbows, lowering the weight to just under your nipples, always keeping your elbows pointed out. Hold for a second and, with control, press the barbell back up, extending it to arm's length.

Dumbbell Flies

RATING: DIFFICULT

Flies are one of the best exercises for developing the middle of the pectoralis major muscles—the big fan-shaped muscles on either side of the breastbone, which cover most of your chest. This exercise also works the minor pecs (underneath the major pecs), the outer deltoids (shoulder), the coracobrachialis (inner upper arm), and the serratus anterior (upper and outer rib cage) muscles.

Holding a dumbbell in each hand, lie on your back on an exercise bench, legs spread and feet flat on the floor. Extend your arms above your chest, perpendicular to the floor, palms facing one another. The dumbbells should be almost touching.

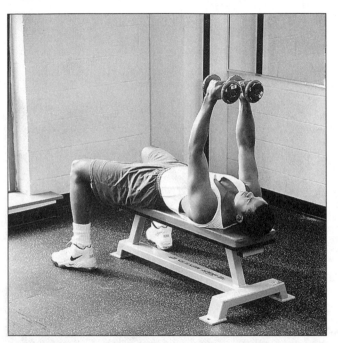

Bending your arms slightly at the elbows, slowly lower the dumbbells to each side of your chest in a semi-circular motion. At the bottom of the lift, the dumbbells should be at shoulder level or slightly lower and in line with your ears. Hold for a moment, then slowly return the dumbbells to the starting position.

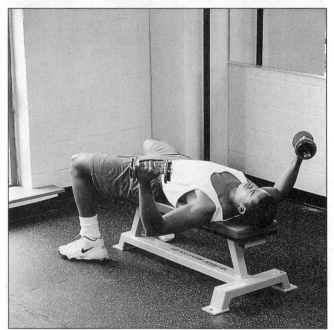

Barbell Overhead Pulls

RATING: DIFFICULT

Although the position for this exercise looks similar to the lying triceps extension, it works different sets of muscles. Specifically, it works both the pectoralis major and minor (chest) muscles, the latissimus dorsi (mid and lower back), and the teres major (below shoulder blade) and rhomboid (upper back) muscles. Use this exercise to improve your stroke in swimming, rowing, or hammering.

DO IT BETTER

• Using a curl bar makes this exercise more comfortable and easier to control.

• To get the maximum amount of stretch in your rib cage, keep your arms as straight as possible when bending them back behind your head.

• To reduce uncomfortable (and potentially dangerous) stress in your arms, bend your elbows a bit more.

• Wearing a weight belt or switching to a lower weight will help keep the back from arching.

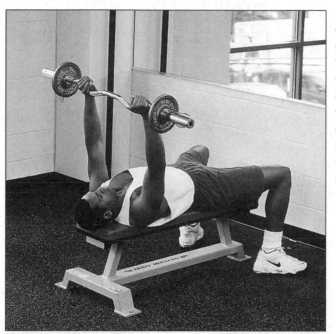

Lie flat on the bench with your feet on the floor on either side. With your palms facing your feet, lift the barbell above your chest until your arms are perpendicular to the floor, keeping your elbows unlocked and slightly bent.

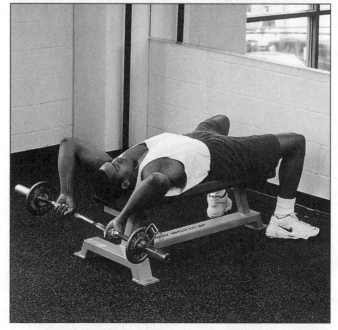

Slowly lower the barbell behind your head in a semicircular motion until your upper arms are parallel to the bench or lower. Hold for a second, then pull the barbell back over your head to the starting position.

Bent-Arm Pullovers

RATING: DIFFICULT

Unlike most exercises using a weight bench, which require you to lie lengthwise, this one has you lying crosswise—quite a challenge to your balancing skills. The change of position puts additional stress on the lower chest and back. Specifically, this exercise works the lower pectoralis major (chest) muscle, and its opposing muscle, the latissimus dorsi (mid and lower back). It also works the teres major (below shoulder blade) muscles, which assist the lats, and the triceps (back of upper arm) muscles.

Lie crosswise on the bench with your head just off the end. Keep your torso straight and your feet flat on the floor. Hold a dumbbell by the end, palms up and thumbs around the bar. Your arms should be extended above your chest, elbows slightly flexed.

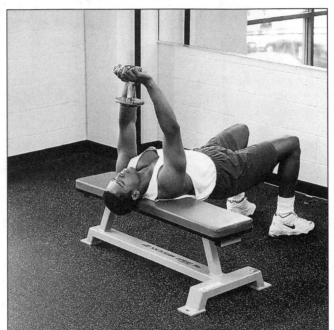

Slowly lower the dumbbell backward over your head until your upper arms are parallel with the floor. Pause for a second, then slowly raise the bar back to the starting position.

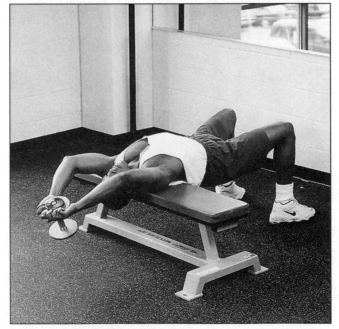

Cable Crossovers

RATING: MODERATELY DIFFICULT

In bodybuilding contests you'll see a pose called the most muscular, which is similar to the ending position for this exercise. It works the pectoralis major and minor (chest) muscles as well as the serratus anterior (upper and outer rib cage) muscle, the anterior deltoids (shoulder), and the coracobrachialis (inner upper arm) muscles. To do cable crossovers, you'll need two overhead cable pulleys.

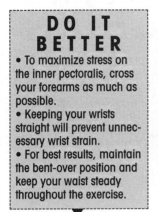

DO IT BETTER

• To maximize stress on the inner pectoralis, cross your forearms as much as possible.
• Keeping your wrists straight will prevent unnecessary wrist strain.
• For best results, maintain the bent-over position and keep your waist steady throughout the exercise.

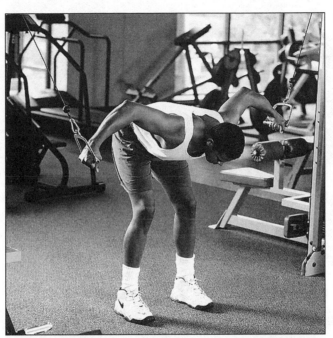

Stand between the overhead pulleys. With your feet shoulder-width apart, grip the handles with your palms down. Bend at the waist so that your upper body is parallel to the floor. Keeping your elbows slightly bent, pull the handles down until they are in line with your shoulders. This is the starting position.

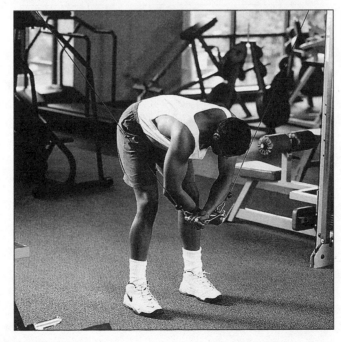

Slowly pull the handles down and in until they cross in front of your chest. Pause for a second, then slowly return to the starting position.

Push-Ups

RATING: MODERATELY DIFFICULT

A classic that will never go out of style, push-ups are perhaps the most comprehensive upper-body exercise you can do. They strengthen the chest, shoulders, arms, wrists, and upper back. They also have the advantage of being completely portable; you can do them anywhere, without fancy equipment—just you and gravity.

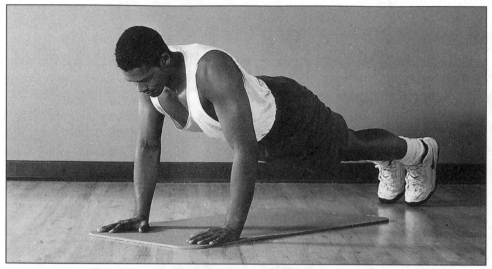

Lie facedown on the floor, balancing your weight on the balls of your feet and the palms of your hands. With your hands shoulder-width apart, extend your arms until your body is at a 45-degree angle to the floor. Your legs should be together and fully extended. Keep your elbows slightly bent and your fingers pointing forward. Keep your legs, back, and neck in a straight line and your eyes on the floor.

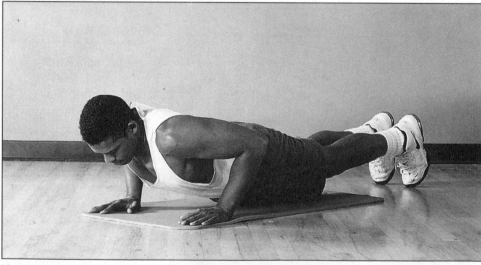

Keeping your body straight, bend your arms, lowering yourself until your chest is almost touching the floor. Hold for a second, then slowly return to the starting position.

DO IT BETTER

• To concentrate stress on the chest muscles, move your hands to slightly more than shoulder-width apart.
• Bringing your hands together so that the thumbs and index fingers touch (forming a diamond pattern) puts additional stress on the triceps and back.
• To increase finger strength, rise up on the fingertips instead of resting on the palms.
• To increase difficulty, have a partner place a weight plate on your upper back.
• To increase difficulty even more, do one-handed push-ups by putting one hand behind your back.
• To decrease difficulty, keep your knees bent and in contact with the floor, with your feet in the air.

Bench Push-Ups

RATING: EASY TO MODERATELY DIFFICULT

Slightly easier than traditional push-ups, these push-ups are commonly used early in a training program. Once you can do these easily, you'll graduate to the more difficult variety.

DO IT BETTER

- If you don't have a weight bench, this exercise can be done using a sturdy chair or even the bottom step of a stairway.
- To work your chest muscles more, move your hands to more than shoulder-width apart.
- To work your triceps and back more, bring your hands together so that your thumbs and index fingers are touching to form a diamond pattern.
- To increase difficulty, have someone put a weight plate on your upper back when you are in the push-up position.
- To decrease difficulty, don't drop all the way to the floor. Do shallower dips until your arms get stronger.
- An easier variation of this exercise is the inclined push-up: Stand 2 to 3 feet away from a wall and lean forward, putting your arms out and your palms flat on the wall. Bend your elbows while leaning into the wall, then push yourself out again.

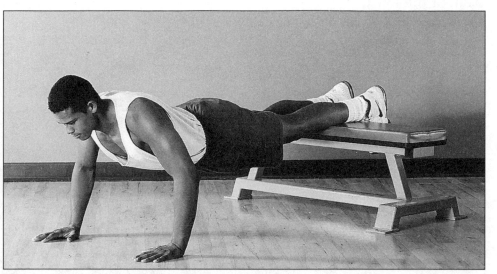

Assume the standard position, with your legs together and your arms and legs fully extended. But instead of putting your feet on the ground, rest them on a weight bench. Keep your elbows slightly bent and your fingers pointing forward. Keep your eyes on the floor and your legs, back, and neck in a straight line.

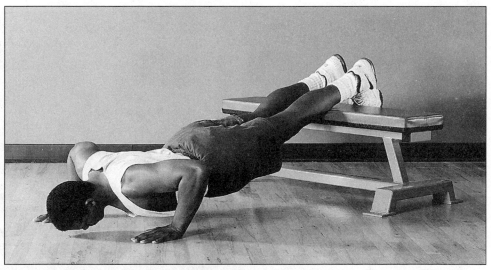

Keeping your body straight, bend your arms, slowly lowering yourself until your chest is almost touching the floor. Hold for a second, then slowly return to the starting position.

Neck Pull-Downs

RATING: EASY

Most men don't think about strengthening the neck muscles, but they should. If the neck muscles are weak, they're likely to be injured when stress is put on the shoulders. This simple exercise uses hand pressure to create resistance, strengthening muscles in the back of the neck.

Sit on the end of a bench with your back straight, head up, and feet flat on the floor. Interlace your fingers behind your head at about ear height.

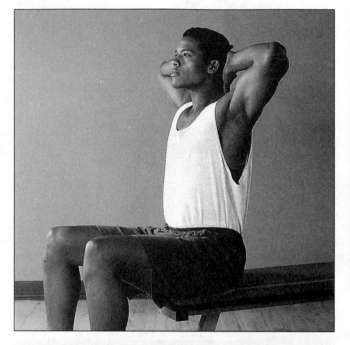

DO IT BETTER

• To prevent muscle strain, warm up with neck rotations (see page 290) before doing this exercise.
• Don't pull your head down farther than is comfortable.
• To increase difficulty, do this exercise using a head harness attached to a weight plate.
• Neck muscles generally aren't as strong as other muscles in the body, so plan on using light weights and a higher number of repetitions.

While resisting with your neck, slowly pull your head forward and down with your hands as far as it will comfortably go. Hold for a second, then return to the starting position—this time, using your hands to resist the motion.

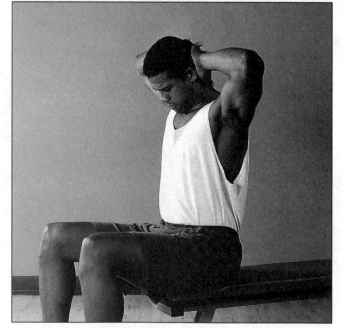

Neck Push-Ups

RATING: EASY

This exercise sounds torturous, but it is really quite simple. It's also essential since it works the muscles at the front and sides of the neck—muscles that come into play any time you twist your head, whether you're playing golf or baseball or simply talking to the person next to you.

DO IT BETTER

• To keep your shoulders relaxed and prevent muscle strains, do a few shoulder rolls or shrugs before you start.
• To work the muscles in the front of the neck, use your fists to offer resistance when returning your head to the starting position.
• Position your fists so that the pressure is on the jaw and not on the soft (and easily injured) tissue of the neck.
• Keeping your movements smooth will help prevent muscle and ligament strains.
• Keep your eyes open to maintain better balance.

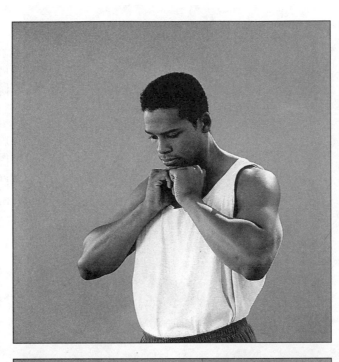

Stand with your back straight, knees relaxed, and feet shoulder-width apart. Allow your head to drop to your chest. Put your fists under your jaw so that they support your head. Keep your arms away from your chest, pointing your elbows outward slightly.

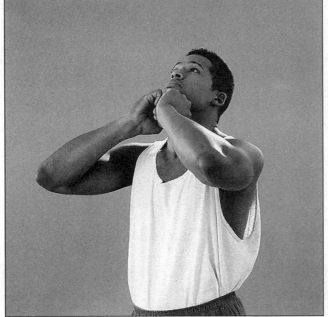

Resisting with your neck, gradually push your head up until your neck is fully extended or as far as it will comfortably go. Do not lean your body backward. Hold for a second, then release pressure and return to the starting position.

Neck Rotations

RATING: EASY

This stretch energizes the nervous system and eliminates stiffness in the neck and upper shoulders. It strengthens the neck muscles, which will increase flexibility and improve posture. If you have neck or upper back problems, however, you should avoid this exercise.

Stand upright with your feet shoulder-width apart, knees and shoulders relaxed. Allow your head to drop to your chest as far as comfortably possible.

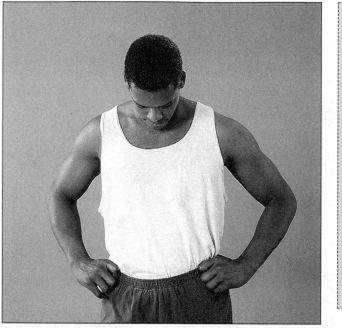

DO IT BETTER

• Don't do this exercise with your eyes closed. It makes some people dizzy.
• Keep the movement smooth and continuous—but don't force it if you feel stiffness or resistance.
• To relax stiffness, hold the stretch for a few seconds at each side.
• For a variation, place the middle of a rolled-up towel against the front of your head. While leaning forward, pull back on the towel slightly to create resistance. Moving the towel will create resistance for each head position.

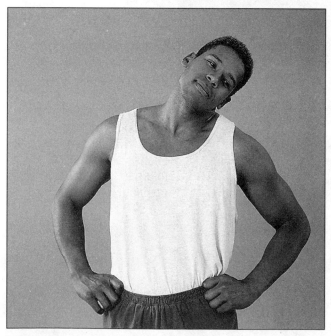

Slowly roll your head to the left until your ear almost touches your shoulder.

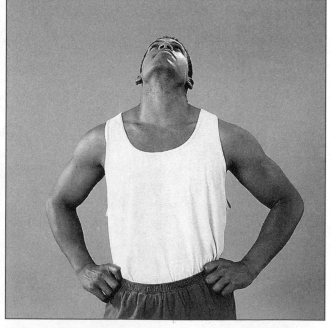

Roll your head slowly backward. Don't force this movement or let your head hang so far back that it rests on your shoulder. Roll your head to the right and then forward. Repeat the movement, rolling the other way.

Head Twists

RATING: EASY

The two most prominent muscles in the neck are the sternocleidomastoids. These are the two main neck muscles, which you use for nodding or turning your head. Head twists are an excellent exercise for building them to substantial proportions.

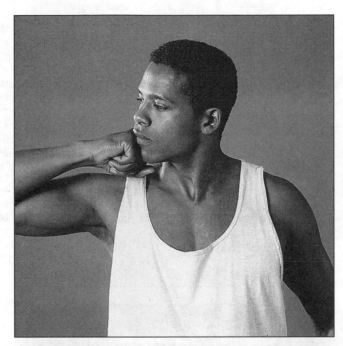

Stand with your legs shoulder-width apart and your knees slightly bent. Make your right hand into a fist and place it at the right side of your chin, keeping your elbow and forearm parallel to the floor. Using your fist for resistance, rotate your head to the right until your chin touches your right shoulder.

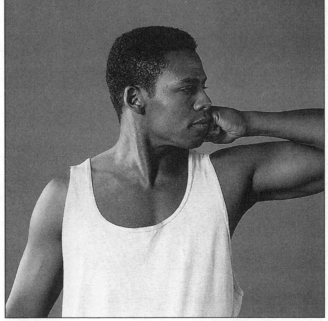

When your chin reaches your shoulder, return to the starting position and repeat on the left side.

Overhead Presses

RATING: DIFFICULT

Also called standing military presses, this exercise strengthens the front and outer deltoids (shoulder).

Stand with your back straight, feet shoulder-width apart, and knees slightly bent. Using an overhand grip, hold a barbell with your hands shoulder-width apart or slightly wider. Bend your elbows and raise the bar to shoulder level. Keep your elbows pointing down, keeping your chest high.

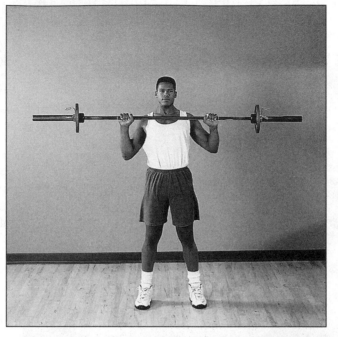

DO IT BETTER
- This exercise puts a lot of strain on the lower back, so it is a good idea to wear a weight belt.
- Keeping your wrists straight will help protect the joints.
- Don't bounce the bar off your chest in order to gain momentum. This increases the risk of back injury and reduces the effectiveness of the exercise.
- If you find yourself swaying when raising the bar, use a lighter weight until you can lift it with complete control.

Slowly lift the bar straight over your head. Hold for a second, then slowly lower it to chest level.

Behind-the-Neck Presses

RATING: VERY DIFFICULT

This is an excellent, all-purpose exercise. It works the front and rear deltoids (shoulder). It also works the trapezius (upper back and neck), supraspinatus (upper back), pectoralis minor (chest), serratus anterior (upper and outer rib cage), and triceps brachii (back of upper arm)—all muscles that work with your shoulders. This exercise can be tough to control, so use lighter-than-usual weights when first learning the movement.

DO IT BETTER

• To decrease difficulty, do this exercise while sitting.
• Wearing a weight belt will help support your lower back.
• Warm up shoulder and neck muscles with neck rotations and shoulder rotations without weights (see pages 290 and 305) before beginning this exercise.

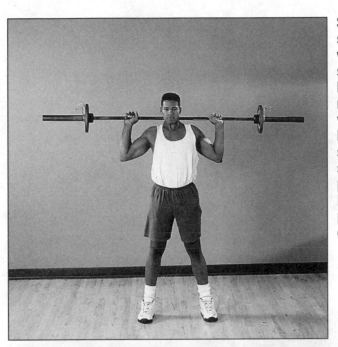

Stand with your back straight, feet shoulder-width apart, and knees slightly bent. Hold a barbell behind your neck across the top of your shoulders. Your hands should be slightly more than shoulder-width apart, palms facing forward. Keep your elbows pointing down and your chest high.

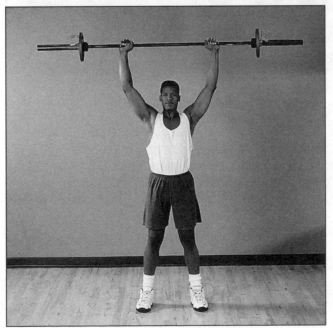

Slowly raise the barbell straight up, keeping your elbows pointed outward. Pull your head slightly forward to allow space for the bar to move. Hold for a second, then slowly lower the bar to the starting position.

Dumbbell Military Presses

RATING: DIFFICULT

You can be sure that any exercise called military isn't going to be easy. This one is no exception. It mainly works the front and outer deltoid (shoulder), triceps (back of upper arm), and trapezius (upper back and neck) muscles. If you want to build massive shoulders, this exercise is a must.

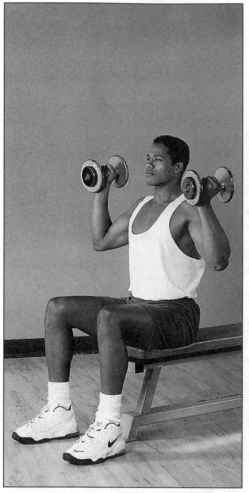

Sit on the end of a bench with your back straight. With your palms facing your body at shoulder height, hold a dumbbell in each hand.

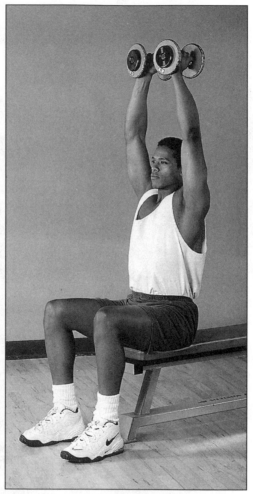

Slowly raise both dumbbells overhead until they almost touch. Extend your arms fully, but don't let your elbows lock. Pause for a second, then slowly lower the dumbbells to the starting position.

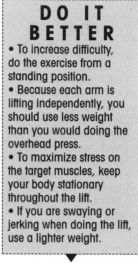

DO IT BETTER

• To increase difficulty, do the exercise from a standing position.
• Because each arm is lifting independently, you should use less weight than you would doing the overhead press.
• To maximize stress on the target muscles, keep your body stationary throughout the lift.
• If you are swaying or jerking when doing the lift, use a lighter weight.

Curling Overhead Dumbbell Presses

RATING: MODERATELY DIFFICULT

This compound exercise, which puts two exercises back-to-back, is sometimes recommended for shoulder rehabilitation. It works the biceps (front of upper arm), triceps (back of upper arm), brachialis (outside of upper arm), and deltoid (shoulder) muscles.

DO IT BETTER

- Do not pause at the end of the curl or overhead press, but keep the movement smooth and continuous.
- To avoid muscle strains, keep your back straight and stable.
- Don't shrug your shoulders as you lift overhead. Keeping them relaxed at all times will help prevent neck and shoulder strain.
- To increase difficulty, do this exercise while standing.

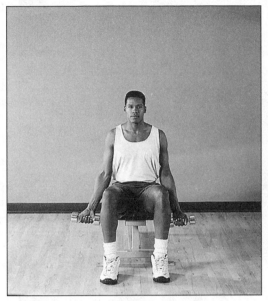

Sit at the end of a bench with your feet flat on the floor and shoulder-width apart. With a dumbbell in each hand and palms facing forward, extend your arms at your sides.

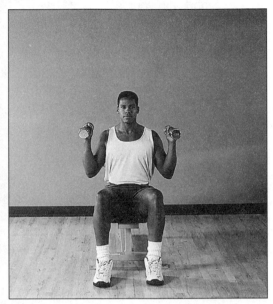

Keeping your upper arms stationary, curl your forearms up to your shoulders. As you lift, rotate your wrists so that your palms are facing each other.

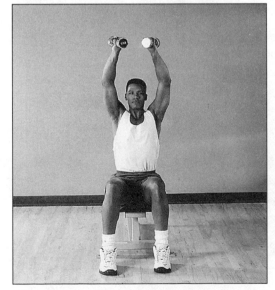

Raise the weights over your head until your elbows are almost completely straight, but not locked. As you lift, rotate your wrists so that your palms are facing outward.

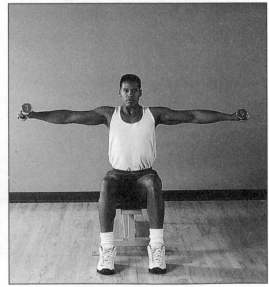

Using a semicircular motion, slowly lower the dumbbells to the starting position, keeping your arms straight and out to your sides.

Upright Rows

RATING: MODERATELY DIFFICULT

As the name suggests, this exercise works the muscles used when rowing a boat—the front deltoid (shoulder) and trapezius (upper back and neck) muscles as well as the forearm and chest muscles.

Stand with your feet shoulder-width apart. Using a narrow, overhand grip, hold a barbell with your arms fully extended. The bar should be resting on your upper thighs. Lean forward slightly at the waist and allow your shoulders to droop forward just a bit, but keep your back straight.

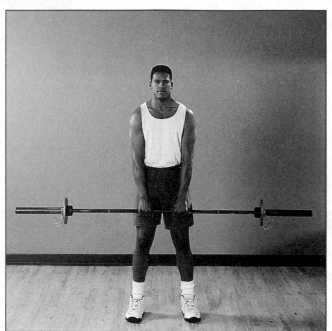

DO IT BETTER
• To decrease difficulty and balance problems, do this exercise with a low pulley.
• It's important not to lean back or sway when lifting the bar, since this reduces the effectiveness of the exercise.
• To increase difficulty, use dumbbells instead of the barbell.

Keeping the bar close to your body, slowly lift until it is at the height of your collarbone. Your elbows should be pointing outward and above the barbell. Hold for a second, then slowly lower the bar to the starting position.

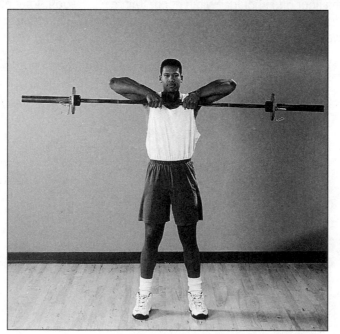

Dumbbell Raises

RATING: DIFFICULT

This is an excellent overall exercise for strengthening the upper body. It works the biceps (front of upper arm), upper pectoralis (chest), outer deltoid (shoulder), trapezius (upper back and neck), and rhomboid (upper back) muscles.

DO IT BETTER

• Keeping your torso straight will help prevent strain on your neck and shoulders.

• To keep from straining muscles in your upper back, don't jerk at the top of the lift.

• To maximize the benefits to the target muscles, keep your wrists straight while raising the weights.

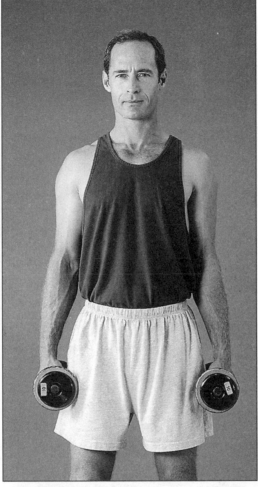

Stand with your legs shoulder-width apart and your knees slightly bent. Hold a dumbbell in each hand, with your arms hanging down and your palms facing your body.

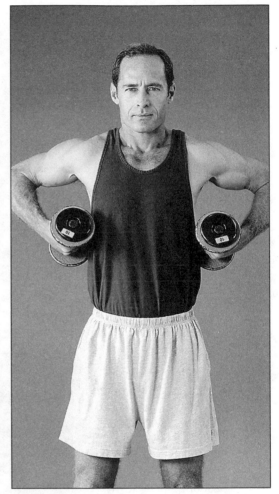

Slowly raise the weights as far as you can toward your armpits. Keep your elbows pointing outward and the weights close to your body. Hold for a second, then slowly lower your arms to the starting position.

Standing Lateral Raises
RATING: MODERATELY DIFFICULT

This is a simple but highly effective exercise that works the deltoid (shoulder) muscles. You need strong deltoids for virtually all sports, but they're particularly helpful for activities requiring a lot of arm motion, like rock climbing, baseball, golf, and swimming.

Stand straight with your feet shoulder-width apart and your knees slightly bent. Hold a dumbbell in each hand, with your arms hanging down and the weights facing your body. Lean forward slightly at the waist, keeping your shoulders back and your back straight.

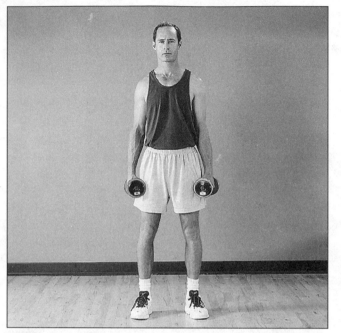

DO IT BETTER
- To prevent neck strain, keep your head in line with your spine.
- To maximize stress on the target muscles, concentrate on squeezing the deltoids as you raise your arms.
- Keep the movements smooth and controlled; swinging your arms will reduce the effects of the exercise.
- Lower the weights at the same pace used when raising them.
- Doing this exercise while seated makes the movements easier to control.

With your elbows slightly bent, slowly raise your arms up and out to your sides until the dumbbells reach shoulder level. Your hands should be facing the floor. Hold for a second, then slowly lower your arms to the starting position.

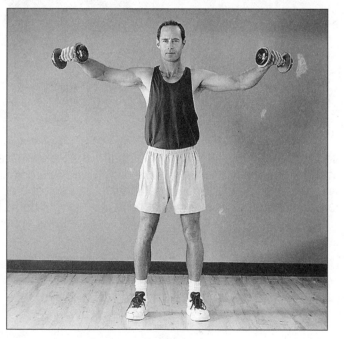

Bent-Over Cable Lateral Raises

RATING: DIFFICULT

While this exercise looks similar to bent-over cable crossovers, it works the opposite muscles. Specifically, this exercise works the middle and posterior deltoids (shoulder), the trapezius (upper back and neck), the rhomboid (upper back), teres minor (outside of shoulder blade), and infraspinatus (shoulder blade) muscles.

DO IT BETTER

- Do not round your back, but maintain the slightly arched position. This helps reduce stress and possible injury to the back.
- To put additional stress on the rear deltoid muscle, bend forward slightly while doing the exercise.
- To put additional stress on the shoulders, lift with only one arm at a time.

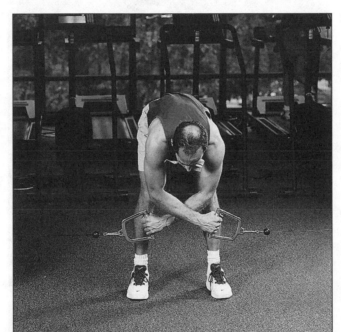

Stand between the two low pulleys with your feet shoulder-width apart and knees slightly bent. With both hands, reach across your body to grasp the pulley handles on the opposite sides. Allow your arms to hang down, with elbows slightly bent and your forearms crossed. Bend forward at the waist, keeping your back slightly arched, until your upper body is parallel with the floor.

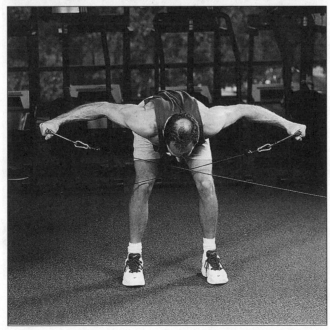

Slowly raise your arms outward and upward as high as you can. Hold for a second, then slowly lower to the starting position.

Front Deltoid Raises

RATING: MODERATELY DIFFICULT

Although similar to standing lateral raises, this simple exercise works the deltoid (shoulder) muscles from a slightly different angle, stressing the front part instead of the side and upper portions. It also works the pectoralis (chest) and trapezius (upper back and neck) muscles as well as the coracobrachialis (inner upper arm) muscles.

Stand straight with your feet shoulder-width apart, knees slightly bent. With a dumbbell in each hand, allow your arms to hang at your sides, with your elbows slightly bent. Your palms should be facing your upper thighs. Lean forward slightly at the waist, keeping your elbows back, chest out, and lower back straight.

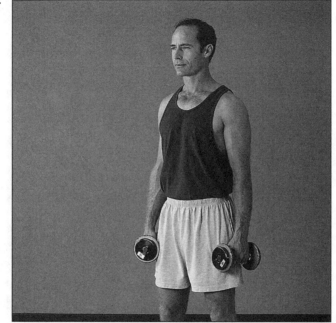

DO IT BETTER
• Although you can do both arms at once, working each arm separately will maximize stress on the target muscles.
• To improve stability while decreasing difficulty, do this exercise from a sitting position. Or use a barbell instead of the dumbbells.

Slowly raise one dumbbell in front of you until it is at shoulder height. The palm of your hand should be facing downward. Don't rock your hips or swing your arms for momentum. Hold for a second, then slowly return to the starting position. Repeat with the other arm.

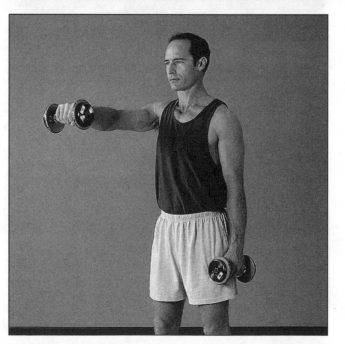

Lying Lateral Raises
RATING: DIFFICULT

This exercise is done on an inclined bench rather than standing straight. The inclined position better isolates the deltoid (shoulder) muscles, making it more rigorous and harder to cheat. It also works the trapezius (upper back and neck), infraspinatus (shoulder blade), teres minor (outside of shoulder blade), and rhomboid (upper back) muscles. Because it's done on a bench, the lower back is supported, reducing the risk of injury.

DO IT BETTER

• To reduce difficulty, raise one arm at a time instead of doing both together.
• Raise your elbows as high as possible during the lift, which puts additional stress on the deltoids.
• Don't let your arms fall on the downward motion; lower the weight slowly and with constant control to maximize muscle contraction.
• Don't let the weights drift behind your shoulders, which brings the upper back muscles into play. Keeping them in line with your shoulders maximizes stress on the target muscles.

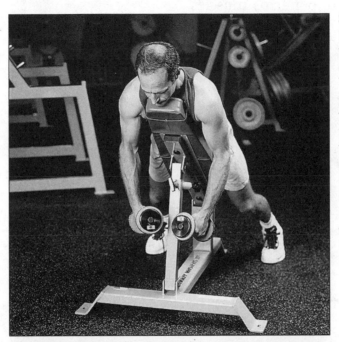

Stand facing an inclined bench, with your chest leaning against the incline. Your legs should be shoulder-width apart, feet on the floor, with your chin just above the top of the bench. Hold a dumbbell in each hand, with your arms dangling below the bench. Keep your elbows slightly bent and your palms facing each other.

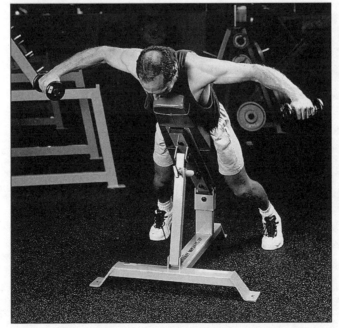

Keeping your elbows relaxed, raise your arms to the sides until they are slightly higher than your shoulders. Hold for a second, then slowly lower to the starting position.

Rotator Cuff External Rotations

RATING: DIFFICULT

The inherent instability of the shoulder joint commonly leads to painful dislocations, particularly for pitchers, bowlers, weight lifters, and even golfers. This exercise strengthens the four tendons and muscles that hold together the joint known as the rotator cuff. It also works the rear deltoids (shoulder), the extensor muscles of the outer forearms, and the brachialis (outside of upper arm) muscles.

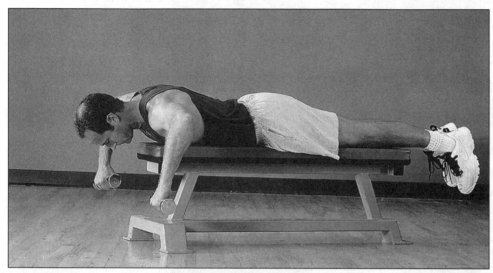

Lie facedown on a bench with a dumbbell in each hand. Start by raising your elbows to shoulder level, letting your forearms hang perpendicularly to the floor. Your palms should be facing your feet.

DO IT BETTER
• If you find this difficult or painful, use hand weights until you have built up the strength of your rotator cuff.
• Don't exaggerate the rotation in the shoulder joint. Pushing it too far can easily result in muscle or tendon strain.
• Maintain a smooth and controlled rhythm to avoid injury to muscles and ligaments.
• If you have difficulty balancing your body on a flat bench, try using a standing inclined bench.

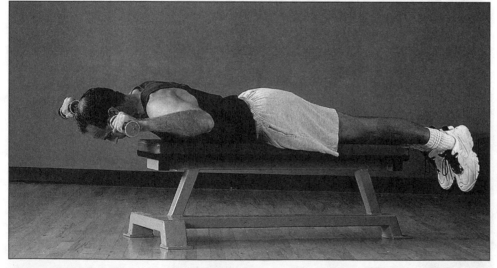

Slowly rotate your forearms up and forward, raising the weights until they are level with your shoulders and parallel to the floor. As you lift, your head and upper body will rise off the bench. Be careful not to arch your back sharply or pull your head back. Keep your head in line with your spine and your eyes on the bench. Hold for a second, then lower your forearms, always keeping your upper arms parallel to the floor.

Swimmer's Breaststroke Imitation

RATING: MODERATELY DIFFICULT

The shoulder is the most flexible joint in the body but inherently unstable. Strengthening the surrounding muscles is the best way to prevent injury. This exercise works muscles and tendons in the rotator cuff, which holds the arm in its socket; the back of the deltoid (shoulder); the trapezius (upper back and neck); and rhomboid (upper back) muscles.

DO IT BETTER

• To maximize stress on the target muscles, keep your arms in the same plane as your body at all times.

• To get the most benefit, fully extend your arms in the overhead motion. Maintain smooth and controlled movements, avoiding jerking or rocking to prevent injury.

• To work more of the inner deltoids, upper pectoralis, and biceps, the same movements can be done while lying on your back on the bench.

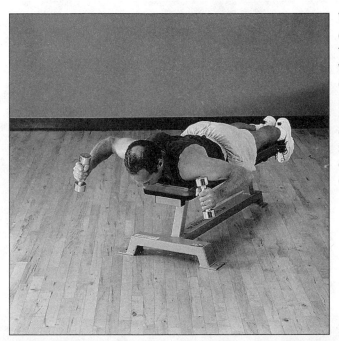

With a dumbbell in each hand, lie facedown on a bench with your arms bent at a 90-degree angle, palms held at shoulder height and facing one another. Your legs should be together and extending over the end of the bench.

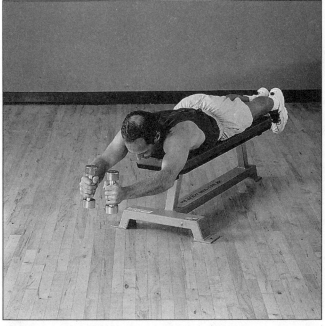

Smoothly extend your arms fully in front of you until the weights almost touch.

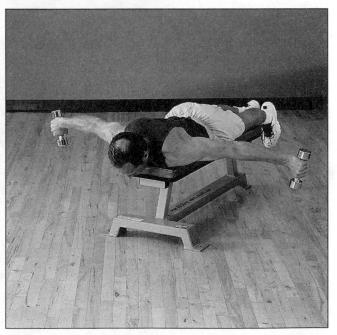

Rotate your palms outward as you "stroke" your arms backward in a semicircular motion until they are fully extended out to the sides, palms facing back. Repeat.

Shoulder Shrugs

RATING: EASY

The upper back is covered by two large, flat, triangular muscles called trapezius muscles, which run down the neck, stretch out to the middle of the shoulders, and extend to a point in the midback. Along with the levator scapulae (beneath the trapezius), they help raise your shoulder blades and make it possible to extend your head. This exercise works each of these muscles, along with the rhomboid (upper back) muscles.

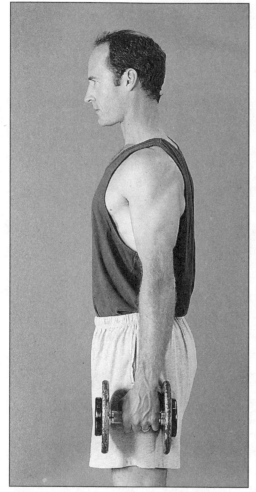

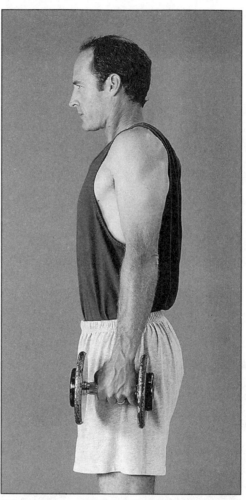

DO IT BETTER
• To prevent strain on the neck, keep your head stationary and chin slightly tucked in.
• To help maintain good control and balance, try holding a single barbell instead of two dumbbells.
• Wearing a weight belt will add support for your lower back.
• To get the most benefit from each movement, concentrate on lifting and lowering the weight at the same rate—slowly and with control.

Stand straight with your feet shoulder-width apart and your knees slightly bent. Hold a dumbbell in each hand, letting your arms hang alongside your body. Your palms should be facing your body. Make sure your shoulders are back and relaxed.

Slowly shrug your shoulders as high as they'll go. Hold for a second, then slowly return to the starting position.

Shoulder Rotations

RATING: EASY

This simple exercise is often used to rehabilitate shoulder joints and neck injuries. It's also good for increasing shoulder flexibility and strength.

DO IT BETTER

• You may want to warm up for this by doing a few shoulder rotations without weights at first.
• Don't drop your shoulders abruptly or jerk as you do any movements as this can lead to neck strain.

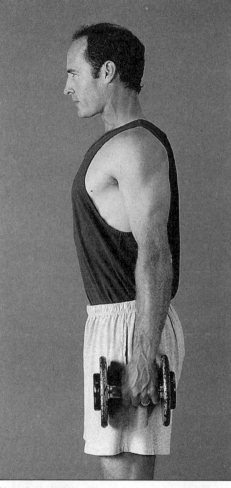

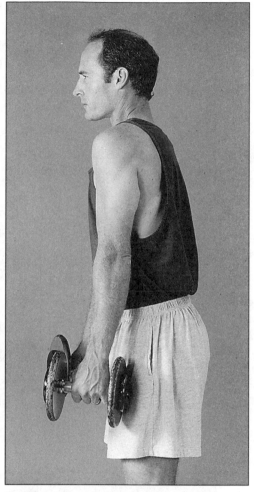

Stand straight with your feet shoulder-width apart and your knees slightly bent. Hold a dumbbell in each hand, letting your arms hang down at your sides. Your palms should be facing your body. Make sure your shoulders are back and relaxed.

Keeping your head and neck relaxed, slowly shrug your shoulders as high as they will go. In a smooth, flowing motion, rotate the shoulders forward, down, back, and then back up again. Repeat this circling movement in this direction to finish set, then reverse course and do the same movement in the opposite direction.

Upper-Body Circuit

According to Dragomir Cioroslan, head coach of the U.S. Weightlifting Federation and the 1996 U.S. Olympic weightlifting team, the following program will provide a great deal of upper-body strength in a relatively short amount of time. Be sure to do the exercises in the order given. To get the best workout, you always want to begin with exercises that use multiple large muscle groups—the bench press is a perfect example—and then move on to exercises that target smaller muscles and joints.

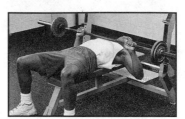

1. Bench Presses (page 277)

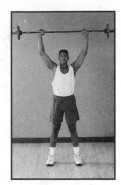

2. Overhead Presses (page 292)

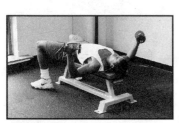

3. Dumbbell Flies (page 282)

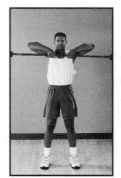

4. Upright Rows (page 296)

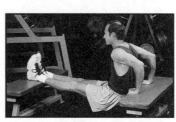

5. Parallel Dips (page 272)

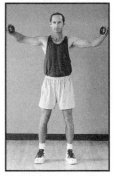

6. Standing Lateral Raises (page 298)

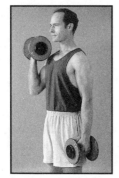

7. Alternating Biceps Curls (page 261)

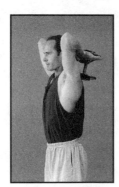

8. Standing Triceps Curls (page 266)

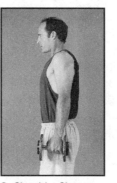

9. Shoulder Shrugs (page 304)

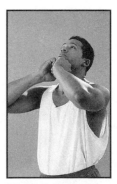

10. Neck Push-Ups (page 289)

PART VIII
LOWER-BODY
WORKOUTS

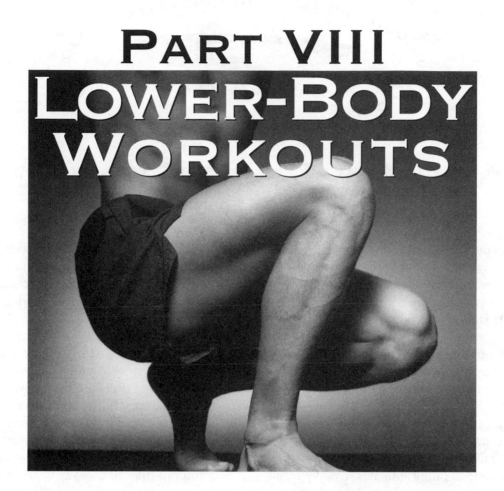

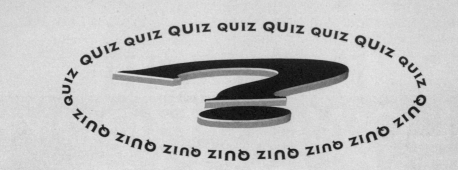

ARE MY LEGS STRONG?

Unless you're a serious runner or bike rider, you probably pay more attention to women's legs than your own.

Maybe it's because men wear pants all the time or because fat doesn't collect in the legs the way it does on the belly. Whatever the reason, we don't give our legs the attention they deserve—which is why at the gym there's always a line at the bench press and never one for the leg-curl machine.

Men's legs simply aren't a hot commodity in our image-driven culture. When you think of Sylvester Stallone, for example, the image that comes to mind is bulging biceps, sinewy shoulders, and prominent pecs. True, he had one movie in which he played a mountain climber in lederhosen, and he showed some pretty good calf muscles, but rest assured, he's not making a zillion bucks a picture because his hamstrings are buffed.

Despite their lack of glamour, strong legs are an invaluable asset—for walking, climbing stairs, and virtually any lifting. How strong are your legs? Take this quiz to see.

1. You're on vacation in New York City, and, naturally, your girlfriend wants to climb to the top of the Statue of Liberty. Assuming that you're there early on a weekday morning and that you can walk right to the top, how long can you keep hiking without stopping for breath?

To a large extent this is a test of cardiovascular fitness, but it's still a reliable indicator of what kind of lower-body strength you have, says Marjorie Albohm, a certified athletic trainer and director of sports medicine at Kendrick Memorial Hospital in Mooresville, Indiana.

Climbing stairs mainly calls on the quadriceps muscles at the top of the thigh, which are responsible for raising the knee toward the chest. And don't forget the walk back down. That calls on the quadriceps' opposing muscles, the hamstrings, which help stabilize the body so that you don't get to the bottom a lot faster than you had planned on.

If you can hike all the way to the top without resting and without being painfully sore the next day, your legs are in good shape.

If you make it to the top, but only after making dozens of excuses to stop (like, "Have you ever noticed how cool the statue looks from the inside?"), your legs are in average condition.

If you never make it to the top and spend the next day hobbling around, your legs are weaker than they should be and need some more work.

2. You're helping your girlfriend move, and you're beginning to wonder why you fall for the brainy type: She has more books than the local library. Worse, she has a third-floor apartment in an old walk-up building. How long will you be able to carry boxes up those stairs before collapsing?

Walking up stairs is one thing. Walking up stairs carrying a 30-pound load is another,

Albohm says. Both situations will test the endurance of your leg muscles, but carrying the box of books will also require sheer strength. Albohm describes this as "an overload test."

If you can get your girlfriend moved and still have time and energy left for a romantic dinner in her new digs, your legs are in good shape.

If you find yourself carrying a load, resting, carrying another load, breaking for pizza, carrying another load, then going home to collapse, your legs are only in average shape.

If you embarrass yourself by moving fewer boxes than your girlfriend, your legs certainly could use some work.

3. You're walking through the park carrying your three-year-old on your shoulders. There are tree branches hanging over the path that you're on, and each time you come upon one, you have to bend your knees so that your child won't get her face scraped. How many times can you bend before making the poor girl walk?

"This is a good test of lower-body strength," Albohm says, "because most of us would probably try to save the stress on our legs by bending forward, which isn't that safe for you or your child."

Essentially, what you're doing in this test is a mini-squat, which puts stress on the quadriceps and hamstrings of the upper leg and on the gluteals of the butt.

If you can comfortably carry your daughter all the way around the park without losing your balance, your legs are in pretty good shape.

If you find yourself almost falling over when your daughter shifts her weight just as you're passing under the branch, your legs are in so-so condition.

If you can walk only 5 minutes before offering to drive your daughter to the store for ice cream, your leg strength needs some serious attention.

4. You're getting dressed for your company's annual Christmas party, a full-blown black tie affair at the biggest hotel in town, when you drop one of your cuff links. You can't see where it went, but you would prefer not ruining the crease in your trousers by getting down on all fours to look. Can you keep yourself balanced in a squat long enough to find the missing link?

If you can search for 5 minutes and still be able to get up and dance the night away, your legs are in good condition.

If you're able to search for 5 minutes, but afterward your knees are sore for the rest of the night, your legs are in average condition.

If, after 5 minutes, you find that you can't stand up until your wife rescues you, your legs need some work.

Incidentally, squatting requires a lot of lower-body strength, so don't feel too bad if you come up short.

5. One car is in the shop and your wife is running errands in the other. You would love to have a couple of beers and some chips for the game that's about to come on, but you'll have to dust off your old three-speed to go get them. There are 2 miles of hilly road between you and the nearest convenience store. How many innings will it take you to get there and back?

Riding 4 miles on a decent bike is an excellent test of quadriceps, hamstring, and calf endurance, Albohm says. The ride is a test of cardiovascular fitness, too.

If your legs are in good condition, you should be able to make the ride and still be back in time to see most of the game.

If your legs are in average condition, you could miss half the game.

If your legs are in poor condition, you'll see virtually the entire game—perched on a stool at the tavern just down the hill from your house. A friend will drive you and your bike home when the game's over.

WHY LEG STRENGTH MATTERS
THE IMPACT OF BIG MUSCLES

With the possible exception of models and a few high-speed athletes, most of us don't spend a lot of time thinking about our legs. They carry us around, sure, but they aren't exactly a hot topic of interest—at least, not consciously.

But on some deeper level, our legs possess a profound, symbolic significance. Just look at our language. When a movie keeps drawing crowds, for example, we say it "has legs." A defendant with a weak case "doesn't have a leg to stand on." If you're in business, you spend your days getting "a leg up" on the competition. Has a colleague lost power in the office recently? He's had his "legs cut out from under him."

Clearly, a man's legs aren't merely the means to a rudimentary form of locomotion. Yet, despite their psychological (and physical) significance, men don't do nearly enough to keep their legs strong. In fact, when it comes to working out, most of us treat our legs like second-class citizens.

There are several reasons for this benign neglect. Most of us assume that our legs get all the exercise they need simply by walking around, says Ed Burke, Ph.D., associate professor of exercise science and an exercise physiologist at the University of Colorado in Colorado Springs. There is some truth to this. If you have even a moderately active lifestyle, your legs do get something of a daily workout, Dr. Burke says. But having legs that are moderately toned isn't the same thing as having legs that are strong and in shape.

Even men who are serious about staying in shape tend to overlook their legs. That's partly because most men focus more on developing their upper bodies. But there's another, less-noble reason as well.

"The leg muscles are the largest muscles in the body, and large muscles tend to take a toll when you're working them," says Harvey Newton, a certified strength and conditioning specialist and the executive director of the National Strength and Conditioning Association in Colorado Springs, Colorado. In addition, since the legs are farther from the heart than the chest and arms, the body has to work a lot harder keeping them supplied with blood and oxygen. In other words, men often neglect their legs because not neglecting them is such hard work.

It can also be pretty boring, Newton adds. "Leg exercises are all pretty similar—extensions and squats, for the most part. With the upper body you have much more variety."

Mobility and More

In short, most men would rather spend an hour on the bench press than 10 minutes doing leg workouts. Yet this attitude, while understandable, is also shortsighted. Whether you're trying to get your whole body into shape or are simply looking to stay fit and healthy, having good leg strength is of critical importance. Here are some of the reasons why.

Strong legs keep you moving. Even apart from the role they play in walking, strong legs are key players in virtually any aerobic workout you can name. "Almost any kind of cardiovascular training involves your legs," says Frank Eksten, strength co-ordinator in the Department of Athletics and visiting lecturer in kinesiology at Indiana University in Bloomington.

In fact, if you have a problem with your legs—they're not strong, say, or they don't have much endurance—you're going to have a problem doing any activity long enough to derive an aerobic benefit, be it tennis or mowing the lawn. This is particularly true once you're in your thirties and beyond. The saying "the legs go first" in many ways is true. Even if you don't like working out, maintaining good leg strength is essential just to continue doing the things you enjoy.

Strong legs make you a better competitor. The next time you're watching the game—be it baseball, tennis, basketball, whatever—check out the legs on those guys. They're big. There's a good reason for this. In virtually every sport, power is generated from the legs, especially the hips and quadriceps.

"Keeping them strong can improve your overall performance in whatever sport you play," says Brett Brungardt, former strength coach for the University of Houston and co-author of *The Complete Book of Butt and Legs*.

Strong legs keep you healthy. Another overlooked service that our legs provide is helping us pick things up. One of the most common health problems in America is a bad back, and a lot of those injuries come from using arm and shoulder muscles instead of the legs when lifting heavy objects.

"The lower body is very important when we look at what constitutes efficient body mechanics and efficient movement," says Marjorie Albohm, a certified athletic trainer and director of sports medicine at Kendrick Memorial Hospital in Mooresville, Indiana.

"When we're lifting, the support should come from the hamstrings and quadriceps in the thigh. Those are two of the largest muscle groups we have. Men who have strong arms and shoulders think that they can get away with lifting with their upper bodies, and sometimes they can. But it's much more efficient and much safer to use your legs."

Strong legs can save your knees. The knee is a marvelous joint, providing excellent leverage, flexibility, and speed. It also is responsible for giving us high orthopedic bills. In terms of work-related injuries, knees have surpassed the back and all other parts of the body.

Unlike the hip joint, which is very solidly constructed, the knee is relatively wobbly. Although it is held together by a crosshatching of ligaments and tendons and covered up by the kneecap, the knee is intrinsically unstable. That's what makes it agile—and vulnerable.

Strong legs play a large role in keeping the knee safe. The stronger your leg muscles, the better able they are to withstand shocks that otherwise would travel straight to the joint. Further, strong legs will help stabilize the knees, helping them sustain sharp jolts and abrupt movements without going down.

Strong legs look good. The most compelling argument in favor of strong legs, for most of us, at least, is that they look good. "A lot of people pay all their attention to the upper body when they're working out, but that's certainly not true of anybody who knows anything about bodybuilding," says Art Drechsler, former board member of the U.S. Weightlifting Federation. "Symmetry is important."

There are some surprising connections between leg strength and the flatness of your belly, too. Take the powerful hamstring muscles along the back of your thigh. If they're not strong and fit, they frequently get tight. This means that muscles in your lower back have to work a lot harder just to keep you upright. Eventually, most men with weak hamstring muscles begin to slouch, which in turn makes the belly stick out and look larger. So keeping your legs strong will help your belly look smaller.

Strong legs burn more fat. All muscles burn calories, and large muscles burn considerably more calories than small ones. Since the legs contain the biggest muscles in your body, making them larger and stronger can increase the number of calories you burn.

Indeed, when you're trying to whittle down your belly, it makes a lot more sense to focus on the big muscles, like those in the legs, than the target muscles in the abdomen.

"The abdomen is a relatively small muscle," says Alan Mikesky, Ph.D., director of the Human Performance and Biomechanics Laboratory at Indiana University–Purdue University in Indianapolis. "If you want to get the full weight-loss effect from developing muscle tissue, you have to develop the bigger muscles as well."

WHAT TO BE CAREFUL OF
PROTECTING THE STRONGEST

A strange thing about leg muscles: Their very size and strength can get you in trouble.

When you do leg workouts, you're probably moving a lot of weight. This isn't surprising since the leg muscles are the largest muscles in the body. If you don't lift carefully, however, the large weights involved can exert a lot of strain, and not just on the muscles being worked.

"When you're working the lower body, you must pay attention to the knee, the ankle, the hip, and the lower back," says Dragomir Cioroslan, head coach of the U.S. Weightlifting Federation and the 1996 U.S. Olympic weightlifting team.

This is particularly true for men whose high school days are behind them. "If you're in your thirties, you're going to be less flexible than someone in his twenties," says Frank Eksten, strength coordinator in the Department of Athletics and visiting lecturer in kinesiology at Indiana University in Bloomington. "There are some age-related limitations that will improve with time, but you have to give them a few weeks to develop."

Lifting injuries don't have to happen, he adds. If you pay attention to the basics of lifting—like staying focused and not heaving too much weight—you're unlikely to get hurt.

BUILD SLOWLY. Trying to lift large amounts of weight when you're just getting started isn't ambitious. It's stupid. Few things are more humiliating or dangerous than loading the bar with weights—when doing squats, for example—and discovering at the bottom of the lift that you can't stand up again.

"We call that a failure of exercise, and it can be a problem," says Harvey Newton, a certified strength and conditioning specialist and the executive director of the National Strength and Conditioning Association in Colorado Springs, Colorado.

Experienced lifters always start with relatively light loads and work up from there. If you're struggling to complete your first set—or merely to keep your balance—you know that you have put on too much weight and should back off, says Newton.

GO ALL THE WAY. To get the most benefit from a lower-body exercise and to reduce the risk of injury, you want to move smoothly through its full range of motion. Indeed, many injuries result from the mistaken belief that it's possible to save wear and tear on the knees by doing a half-squat or quarter squat—and making up the difference (foolishly) by doubling the weight, Newton says.

USE A SPOTTER. The heavy weights used when working the legs mean that additional caution is called for. When working with free weights, it's a good idea to have a spotter on hand to help out if you get into trouble, says Newton.

For home gyms, Newton recommends getting a special type of squat rack called a power rack. It comes equipped with extra support devices that allow you to get out from under the barbell in a hurry if your strength should give out.

STAY IN BALANCE. Large muscle groups that oppose one another are like large nations that share a border: A balance of power helps maintain the peace. Newton has seen lots of men exercise the quadriceps muscles in the front of their thighs but neglect the hamstrings in the back. As the quads get stronger, they tend to pull the hamstrings out of balance, which often results in muscle strains—or worse. So take the time to work muscles and their counterparts evenly.

Squats

RATING: DIFFICULT

Squats are the number one exercise used by elite athletes for conditioning large muscle groups—specifically, the quadriceps (front thigh), gluteal (butt), and hamstring (back thigh) muscles. Squats also work the calves and shins, along with muscles in the shoulders, back, and arms. Essentially, squats provide a whole-body workout.

DO IT BETTER

- When starting out, practice the movements using an unweighted bar or broomstick.
- Keeping your feet flat at all times will reduce pressure on the toes and help prevent knee and ankle injury.
- Preventing your knees from extending over your toes will focus stress on the target muscles.
- To keep your back in line and your torso straight, look at a point in front of you that is slightly above eye level.
- Turning your toes out will bring more of the inner thigh muscles into play.
- To put more stress on the quadriceps, bring your feet closer together.
- To put more stress on the hamstrings and outer thighs, stand with your feet farther apart.
- To put more stress on the gluteal muscles, stand with your heels on a raised platform that is 1 to 2 inches high.

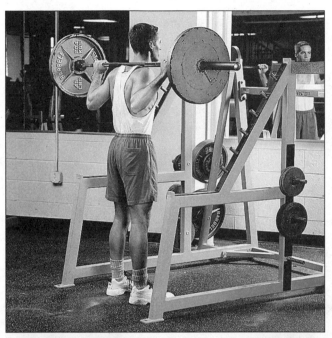

Place a barbell at shoulder level on a squat rack. Grip the bar with your hands slightly more than shoulder-width apart, palms facing away from your body. Step under the bar so that it is positioned evenly across your upper back and shoulders. Stand up straight with your feet hip-width apart, toes pointing slightly out. Don't drop your head; it should be in line with your torso, with your eyes looking ahead.

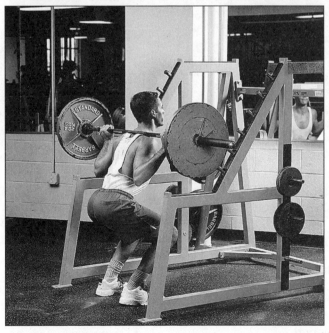

Keeping your feet flat and torso straight, bend your knees slightly and squat down. Do not allow your knees to extend past your toes. Continue the movement until your thighs are parallel to the floor. Slowly rise to the starting position, then repeat.

Front Squats

RATING: VERY DIFFICULT

Front squats are more difficult than traditional squats because they specifically target areas of potential injury. Athletes at any level can appreciate the benefit of strengthening these problem areas—the knees, the hips, and the erector spinae (lower back) muscles. In addition to injury prevention, front squats also aid in developing the quadriceps (front thigh), hamstring (back thigh), and gluteal (butt) muscles.

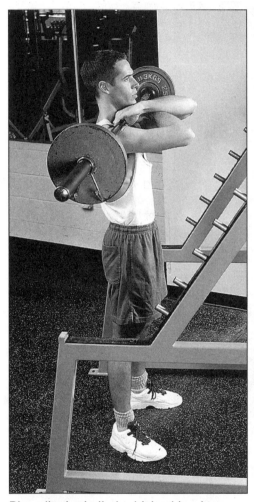

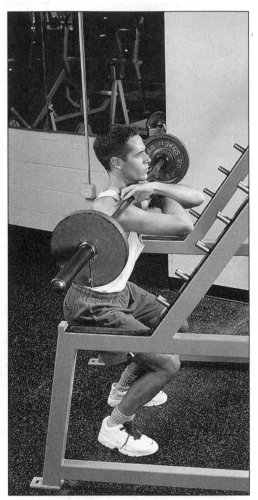

DO IT BETTER

• Keeping your elbows high will help prevent the torso from leaning forward.
• Use less weight than you would for a traditional squat because front squats require more balance and coordination.
• Placing your heels on a low platform that is 1 to 2 inches high will put additional stress on the quadriceps and gluteal muscles.
• Turning your toes out slightly will work the inner thighs more.

Place the barbell at midchest level on a squat rack. Walk in toward the bar until it is resting on top of the front of your shoulders. Cross your arms, using your right hand to grip the bar at your left shoulder, and your left hand to grip it on the right. Stand up straight until the bar is fully supported by your shoulders and arms, keeping your elbows high. Take one step back away from the rack. Your feet should be flat on the floor and shoulder-width apart. Keep your upper body straight and your head in line with your body.

Slowly squat down until your thighs are parallel to the floor. Do not let your knees extend over your toes. Keep your torso straight, eyes looking ahead. Slowly rise to the starting position, then repeat.

Hack Squats

RATING: MODERATELY DIFFICULT

The advantage of this exercise is that it's less complicated than traditional squats and it puts less pressure on your knees and lower back. It's also easier to control. Some gyms have hack-squat machines, but you can do it at home using just a barbell. These squats are good for strengthening the knees and the hamstring (back thigh), quadriceps (front thigh), and gluteal (butt) muscles.

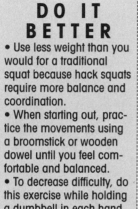

DO IT BETTER

• Use less weight than you would for a traditional squat because hack squats require more balance and coordination.
• When starting out, practice the movements using a broomstick or wooden dowel until you feel comfortable and balanced.
• To decrease difficulty, do this exercise while holding a dumbbell in each hand. The dumbbells should be held behind your thighs.

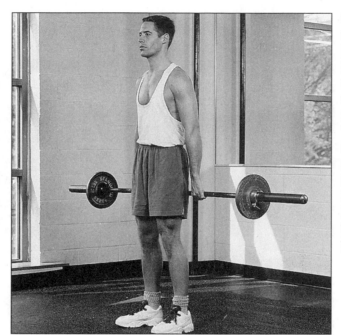

With your feet hip-width apart, stand with a barbell placed directly behind your heels. Squat down and grip the bar with your palms facing away from your body. Your hands should be slightly more than shoulder-width apart. Stand up, holding the bar at arm's length behind your thighs. Keep your head in line with your body.

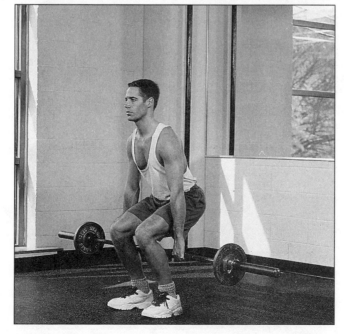

Squat down until your thighs are close to parallel with the floor. Do not allow your knees to extend over your toes. Then rise, keeping your arms fully extended, and repeat.

Lateral Squats

RATING: DIFFICULT

Quick movements are essential for most sports and a lot of daily activities. These squats will help keep your joints, tendons, and ligaments strong and agile. Unlike many lifts, they require little weight to strengthen the quadriceps (front thigh) muscles. They also work the hip flexor (front hip) muscles of the leg as well as the gluteal (butt) muscles, which are used to step sideways, and the tensor fascia latae (a band of muscle down the side of the thigh).

Adjust the squat rack so that the bar is at shoulder level. With your palms facing away from your body, grip the bar with your hands slightly more than shoulder-width apart. Step under the bar and place it evenly across your upper back and shoulders. Stand up straight and take one step back from the rack. Place your feet in a wide stance, toes pointed out, and keep your head in line with your body.

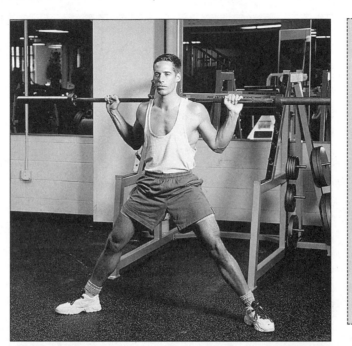

DO IT BETTER

• If you are just starting out, you can do this exercise using dumbbells instead of a bar.
• To decrease difficulty, do a complete set on one side of your body before switching to the other side.
• Another way to decrease difficulty is to do this exercise without weights. Raise your arms over your head, elbows slightly bent, fingers interlaced and palms up. As you squat, fully extend your arms. This helps keep your torso upright and provides a good whole-body stretch.

Drop down by bending your right leg until the thigh is parallel to the floor. Do not allow your right knee to turn in or to move over the toes. Put most of your weight on your right leg, keeping your left leg extended, knee slightly bent. Hold for a second, then return to the starting position by extending your right leg and bringing your torso back to the center. Repeat to the left side without resting.

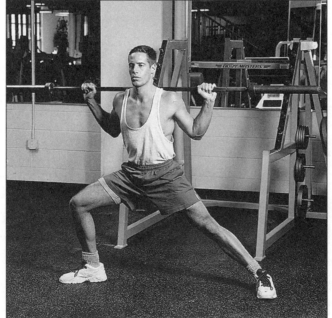

Freehand Squats

RATING: EASY

The easiest of all the squats, this exercise strengthens the hip flexor (front hip), quadriceps (front thigh), and gluteal (butt) muscles. It also works the erector spinae (lower back) muscles. The advantage of these squats is that they can be done without equipment and in any location.

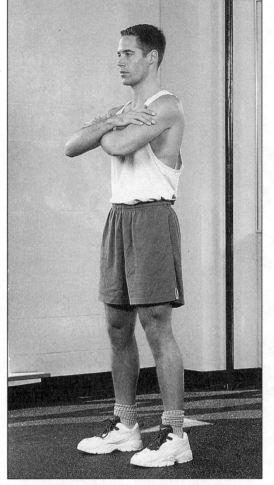

Stand with your feet flat and positioned slightly more than hip-width apart. Cross your arms over your chest and align your head with your upper body.

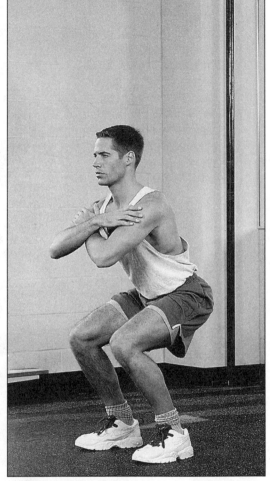

Slowly squat until your thighs are parallel to the floor or as close to parallel as you can comfortably get them. Keep your torso straight and don't let your knees extend over your toes. Hold for a second, then return to the starting position.

Vertical Leg Presses
RATING: MODERATELY DIFFICULT

Squats can be difficult for people who don't have a lot of flexibility or who have back problems. Vertical leg presses are a good alternative. More effective than the traditional horizontal leg presses, this exercise is ideal for working the hamstring (back thigh), quadriceps (front thigh), and hip flexor (front hip) muscles.

Sit in a vertical leg-press machine, making sure that the seat is adjusted so that your knees are bent at a 90-degree angle or slightly less. Place your feet shoulder-width apart, toes turned out slightly. Grip the handlebars and press your lower back to the pad.

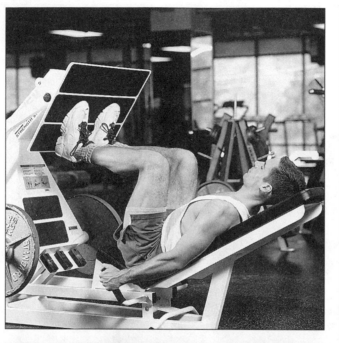

Push forward on the foot plate to straighten your legs, keeping your knees unlocked. Slowly return to the starting position, then repeat.

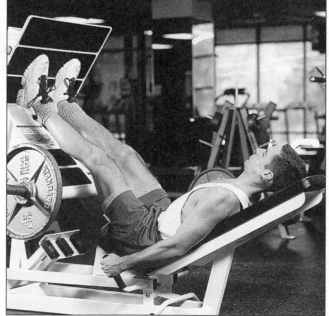

DO IT BETTER

• Putting your feet and legs closer together will put extra stress on the quadriceps.

• Placing your feet more than shoulder-width apart gives more of a workout to the hamstrings and hip flexors.

• Try working one leg at a time. You can turn your toes out to work more of the inner thigh or turn your toes in to work the outer thigh. Be sure to use less weight than you would for the original version.

• You can use this machine to work your calves between leg-press sets. Lower your feet so that the heels hang off the foot plate. Extend your legs, knees bent, and flex and extend your feet.

Leg Extensions

RATING: EASY

Leg extensions are popular for strengthening and conditioning the quadriceps (front thigh) muscles and the ligaments and tendons of the knee, particularly for rehabilitation. Unlike free weights, which work several muscle groups, machines typically isolate one or two groups. This exercise is often recommended for sports in which knee injuries are common, like skiing, running, or football.

DO IT BETTER

• Maintaining a constant speed throughout the exercise increases effectiveness by placing constant tension on the muscles.
• You can do this exercise using ankle weights. Follow the same movements while sitting on a chair or bench, with your legs bent at a 90-degree angle.
• For maximum burn, hold for 4 seconds at the top of each movement, then release slowly.
• To isolate the muscles more efficiently, work one leg at a time.
• To increase difficulty, use both legs to raise the weights, then lower them using one leg.
• Turning your toes out will work more of the inner quadriceps muscles.
• To work more of the outer quadriceps, turn your toes in.

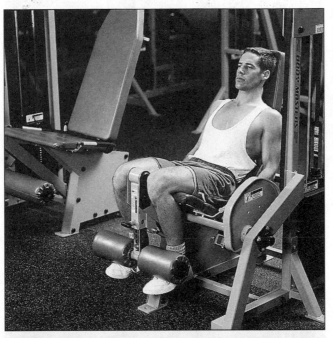

Sit in a leg-extension machine with your legs behind the padded lifting bars. Your back should be pressed against the back pad, with your hands gripping the handles. Your feet should be flexed, and your knees bent at slightly more than a 90-degree angle.

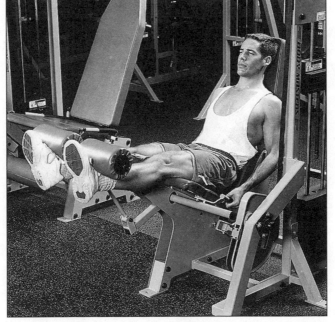

Keeping your lower back pressed to the pad, straighten your legs by raising the padded lifting bars. Extend your legs fully, keeping your knees unlocked. Hold for a second at the top of the movement. Slowly return to the starting position and repeat.

Leg Curls

RATING: EASY

The main purpose of this exercise is to work the hamstrings, those long muscles in the back of the thighs. Compared to quadriceps (front thigh) muscles, hamstrings are somewhat difficult to work, which explains why they are prone to pulls and strains.

Lie on your stomach on the leg-curl machine, hooking your ankles behind the pads, with your knees just over the edge of the bench. Grip the handles or the side of the bench. Your legs should be fully ex-tended, knees slightly bent.

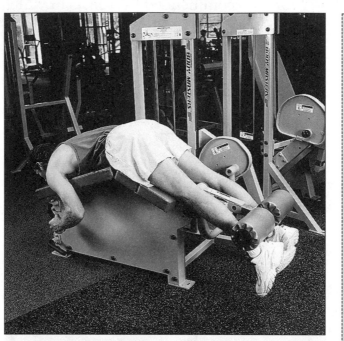

Keeping your pelvis against the bench and using the handles for support, raise your heels toward your butt until your legs are at an angle slightly less than 90 degrees. Return to the starting position, keeping your hamstrings tense throughout the entire range of motion.

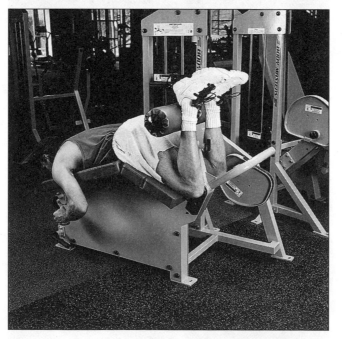

DO IT BETTER

• Hamstrings are relatively weak, so use less weight than you would for leg extensions.
• Turning your toes out will work more of the outer thigh area of the ham-strings.
• Turning your toes in, with your feet flexed, works more of the inner thighs in the hamstring area, while pointing your toes involves the calf muscles.
• To increase difficulty, do this exercise with one leg at a time.
• To increase difficulty even more, raise the weights with both legs, then lower them using just one.
• You can do this exercise at home by using ankle weights and following the same movements.

Walking Lunges

RATING: DIFFICULT

More difficult than alternating leg lunges (see page 235), these lunges work the hamstring (back thigh), quadriceps (front thigh), gluteal (butt), hip flexor (front hip), and calf muscles. This exercise is good for increasing flexibility and strength of all leg muscles and joints. The greatest challenge is balance, especially when using dumbbells.

DO IT BETTER

• For maximum effectiveness, concentrate on keeping your torso upright at all times. You should be pushing your hips down and not forward when in the lunge position.

• To decrease difficulty, do the same movements without using weights. Or do it while wearing wrist weights.

• Another way to decrease difficulty is to do multiple lunges on one leg rather than alternating legs.

• To increase difficulty, replace the dumbbells with a barbell held behind your neck, across your shoulders.

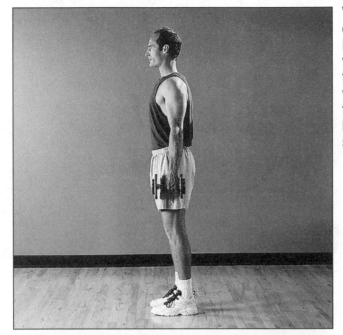

With your feet hip-width apart, hold a dumbbell in each hand, keeping your arms fully extended, palms facing your sides. Keep your torso straight and your head in line with your spine.

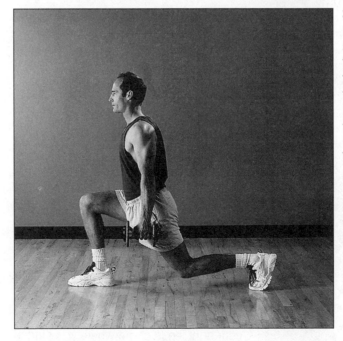

Step forward with your right leg, taking a long stride, landing heel to toe. Lower your right thigh until it is parallel to the floor, with the left knee just short of touching the ground. Hold for a second, then rise, pulling forward and up with your right leg as you bring your left leg forward and into the starting position. Repeat on the left side. Continue alternating legs as you walk across the room.

Step-Ups
RATING: DIFFICULT

This is a good dual-purpose exercise that conditions you aerobically while increasing strength and flexibility in the hamstring (back thigh), hip flexor (front hip), quadriceps (front thigh), gluteal (butt), and adductor (inner thigh) muscles.

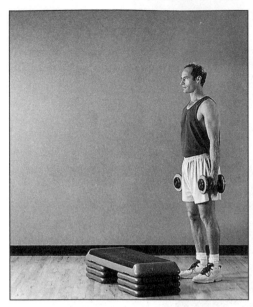

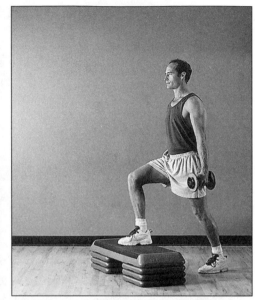

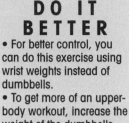

DO IT BETTER
• For better control, you can do this exercise using wrist weights instead of dumbbells.
• To get more of an upper-body workout, increase the weight of the dumbbells.
• To increase difficulty, hold a barbell behind your neck across your shoulders, which will increase the number of muscle fibers being used and will increase heart rate.

Hold a dumbbell in each hand, arms down at your sides, palms facing your body. Stand upright with your shoulders back, chest out. You should be standing about 1 foot away from a sturdy box or platform that is 12 to 18 inches high or aerobic steps of equivalent height.

Keeping the dumbbells at your sides and your upper body straight, step forward with your right foot, placing it on the center of the box.

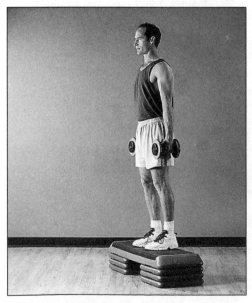

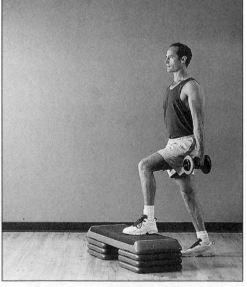

Complete the step by bringing your left foot next to your right.

Step backward with the right foot so that your right leg is about where you started. Step down with the left foot to bring it back to the starting position. Repeat the steps, this time leading with the left foot.

Bench Lateral Step-Ups

RATING: DIFFICULT

This exercise is a favorite of the U.S. Olympic ski team. It's excellent for building the hamstring (back thigh) and quadriceps (front thigh) muscles as well as those used to pull the thighs to the sides—two of the three gluteal (butt) muscles and the tensor fascia latae (a band of muscle down the side of the thigh). Skiers use these step-ups to get in shape for slaloms, jumps, and other moves.

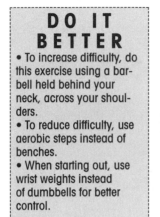

DO IT BETTER
- To increase difficulty, do this exercise using a barbell held behind your neck, across your shoulders.
- To reduce difficulty, use aerobic steps instead of benches.
- When starting out, use wrist weights instead of dumbbells for better control.

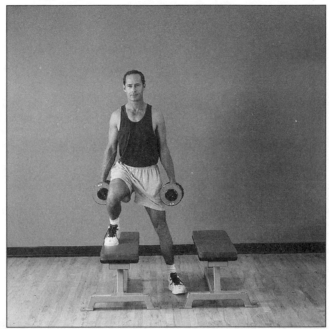

Begin with two benches placed slightly more than shoulder-width apart. With a dumbbell in each hand, stand between the benches, arms extended down, palms facing your sides, feet shoulder-width apart.

Step up with your right leg and place your foot to the far right on the bench. Be sure there is enough room for your left foot, which will shortly follow.

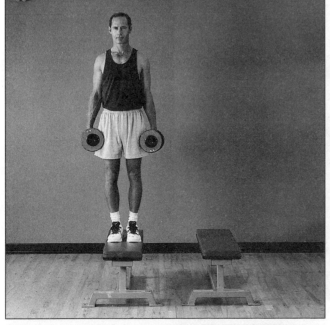

Shift your weight from the left to the right leg. Extend your left leg and place the foot on the bench next to your right foot.

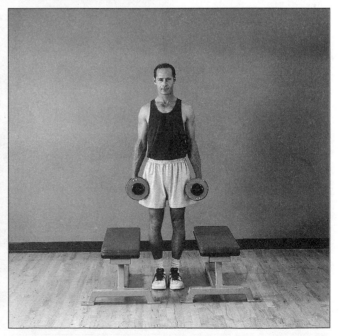

Step down, slowly extending the left leg toward the floor. When your weight is on your left leg, bring the right foot back to the starting position. Repeat on the left side.

Phantom Chairs

RATING: MODERATELY DIFFICULT

It's been said that the simpler a movement is, the more powerful it can be. This certainly applies to this exercise, which is nothing more than a simple wall squat (hence the term phantom chair). It provides a superb workout for the hip extensors (hamstrings and butt muscles) at the back of the thighs and for the knee extensors (quadriceps) at the front of the thighs. The great advantage of this exercise is that you can do it anywhere there is a wall.

Stand leaning your back against a wall. Your feet should be a little more than shoulder-width apart, 1½ feet out from the wall, with the toes pointed out slightly. Keep your shoulders back and your chest out.

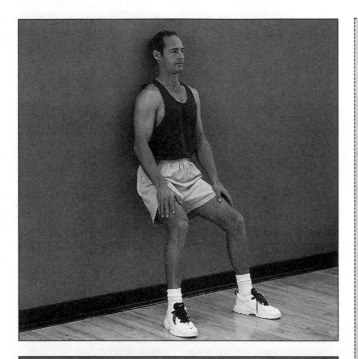

Slowly bend your knees, lowering yourself until the tops of your thighs are parallel to the ground. Don't go so far down that your knees extend over your toes. Hold until your muscles are fatigued, then slowly straighten your legs and return to the starting position.

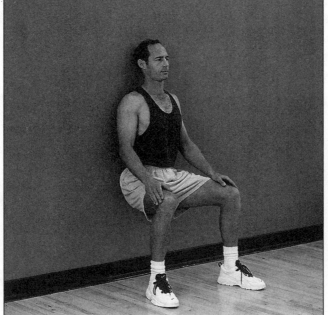

DO IT BETTER

• Leaning forward and resting your elbows on your thighs takes stress off the thighs, making the exercise less effective. To get the best results, keep your lower back firmly pressed against the wall.

• To increase difficulty, hold a dumbbell in each hand. Or do the exercise while standing on one leg.

• Another way to increase difficulty is to do this exercise in continuous, fluid motion, rather than holding the squat position.

• Changing the position of your feet will work different parts of the quadriceps. Putting your feet close together, toes straight ahead, isolates more of the outer thigh. Putting your feet wider apart, toes pointed out, stresses the inner and front thigh.

• To work your calves as well as your quadriceps and hamstrings, support your weight on the balls of your feet.

Lying Inside Leg Raises
RATING: EASY

If you have ever pulled a groin muscle, you know where the adductor muscles are. The adductors, consisting of three separate muscles, lie along the inner thigh. You use these muscles whenever you press your legs together, such as while riding a horse. This exercise not only works the adductors but also the part of the quadriceps that runs along the inner thigh.

DO IT BETTER

• To increase difficulty, use an ankle weight on the leg you are raising. The inner thigh muscles fatigue quickly, so you'll want to be in good shape before adding resistance.

• Another way to add resistance is to use your free hand to press on the inner thigh of the leg that you are raising.

• Raise and lower the leg slowly and with control. Moving too quickly or jerking the leg reduces the effectiveness of the exercise.

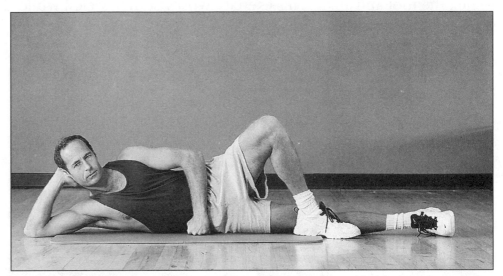

Lie on your side, supporting your head by placing your hand behind your ear. Put the free hand on the floor in front of your chest. Bend your top knee, placing the foot of that leg in front of your other knee, which should be fully extended and resting on the ground.

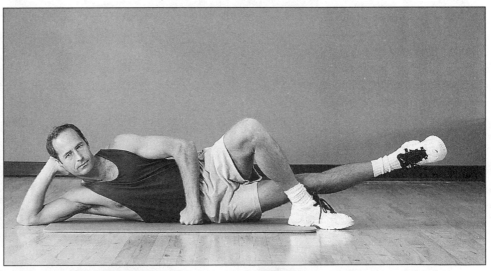

Slowly raise the straight leg as high as possible without moving the rest of your body. Hold for a second, then lower it to just above the floor. Repeat to finish the set, then change positions and repeat with the other leg.

Toe Presses
RATING: EASY

Most people don't know that they have triceps muscles in their legs as well as their arms. The triceps in the legs are called triceps surae, and they actually consist of two (not three, as in the arms) muscles: the gastrocnemius and soleus. The gastrocnemius is the muscle that makes the calf curve; the soleus lies underneath the gastrocnemius and works with it to flex the foot and ankle. This exercise works both muscles, while also stretching and strengthening muscles in the foot.

Sit up straight on a rotary calf machine, making sure that the small of your back is firmly against the back pad. Adjust the seat so that the balls of your feet rest comfortably on the foot lever, about 4 to 6 inches apart, with your toes pointing upward. Your legs should be slightly bent.

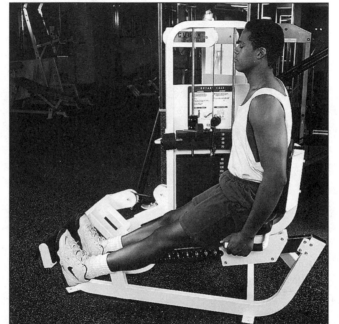

Gradually push down with the balls of your feet, pointing your toes as much as you can. Hold for a second, then slowly allow your feet to return to the starting position.

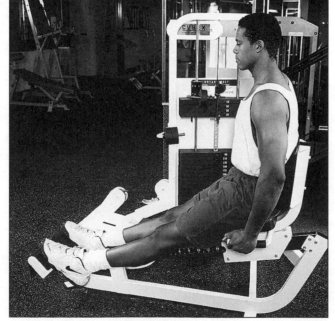

One-Leg Heel Raises

RATING: MODERATELY DIFFICULT

You have probably never noticed, but there's a good chance your calves are different sizes. (Here's an easy check: Time how long you can stand on one leg, then the other. The weaker muscle will be somewhat smaller.) The advantage of this exercise is that it isolates the muscles separately; you can build strength and size right where you want it. Even if your calves are perfectly even, this exercise will make you stronger for any activity involving running, jumping, and walking.

DO IT BETTER

- Always keep your ankle straight. Otherwise it might turn and sprain.
- Keep your back straight throughout the lift. Don't allow your body to sway or bend, which puts un-necessary stress on the calf.
- To increase difficulty, do this exercise while balancing a barbell behind your neck, across your shoulders.
- For best results, work the calves through their full range of motion. If the weight is too heavy to maximize the stretch, lower it.
- If one calf is smaller or weaker than the other, do additional sets to help achieve balance.

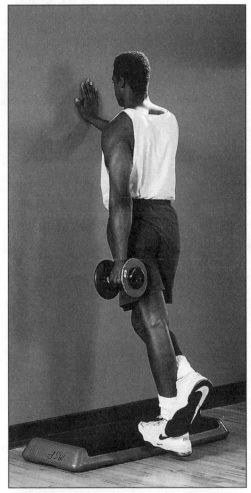

Stand on one leg with your heel off the edge of a stable platform—a stair, for instance—that is 6 to 10 inches high. Your knees should be slightly bent, with your toes pointed straight ahead. Let your heel drop down as far as it will comfortably go. Tuck your other foot behind the calf of the supporting foot. Hold a dumbbell on the same side as the supporting leg, with your palm facing inward. Hold on to a chair, wall, or other support for balance.

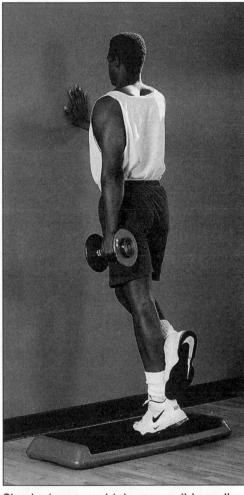

Slowly rise up as high as possible on the ball of your foot. Hold for a second, then slowly return to the starting position. After completing the set, switch legs and repeat.

Seated Heel Raises

RATING: EASY

Calves are considered the most difficult muscle group in the body to develop, especially the lower calves. While this exercise works the entire calf, it puts particular stress on the soleus (below calf) muscle.

Sit up straight on the side of a bench. Rest the balls of your feet on a 6- to 8-inch platform that is in front of you, allowing your heels to stretch down as far as they will go. Your knees should be together and bent at a 45-degree angle. Hold a dumbbell with both hands, resting it vertically on a folded towel on your thighs.

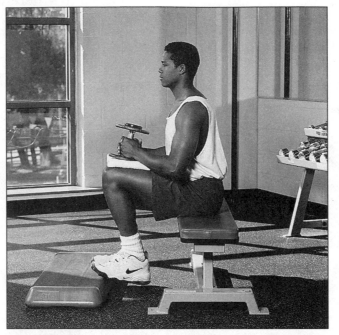

DO IT BETTER

• Rather than using a dumbbell, you may find it more comfortable to balance a barbell across your thighs.
• Keep your movements smooth and under control. Jerking upward or letting your heels suddenly drop brings momentum into play, reducing the effectiveness of the exercise.
• To increase difficulty, do the exercise one leg at a time.
• Turning your toes inward will develop more of the outside of the calves; turning them outward develops more of the inside.

Push up as high on the balls of your feet as you can. Hold for a second, then lower to the starting position.

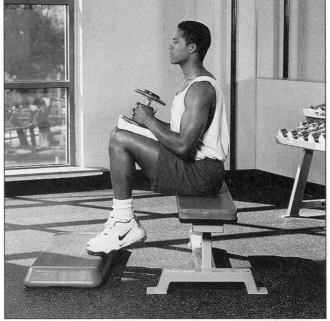

Donkey Calf Raises

RATING: MODERATELY DIFFICULT

This is one of Arnold Schwarzenegger's favorite exercises, as the size of his calves will attest. It works both the gastrocnemius (calf) and the soleus (below calf) muscles, which come together in the Achilles tendon. Strengthening these muscles can help prevent tendon injuries that often occur when running or playing basketball or baseball.

DO IT BETTER

• To increase difficulty, stand on a slightly higher block—say, one that's 4 to 6 inches high—and allow your heels to drop as far as they will go.
• Don't allow the person sitting on you to straddle your lower back, since this can cause serious injury.
• Warming up with alternating leg lunges or inclined heel raises (see pages 235 and 330) will help prevent muscle strain when doing this exercise.
• Changing foot position (moving your feet farther apart, for example) will work different parts of the muscles. Changing the direction of your toes will also work these muscles from different angles.

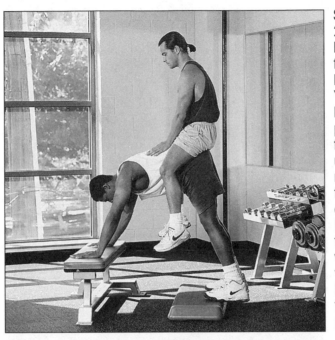

Stand on the edge of a 2- to 4-inch platform (a block of wood will work fine), with your heels hanging off the edge. Your legs should be hip-width apart, toes pointed forward. Bend forward at the waist until your upper body is roughly parallel with the floor. Extend your arms out straight and lean on something in front of you (a bench will do nicely). Keep your knees slightly bent. Then have a friend sit as far back as possible on your hips.

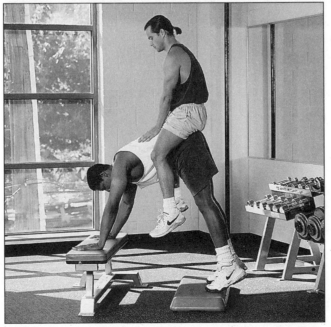

Slowly lift yourself up as high as possible on the balls of your feet. Hold for a second, then slowly lower your heels as far as they will go.

Inclined Heel Raises
RATING: MODERATELY DIFFICULT

This exercise provides an excellent stretch for the Achilles tendon and is a great warm-up for any sport that requires running or jumping.

Stand about 3 feet away from a wall. Keeping your heels in contact with the floor, put your arms straight in front of you and lean forward, putting your palms flat on the wall. Your back should be straight, legs and arms locked.

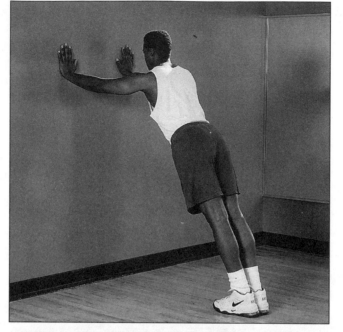

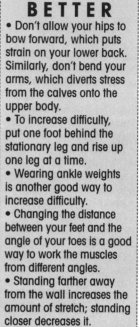

DO IT BETTER

• Don't allow your hips to bow forward, which puts strain on your lower back. Similarly, don't bend your arms, which diverts stress from the calves onto the upper body.
• To increase difficulty, put one foot behind the stationary leg and rise up one leg at a time.
• Wearing ankle weights is another good way to increase difficulty.
• Changing the distance between your feet and the angle of your toes is a good way to work the muscles from different angles.
• Standing farther away from the wall increases the amount of stretch; standing closer decreases it.

Slowly rise up on the balls of your feet, lifting yourself as high as possible. Hold for a second, then slowly lower your heels to the starting position.

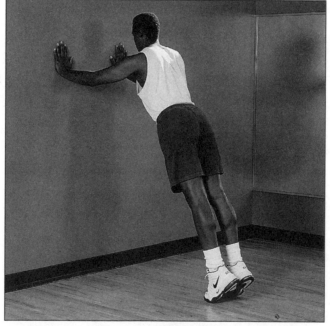

Sideways Dance Walks

RATING: DIFFICULT

Coordination and balance are the keys to this do-it-anywhere exercise, which isn't as easy as it looks. It utilizes many muscles that stabilize the ankle. It's a good choice for people who often sprain their ankles, or for anyone who does a lot of quick shifting on their feet—runners, or basketball, soccer, or tennis players.

DO IT BETTER

• To make this exercise most effective, pull your heels and toes up as far as possible, which maximizes the muscle contraction.
• When you are starting out, hold on to a wall or an upright object to maintain your balance. To increase difficulty, it's best to maintain your balance without added support.
• To decrease difficulty, use both feet at the same time.
• Don't cheat by using the momentum of your hips to swivel your heels and toes outward.

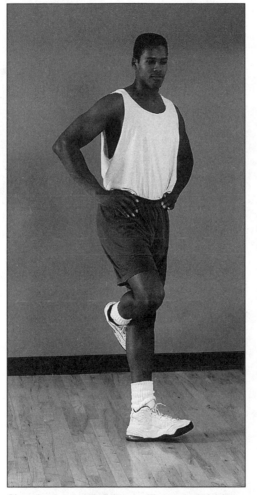

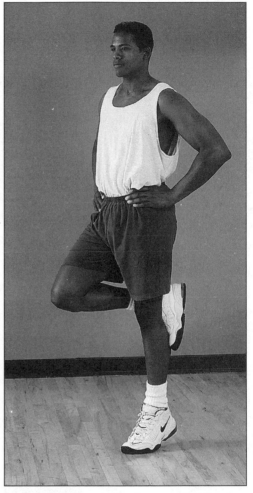

Stand on your left leg, with your right leg bent at a 90-degree angle behind you. You can let the free leg hang there, or you can hold it up with your hand. Raise the toes on your left foot and transfer your weight to your heels. Rotate the toes outward as far as possible.

Lower your toes and raise your heel, transferring your weight to the toes. Pivot your heel outward as far as you can.

Lower the heel and begin again. After you have done this 10 times to the left, do 10 times to the right. Then switch legs.

Feet Flexions

RATING: MODERATELY DIFFICULT

This is probably the best exercise for isolating and working the dorsiflexors of the foot (four muscles that enable you to lift your foot and toes). This exercise is recommended for running and other aerobic sports, which typically call on these muscles for spring and sprinting power.

Sit on the end of a bench with your legs together and your feet flat on the floor. Your knees should be bent at a 90-degree angle. Keeping your back straight, lean forward slightly at the waist, holding in place a weight plate resting across the base of your toes.

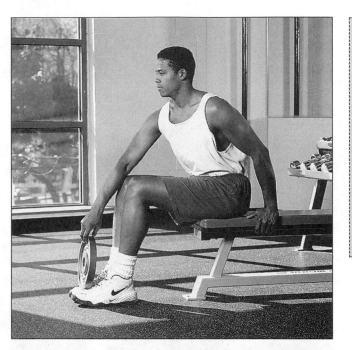

DO IT BETTER
- To increase difficulty, rest your heels on the end of a 2- to 4-inch platform and lower your toes as far as they will go.
- You can also increase difficulty by doing one foot at a time.
- Keeping the motion smooth and steady will help prevent the weight from jolting your toes.
- To prevent back strain, keep your back straight.

Slowly lift your toes as high as you can, keeping the weight balanced. Hold for a second, then slowly lower the weight to the starting position.

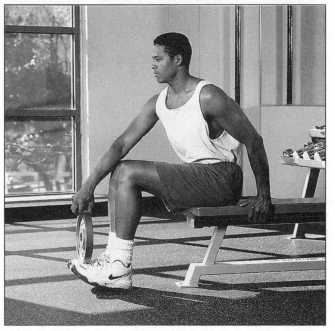

Tennis Ball Ankle Rotations

RATING: EASY TO MODERATELY DIFFICULT

This exercise is often recommended for people who have sprained an ankle. It strengthens and protects the many muscles, tendons, and ligaments that cover and attach in the ankle, particularly the muscles that point your toes and turn your foot outward. It also works the muscle that allows you to pull your toes up.

DO IT BETTER

• If you have trouble holding on to the ball, do the exercise without it.
• A variation of this exercise is to hold the ball between the arches of your feet while keeping your heels on the ground. Without letting go, move your toes up, down, and side to side.
• To increase difficulty, wear ankle weights while rotating your ankles.

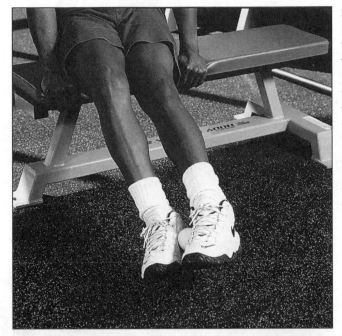

Sit up straight on a bench or chair with your feet flat on the floor. Hold a tennis ball between the arches of your feet. Raise and extend your legs so that your feet are about 3 inches off the ground. Slowly rotate your ankles clockwise, holding the ball between your feet.

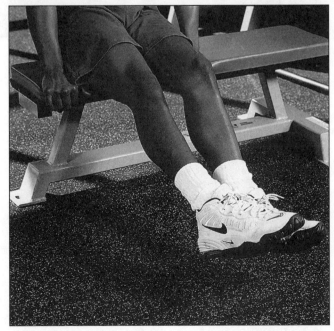

Repeat circles in one direction to complete set, then change course and go the other way.

Lower-Body Circuit

Ironically, although the legs contain some of the largest muscles in the body, they are often neglected in workout routines. The reason is simple: Their size demands a larger amount of energy than do routines for the upper body and midbody. This circuit, designed by Dragomir Cioroslan, head coach of the U.S. Weightlifting Federation and the 1996 U.S. Olympic weightlifting team, provides a total leg workout. Be sure to do the exercises in the order given: It's best to begin a workout with exercises that stress large numbers of big muscle groups, then move on to exercises that work smaller muscles and joints.

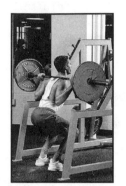

1. Squats (page 313)

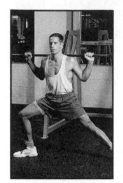

2. Lateral Squats (page 316)

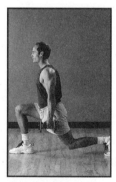

3. Walking Lunges (page 321)

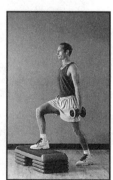

4. Step-Ups (page 322)

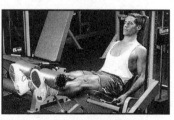

5. Leg Extensions (page 319)

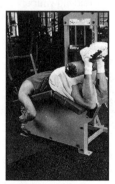

6. Leg Curls (page 320)

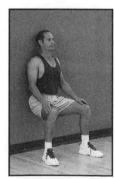

7. Phantom Chairs (page 324)

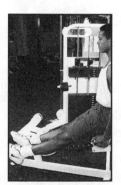

8. Toe Presses (page 326)

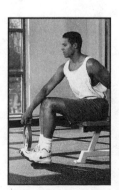

9. Feet Flexions (page 332)

PART IX

FLEXING AND STRETCHING

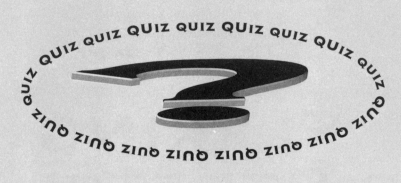

AM I LIMBER?

Flexibility is a hard sell. Few of us need to be convinced that it's good having the strength to bench-press our own weight or the endurance to run a 10-K without collapsing. This is the kind of stuff that makes us feel like small-time champions. But, oh, to be able to touch your toes—now there's a fitness goal to aspire to! The accomplishments of a limber body simply lack visceral drama, which is why there's no Olympic event in contortion.

But flexibility is just as important to fitness as muscular power or endurance—some might say more important. Without flexibility you're likely to get hurt. This is true even if you don't engage in exercise, says Frank Eksten, strength coordinator in the Department of Athletics and visiting lecturer in kinesiology at Indiana University in Bloomington.

Languishing muscles are like dogs: If you rouse them suddenly, they're liable to snap at you. By force of habit—going through the same limited range of motion day after day—we keep muscles penned up when they're dying to get out and play. After a while, restraint makes them surly and mean-spirited. How do you know if your muscles are verging on a show of teeth? Judge them on the following moves.

1. The kayaker stretch: You're paddling in a glassy calm off Baja, sitting upright in the cockpit of your craft, with your legs straight ahead of you and your feet together. Suddenly a gelatinous white bomb from a gull lands on your sparkling new, custom-fitted, paid-through-the-nose fiberglass deck, just beyond where your toes are. You try
splashing, scraping with the oar. Won't come off. Finally, you take the bandanna off your head and lean forward. . . . Can you reach it, or will you have to look at that offensive bit of business until landfall?

To find out, strike the pose, sitting down, legs extended, feet together, back against a wall. Keeping your back straight, lean forward and "walk" your hand along your leg. This tests the limits of your hamstrings, hip, and lower back. "If you can't reach your mid-shin, you have serious flexibility problems," says Eksten. "If you can reach your ankle, you're about average but should be better. If you can reach your toes or farther, that's what's required for adequate fitness."

2. The 24-bottle pickup: The barbecue coals are glowing, raw patties and franks are marshalled on plates, condiments are baking in the sun. Everything is set, except—you forgot beer! Off to the store, where you haul a case off the floor. How do you feel as you lift?

"You should be able to do this without any discomfort," says Eksten. "You might tighten your abdomen and bend your knees, sure, but there shouldn't be any pain, especially in the back or legs."

3. The lawn mower man stance: After mowing the lawn, pay attention to how your lower back feels as you bend over to untie your shoes from a seated position. Feel some tightness there?

That's probably because lack of limberness in your hamstrings or lower back combined with fatigue caused your hips to rotate in an awkward pivot while behind the lawn mower.

4. The "Honey, the light's out" reach: It's our nature to keep things within easy reach, which means we almost never reach over our heads—until it's time to replace a ceiling bulb, a task that women seem to feel men are genetically superior at accomplishing. We're not, which is why we invented step stools.

Fold your stool in a corner for the moment and try this: Reach over your head loosely with both hands, interlocking your fingers with both palms facing the ceiling. Now extend your arms as straight as you can toward the ceiling, suggests Eksten. If you can lock your elbows, you're reaching for the stars flexibility-wise. If you can't go any farther than a bent-elbow position or have to push your way past it, this area could stand some limbering.

5. The "Daddy, I dropped it" twist: Among the crash-test-dummy crowd, child safety seats are no doubt a pinnacle of lifesaving progress, but in the real world they can do you in. Why? Because when your kid drops her Happy Meal toy on the floor of the backseat, it falls to you to retrieve it from the belted-in confines of the front seat. You must execute this move with grace and finesse or be prepared to understand the absurdity of risking the health of your lower back over a 19-cent trinket.

To evaluate your level of training for this maneuver, test your abdominal, oblique, and lower back muscles. Sit upright in a chair, then twist your torso to one side. You should be able to rotate so that a line connecting one shoulder to the other would cross a line connecting one side of your hips to the other at a 90-degree angle, forming a †. "If you can do that, you can reach any point behind you, and that would be a measure of adequate torso flexibility," says Eksten.

6. The toenail touch: Cutting cuticles is a dainty matter, one that men reserve for moments of closed-door privacy such as the steamy aftermath of a shower. It's not something that you really want help with, unless living in a nursing home is your idea of fun. But you'll need help soon if your hips, gluteals, lower back, and upper hamstrings won't put your pinkies within striking distance of a self-performed hangnail-ectomy.

Here's the test: While sitting, can you put your foot in front of you on the chair and bring your heel to your butt without help from your hands so that you can touch your chin on your knee? If not, you're headed for Geezerville two or three decades ahead of schedule.

7. The mouse-mover pose: Pity Generation X, a span of humanity denied the elegance of drafting pencils, slide rules, and ledger books—all sacrificed to the expediency of mouse-driven computers. Which, of course, we all hunker over these days. The question is, how hunkered are you? If it's too much, all this turn-of-the-millennium technology may be lending you the appearance of a certain medieval bell ringer from Paris.

Ask yourself if you tend to walk with your chest out and shoulders back. No? Shoulders a bit stooped? That's probably causing you to crane your neck as well, since we're always aiming our eyes at the horizon. Thus, if your upper back is tight, you'll recognize it in a number of ways beyond looking in the mirror. "If you have soreness in the shoulders, neck, and even the arms—because nerves from the neck to the arm can become impinged at the shoulders—then lack of movement may be a problem for you," Eksten says.

8. The how-low-can-you-go squat: You're bouncing on your toes, ready for a return volley, your opponent is swatting the tennis ball to your left, you spring off—!

We'll let you supply the sad sound effects; some noises, like the cry of a maimed bunny, you just don't want to hear. "It has happened to a number of friends of mine that a sudden, quick change of direction or bouncing on the toes has ruptured the Achilles tendon," Eksten says. "It's debilitating. You're in a cast for six weeks."

The problem is tightness in the calf muscles or the Achilles tendon itself. Fortunately, before things blow, there are warnings, such as an inability to do this: From a standing position, with feet shoulder-width apart, lower yourself on your haunches so that your butt rests on the back of your ankles, while keeping your heels flat on the floor. If you can't do this, please—for us—do some stretching the next time you play tennis, basketball, or volleyball. In the next chapter, we'll tell you how.

FLEXING AND STRETCHING
ALL ABOUT TECHNIQUE

Consider the case of a man we'll call Jeff, since that's his name. Jeff played football in high school. Now in his mid-thirties, he still has the stocky build of a lineman. He's a great outdoorsman and spends a fair amount of time (less than he would like) in the backwoods.

In other words, he's a guy who once had glory-days athletic prowess and still occasionally asks his body to go on vigorous missions, should his body choose to accept them. But despite appearances, Jeff recently realized that he was not in the greatest of shape. His body was, in effect, balking at some of the missions he asked of it.

So he hired a personal trainer to whip him back into the kind of man he knew he should be. The trainer, in an initial test, confirmed the worst of what Jeff suspected. Over a beer in a steak joint, Jeff confessed to us the thing that most captured his attention: When the trainer had him sit down on the floor and put a yardstick between Jeff's outstretched legs (with the 15-inch mark at his heels) and asked him to reach as far as possible up the yardstick, he couldn't even bend far enough to touch the tip closest to him. He still remembers what the trainer wrote on the test paper: a big, fat zero.

The First Thing to Go

Shocking as that was to Jeff, this kind of "flex-lessness" should not come as a surprise to any middle-aged man. "Flexibility peaks when you're somewhere between 10 and 15 years old," says Frank Eksten, strength coordinator in the Department of Athletics and visiting lecturer in kinesiology at Indiana University in Bloomington. That makes decreased flexibility one of the first age-related physical declines to make itself known, kicking in a good 15 years or so ahead of drops in muscle mass, oxygen uptake, or metabolism. If you're over 35, you have probably already found yourself occasionally saying things like, "My joints feel a little stiff and creaky today." Part of you still thinks that you're a college kid—but another part of you is saying that you're more like a grandpa.

But it doesn't have to be this way. Loss of flexibility is mostly a function of how we move—or don't. Age itself doesn't make stiffness happen; we make it happen by constraining our muscles and, over time, causing them to shorten and resist being taken through a full range of motion. This loss of limberness is reversible: If you systematically move and stretch, you will also systematically expand your range of motion. Just ask our friend Jeff. At the end of eight weeks, which included a stretching regimen, he could reach the 11-inch mark on the yardstick.

This has significance beyond an arbitrary line on a slat. If you're more flexible, you'll have a bigger, more powerful arc in your golf or kung fu swing. You'll be more coordinated when using your muscles for small, precise motions like throwing darts or deflecting projectiles. And you'll be able to contract muscles more quickly, which, in conjunction with a longer stride, may pay off by making you a faster runner or a better solar-plexus kicker. Without flexibility, the wise, kick-butt monk Kwai

Chang Caine would just be a dusty, lost man, more like a latter-day David Carradine.

The question is how to go about improving yourself flexibility-wise. Stretching isn't complicated, isn't competitive, and isn't difficult. It's the easiest part of your workout, which may explain why it's so often neglected. (After all, can something so easy be truly worthwhile?) But it does require a bit of know-how. Stretching is partly science and partly art: Surprisingly, little definitive research has been done on it. Much of what's accepted about stretching is based on common sense and experience with athletes. But there is almost universal agreement that it's worthwhile. "In all our sports, flexibility is critically important," says Eksten.

Flexing Fundamentals

Understanding the merits of different techniques for stretching (there are several basic methods) requires a little pre-mission briefing on what happens when you hit targeted muscles.

Obviously, the muscle fibers being stretched become elongated or lengthened. Lengthening a muscle is the opposite of contracting (or shortening) it, which is what happens when a muscle exerts force. So stretching a muscle means relaxing it. The critical fact here is that positioning yourself to relax one set of muscles usually requires contracting a set of muscles opposite those that you have targeted. It's called an agonist/antagonist relationship. To stretch your quadriceps, you contract your hamstrings. To stretch your chest, you contract the upper back. To stretch your lower back, you contract your stomach.

Why is this important? Because strength in opposing muscle groups may improve flexibility when you're doing certain kinds of stretches. We'll explain how that can come into play in a moment, but part of the take-away is this: Building muscle does not make you muscle-bound. In fact, the opposite is true. Building muscle can help improve flexibility if you stretch in conjunction with strength training.

A second point is that although stretching is not a vigorous activity, the targeted muscles don't just passively sit there. When you lengthen muscles beyond what they're accustomed to, an automatic and involuntary reaction called the stretch reflex takes place. The body actually resists overstretching as a matter of injury prevention, like when you jerk your hand off a hot stove. While you're trying to lengthen muscles,

they're working against you by trying to shorten.

"If you hold a stretch for a prolonged period of time, your muscles will adapt to the stretch reflex, tend to relax more, and thus your stretching is enhanced," says William D. Bandy, Ph.D., associate professor of physical therapy at the University of Central Arkansas in Conway. All of which has to do with why proper technique is important for improving flexibility and why lack of technique can lead to injury.

Stretching Options

Although there are several different ways to stretch the body, they don't all have equal standing for most people. Really, there's one basic method, with a few options for people in specific circumstances. Here is the range of approaches, starting with the one you most likely should employ, says Eksten.

Static Stretching

Static stretches are done slow and easy, using very little force—often through some combination of gravity and body weight—to push muscles just a little past their usual range of motion. Targeting a hamstring by propping one foot on a chair and reaching for the toes of the elevated leg is a static stretch. It's hard to go wrong with a static stretch if you follow these simple guidelines.

WARM UP FIRST. There's some debate about whether this is necessary, but the reasoning is sound: If you engage in a few minutes of activity before stretching (enough to break a light sweat), muscles will be warmer and more pliable. That allows you to lengthen them farther without their complaining and possibly getting hurt either during stretching or later in your workout.

Do you need to do it? "Nobody I know exercises without a warm-up," says Bryant Stamford, Ph.D., director of the Health Promotion Center at the University of Louisville. Think of it this way: If warm-up proponents are wrong, there's no harm done; if skeptics are wrong, you could injure yourself. You decide which way to go.

MOVE GENTLY. You're not out to surprise your muscles; move in slow, controlled motions. You also don't want to force muscles beyond a point they don't really want to go; stretch only until you feel a slight tug on the targeted muscle.

HOLD FOR 30 SECONDS. Holding is important because it gives muscles time to overcome the stretch reflex. After a moment of initial alarm, muscles tend to relax and become more susceptible to lengthening. How long should you hold? In a study using hamstring stretches, Dr. Bandy found that 30 seconds is ideal, providing significant, measurable weekly improvements in flexibility. Holding for less than 15 seconds was not much better than not stretching at all, while longer than 60 seconds provided no additional benefit.

Dynamic Stretching

It's called dynamic because there's movement involved. The idea here is to use antagonist muscles (those opposite the ones targeted in the stretch) to briefly power the body into a position that will expand range of motion. Targeting a hamstring by raising an extended leg high enough to produce a stretch—but not resting the foot on something—then lowering it again is a dynamic stretch.

"It's the kind of thing a lot of people do automatically," says Eksten. "If you're going to throw a ball, you might swing your arms around a little first." Part of the theory is that when antagonist muscles contract, agonist muscles (the ones you're stretching) relax more, becoming more pliable. Here's where the value of strength comes in: If the muscles powering the stretch are in good condition, contraction/relaxation movements can be controlled and sustained better.

By their nature, dynamic stretches are done quickly, which is verboten in the world of static stretching. That's because dynamic movement raises the risk of propelling muscles too far beyond their customary range of motion, producing soreness or injury.

"Dynamic stretching is dangerous if misused, and it's probably not within the scope of most people's needs," Eksten says. "It's most appropriate when you're training for a specific sport that actually involves sudden, forceful movement, such as sprinting or pitching."

Ballistic Stretching

This is dynamic stretching taken a step further: The movement is quicker and more violent, so that the stretch is accomplished partly through momentum. This is inherently dangerous and is usually done only to prepare for activities where flexibility is important, and with people who already are extremely pliable—gymnasts or ballet dancers, for example.

PNF Stretching

It's called PNF because who can say "proprioceptive neuromuscular facilitation"? This kind of stretching takes two people: Targeting your hamstring (for which it's often used) would have you lying on your back on the floor, raising an extended leg toward the ceiling while a partner helps move the leg through its range of motion.

It's the agonist/antagonist thing again: The targeted hamstring may be passively stretched for 10 seconds; then, while your partner holds your leg in place, you tense up the hamstring. Then you stretch the hamstring again. This technique, while demonstrated to be highly effective at improving flexibility, is also not recommended for most people, for two reasons: You need a partner, which robs you of stretching's "anywhere, anytime" appeal, and if your partner is not trained in the method, the potential for injury is high. If you're interested in this method, seek a personal trainer who has had some instruction in it.

What to Be Careful Of
Smart Stretching

If you know how to stretch right, you automatically know how not to stretch wrong. But extrapolating on a few principles may be in order.

First, let's assume once and for all that we're talking only about static stretching, the most versatile and universally useful kind. Because of their dangers and the fact that they're most useful only under specific circumstances, we're completely leaving dynamic, ballistic, and proprioceptive neuromuscular facilitation (PNF) stretching out of the picture. (For more on these stretches, see the Flexing and Stretching chapter on page 338.)

To keep your muscles loose, limber, and uninjured, here's what experts advise.

STAY IN CONTROL. Bouncing increases your risk of stretching muscles farther than they can safely go, which can cause tearing just like the kind you see in a rubber band that is overextended, says Frank Eksten, strength coordinator in the Department of Athletics and visiting lecturer in kinesiology at Indiana University in Bloomington.

To get a sense of how this occurs, try statically stretching your chest by raising your elbows at shoulder level, then easing them back behind you until you feel a slight tug. That's where the stretch should end. Now try the same movement quickly. (Don't try this experiment if you have ever injured your shoulder.) Be honest: Didn't you throw your elbows back farther in the dynamic motion than you did in the static one?

TAKE IT EASY. It seems that every man once had a high school gym teacher whose idea of stretching was modeled on methods of medieval justice—for instance, standing some members of the class against the wall, then forcibly trying to raise every student's legs, one at a time, to a point where his toes could touch the wall above his head. The gym echoed with screams, with those lined up smiling weakly along with the instructor, hoping irrationally that this was indeed somehow funny, while the other members of the class stood by horrified, unable to intervene, knowing their turn would soon come . . .

Excuse us, we get these flashbacks.

"I still see people who seem to think they need to be in the utmost pain while stretching," says Eksten. "Something's wrong there. Stretching should be relaxing, and your body should feel good when you're done."

KEEP BREATHING. Breathing is involuntary, but that doesn't mean that you never have to think about it. None of us are going to asphyxiate ourselves stretching our hamstrings, but it pays to remember that some of the most sophisticated flexibility regimens in the world—namely, the various forms of yoga—make slow, rhythmic breathing an integral part of the movements. This is partly a philosophical matter that you'll need to explore in some other book, but from a physiological point of view, it has merit all its own.

"Breathing helps people relax," says Eksten. And relaxing is the core of stretching. There's no need to make stretching mystical (unless that helps). "I usually just tell people to breathe normally," Eksten says. If you want to hone your technique a bit, try exhaling and relaxing as you move into position. As you hold, breathe easily for 30 seconds, then inhale as you return to your starting position.

MIDBODY STRETCHES
Side Bends
RATING: EASY

Activities such as golf and tennis require a lot of twisting. This stretch will help extend your range of motion while preventing muscle pulls. It works the muscles that run along your sides—specifically, the latissimus dorsi (mid and lower back) and oblique (side abdominal) muscles. It also works the erector spinae (lower back) muscles.

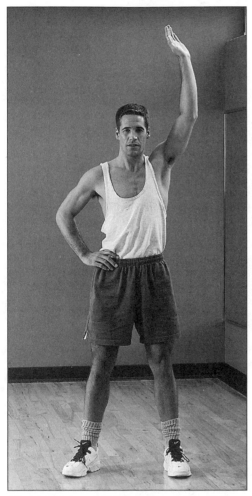

Stand with your feet flat, shoulder-width apart, and your knees slightly bent. Place your right hand on your right hip and extend your left arm straight up, palm facing away from your body.

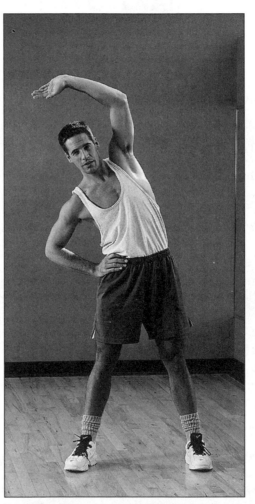

Reach over your head with your left hand, bending at the waist to the right. Moving slowly and with control, reach as far to the right as you comfortably can. Hold for 10 to 15 seconds, then repeat the movements to the left.

DO IT BETTER

• To make the stretch more effective, extend both arms over your head. Gripping your left hand with the right, bend to the right and use your right hand to gently pull the left arm over.

• Extend your right arm down at your side and reach past the knee, or as far as you comfortably can, while simultaneously reaching over your head with the other arm. The farther you reach, the more muscles you will stretch.

• Reach straight up with one hand and hold before reaching to the opposite side. This pre-stretches the muscles, making the second half of the stretch easier.

• To increase difficulty when you're in the full-stretch position, turn your torso to the right and bend at the waist, keeping your back flat. You should be facing the floor. Then repeat to the other side.

Side Twists

RATING: EASY

If you have ever stretched to crack your back, this is probably the movement that you used. These twists are recommended for any activity that involves twisting, from yard work to sports like racquetball or tennis. They primarily stretch the abdominal and back muscles, particularly the latissimus dorsi (mid and lower back) and erector spinae (lower back) muscles.

DO IT BETTER

- To increase the stretch in your neck, look with your eyes all the way to the right when turning right and all the way to the left when turning left.
- To stretch while sitting, twist and reach to the right with both hands until you can grab the side of the chair. Then repeat to the left.
- To incorporate a stretch in your shoulders, extend your left arm across your chest when stretching right. Grab your left elbow with your right hand and pull the left arm to the right. Then repeat to the other side.
- To increase the effectiveness of this stretch, stand about a foot from a fence or wall. As you twist to the right, place both hands on the surface and "walk" both hands as far as you comfortably can. Then repeat to the other side.

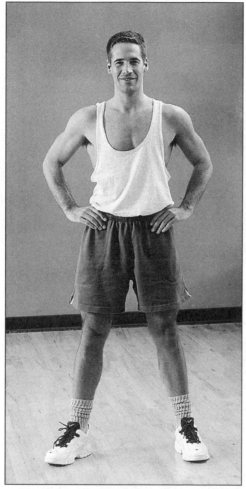

Stand with your feet shoulder-width apart, knees slightly bent. Place your hands on your hips. Keep your head in line with your torso, with your eyes straight ahead.

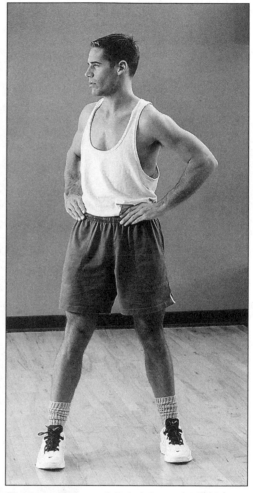

Starting at the waist, twist your upper body to the right, following through by twisting your back and head. Hold for 10 to 15 seconds, then repeat to the left.

Lower Back Leans

RATING: EASY

The bent-over position used in this exercise looks like something you would do in a relaxation class, but it provides a good stretch to the lower back. It is generally considered to be better for cooling down after a workout than for warming up beforehand; it puts the muscles into their relaxed mode, which is where you want them when you're done for the day.

Sit in a chair with your feet flat on the floor and slightly more than shoulder-width apart.

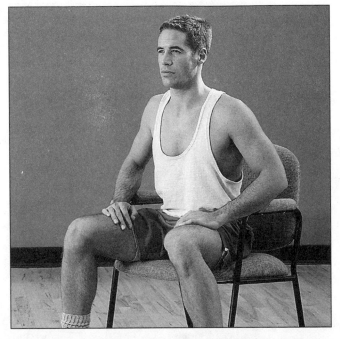

DO IT BETTER

• To stretch the entire back, bend at the waist and reach straight out in front of you. Then relax and lower your upper body between your knees.

• To get an additional stretch in the lower back and midback, reach through your legs and under the chair at the bottom of the movement.

• To reduce tension and improve circulation, be sure to let your head and arms completely relax at the bottom of the stretch.

Lean forward in the chair, letting your upper body, arms, and head slowly fall between your knees. Hold for 30 seconds. Then place your hands on your thighs and gently push back into the upright position.

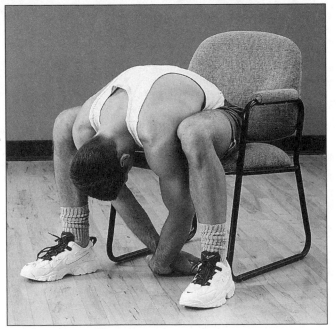

Lying Leg Pulls

RATING: MODERATELY DIFFICULT

This stretch is excellent for relieving lower back pain, which is often caused by poor flexibility of the hips, hamstring (back thigh) muscles, and lower back. It works the hamstring, gluteal (butt), and latissimus dorsi (mid and lower back) muscles. It also stretches the erector spinae (lower back) muscles. The farther you pull your knees in to your chest, the better the stretch.

DO IT BETTER

• To increase the stretch in the lower back, roll your body front to back, keeping your knees tucked into your chest.
• To increase the stretch in your upper back, lower your head to your chest.
• To stretch the shins and calves, alternately point your toes and flex your feet while your knees are pulled into your chest.

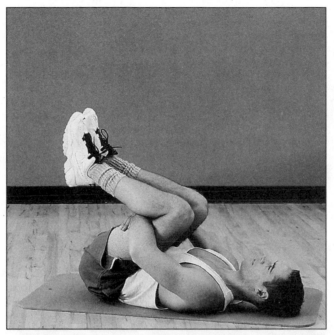

Lie on your back with your arms under your thighs. Pull your knees as close to your chest as they will comfortably go. This stretches the lower back.

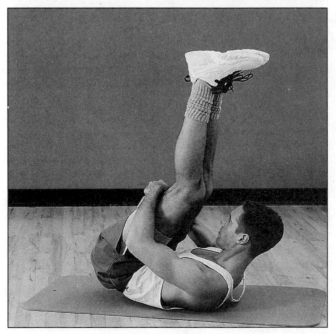

Keeping your knees against your chest, extend your legs over your head. This extends the stretch to include the hamstrings and butt muscles. Hold for 15 seconds, then return to the starting position. Increase to 30 seconds as you feel more comfortable with the stretch.

Legs-Overhead Stretches

RATING: DIFFICULT

This is an advanced midbody stretch that will help loosen the hamstring (back thigh) muscles, lower back, hips, upper back, and neck. Because it's a vigorous stretch, it should be done after you have warmed up with lying leg pulls (see page 345). You'll feel the stretch most in your upper back and neck. If you have any neck problems, it's a good idea to do neck stretches before trying this exercise.

Lie on your back with your arms extended at a 45-degree angle to your body, palms flat on the ground. With your knees slightly bent, roll your legs so that your knees are at your head. Your hips and lower back should be completely off the floor.

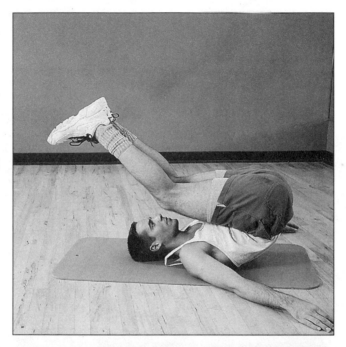

Allow your toes to touch the floor behind your head, with your arms and hands pressed to the floor. Hold for 10 seconds at first and increase to 30 seconds as you feel more comfortable with the stretch.

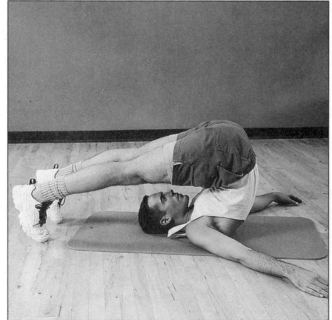

DO IT BETTER

• For good balance, place your hands under your hips as you move your legs over your head.

• To get more stretch in the groin, move your feet apart when your toes touch the floor behind your head.

• To decrease difficulty, bring your feet over your head and hold your legs in position, keeping your middle and upper back on the floor.

• To further decrease difficulty, bring your knees to your chest with your legs bent at more than a 90-degree angle. Hold your legs against your body by placing both hands under your thighs.

• To intensify the stretch in your back, hold on to a stationary object behind your head as you bring your legs up. Then lower your legs very slowly back to the starting position, feeling the vertebrae in your back touch the ground one at a time.

• Assuming you already have strong abs, here's a variation to increase the stretch in your entire torso: Place your hands on the back of your hips, just below your lower back. Push your legs back and up over your head, going farther than just behind your head. Hold your weight on your hands with your elbows bent for support.

Lateral Lower Back Stretches

RATING: MODERATELY DIFFICULT

This is an all-purpose stretch that will prepare your body for just about anything that you'll do in the course of a day, from sitting at a desk to a lunch-hour run. It works the gluteal (butt) muscles as well as the erector spinae (lower back) muscles.

DO IT BETTER

- To increase the stretch in the lower back and hips, use your right hand to press the left knee to the floor. Turning your head to the left will further increase the stretch in your neck.
- To stretch the hamstrings and increase the stretch in the gluteal muscles, extend the left leg straight out on the right side, once the knee is touching the floor.
- Pointing the toes on the right foot will stretch the calf. Flexing the foot will stretch the shin.
- To get more stretch in the buttocks, reach under your left thigh with your right hand and pull it toward your right shoulder, keeping both shoulders flat on the floor.

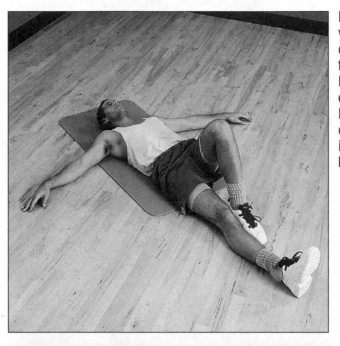

Lie on your back with your arms outstretched at your sides, palms facing the floor. Keeping your right leg extended, bend your left leg, placing the inside of your left foot on the inside of your right knee.

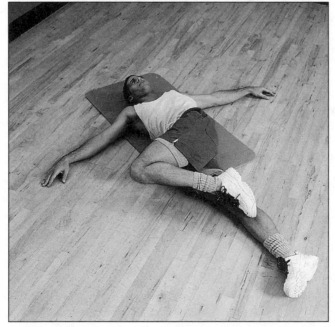

Keeping your arms out, bring your left knee to the floor on the right side—or as close to the floor as you can comfortably reach. As you pull the leg over, press your left shoulder back to the left to stretch the upper back and shoulder. Hold for 15 to 30 seconds.

Lower Back Squats

RATING: MODERATELY DIFFICULT

Sometimes sitting all day can be just as tiring as standing. This is because many of the same muscles—particularly the erector spinae (lower back) muscles—are stressed in both positions. In fact, the only time these muscles truly relax is when you are slumped over. That's the position you will assume when doing lower back squats. This stretch works the lower back, quadriceps (front thigh) muscles, knees, groin, Achilles tendons, and shins. It is not recommended for people with knee problems.

Stand with your feet more than shoulder-width apart, toes angled slightly outward. Keep your head in line with your spine throughout the entire movement.

Squat down, bringing your arms between your legs until your upper arms rest against your inner thighs. Relax your upper back so that you are slumped over with your hands on the ground. Keep your feet flat on the floor and don't let your knees extend past your toes. Relax completely and remain in the slumped-over position for 30 seconds.

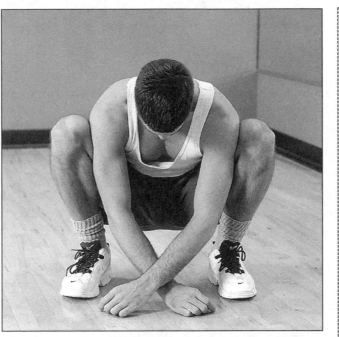

DO IT BETTER

• Holding on to a stationary object will help keep you balanced and will also increase the stretch in the latissimus dorsi muscles.

• Pushing against your inner thighs with your upper arms will increase the stretch in the groin muscles.

• To decrease difficulty, support your back against a wall while in the squatting position.

• To further relax and stretch the back and hamstrings, straighten your legs and stand, keeping your upper body bent over, with your hands touching your feet. Hold this position for 10 to 15 seconds, then slowly stand upright.

Standing Hip Stretches

RATING: EASY

This exercise is perfect for stretching the gluteal (butt) muscles, the hip flexors (front hip), and the iliotibial band (a band of tendon that runs from the hip to the knee). These are the muscles and tendons that often are strained from playing sports that require quick, side-to-side movements, like racquetball, volleyball, and soccer.

DO IT BETTER

- A variation of this exercise is to stand inside a door frame, holding on to the frame with both hands. Push your hip to the right as you simultaneously push your chest through the doorway. This will increase the stretch in your shoulders and back.
- To increase difficulty, keep your weight on the back foot.
- To further increase difficulty, use both hands to hold on to one side of a door frame or a fence, at about shoulder height. Fully extend both arms in the opposite direction of the hip you are stretching. This puts extra stress on the hips and butt, while also stretching the shoulders.

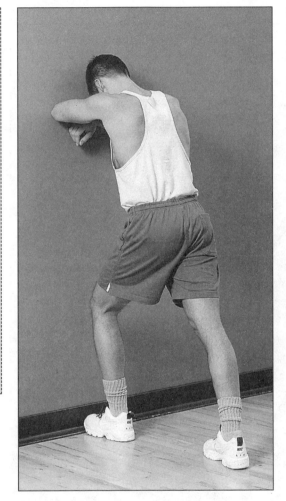

Stand about 2 feet from a wall. Lean on the wall with your forearms; your hands should be crossed and elbows angled to the sides. Rest your head against your hands. Bring your left foot in front of you and put the toes against the wall. Keep your right foot slightly behind you and flat on the floor.

Slowly push your right hip to the right side, allowing your shoulders to move in the opposite direction. This emphasizes the stretch in your right hip. Hold for 30 seconds, then repeat the movements on the left side.

Hip Flexion Stretches

RATING: EASY

By nature, the muscles and tendons in the hip are sufficiently mobile to enable you to raise your leg above your head. Most of us, of course, don't have that kind of flexibility. This exercise, which works the hip flexor (front hip), gluteal (butt), adductor (inner thigh), and abductor (outer thigh) muscles, will help expand your range of motion in your legs.

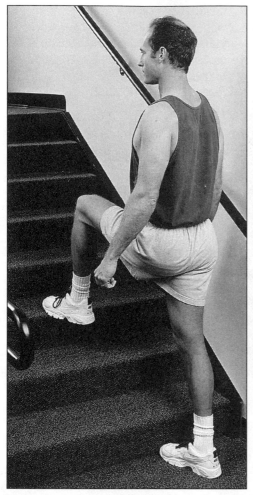

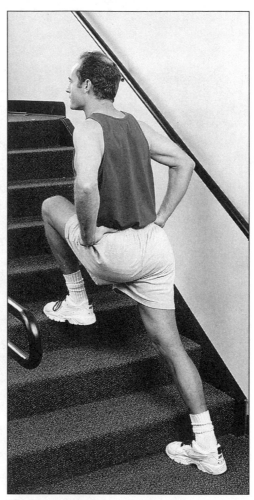

Place the ball of your left foot on a bench (or on the third step of a flight of stairs). Extend your right leg behind you, knee slightly bent.

Place your hands on your hips and lean into your left leg, pushing your hips forward. Keep your torso straight; do not extend your left knee past your toes. Hold for 30 seconds, then repeat on the right leg.

DO IT BETTER
• To stretch more of the groin area when doing this exercise, turn your back foot so the toes are pointing out to the side.
• Rotating your raised leg toward the center of your body will increase the stretch in the outer thigh.
• To add a stretch to your lower back, reach forward and grab the step or bench and pull your torso forward as you stretch your hip and legs.

Knee-to-Chest
Lower Back Stretches

RATING: EASY

The midbody not only supports the torso and head but it also must support any additional weight that you happen to pick up, be it a barbell or grocery bag. As a result, it's the most injury-prone part of the body. This stretch helps loosen all the main muscles in this trouble spot, including the hip rotators (inner thigh), the erector spinae (lower back) muscles, and the gluteal (butt) muscles.

DO IT BETTER

• To get a whole-body stretch while lying down, reach above your head as you simultaneously point your toes.

• To make this stretch more effective, rotate your thigh toward the middle of the body while lifting your knee.

• To save time, bring both knees up to your chest rather than raising one at a time.

• To increase difficulty, grab your right ankle with your left hand and pull the ankle in to your chest, while pushing the raised knee in the opposite direction.

• To get more stretch in the hip rotators and hip flexors, have a partner stand over you and push your ankle toward your body while pushing down on your knee.

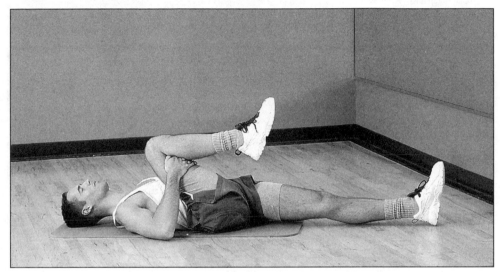

Lie flat on your back. Pull your right knee in to your chest, keeping your lower back pressed to the floor. Hold for 30 seconds, then repeat with the left leg.

Hip Rotator Stretches

RATING: MODERATELY DIFFICULT

This exercise works the hip rotator (inner thigh) muscles and the lower back. If you do any sort of running or jumping, or anything else that stresses the lower body, this exercise is worth doing.

Lie on your back. Bend your right leg at about a 90-degree angle, keeping the right foot planted firmly on the floor. Cross your left ankle over your right knee.

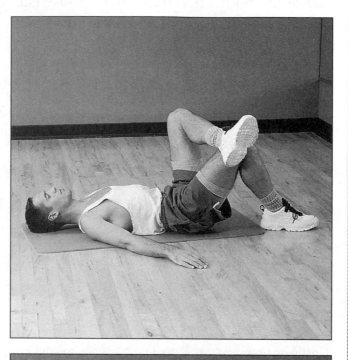

DO IT BETTER

• To increase the stretch in the hip rotator muscles, use your right hand to pull your right thigh in to your body, while pushing in the opposite direction on the left knee with your left hand.

• To decrease difficulty, leave your right foot on the floor and place your left hand on your left knee. Gently push on the left knee, keeping your left ankle on the right leg at all times.

• To increase difficulty, do the stretch as described, but get close to a wall. Put your right foot against the wall and move as close to the wall as you can, with your left ankle crossing your right knee. Gently push on the left knee.

Put both hands behind your right thigh and pull the leg toward your body as far as you comfortably can. Keep your left knee pointing to the outside of your body. Hold for 30 seconds, then switch legs.

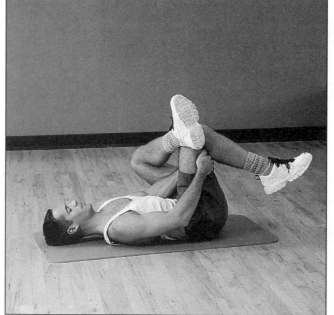

Crossed-Leg Rolls

RATING: DIFFICULT

The midbody is constantly being twisted—when golfing, playing tennis, or picking up around the house. This stretch keeps all the key muscles—particularly the obliques (side abdominals), gluteal (butt) muscles, lower back, and latissimus dorsi (mid and lower back)—relaxed and limber.

DO IT BETTER

- To increase the stretch in your torso, raise your right arm and right shoulder off the ground while rolling your upper body to the left in the opposite direction of your legs.
- In the same crossed-leg position, with your left ankle crossed over your right knee, roll your hips to the left instead of to the right, allowing the side of your left thigh and the inside of your right thigh to touch the floor. This will stretch your gluteal muscles on the opposite side.
- While doing the variation above, raise your left arm and left shoulder off the ground while rolling your upper body to the right—in the opposite direction your hips are going. This will accentuate the stretch in your abdominal and gluteal muscles.

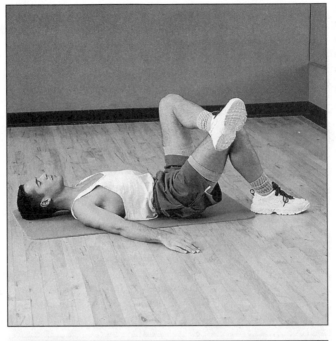

Lie on your back. Bend your right leg at about a 90-degree angle with your right foot planted firmly on the floor. Cross your left ankle over your right knee.

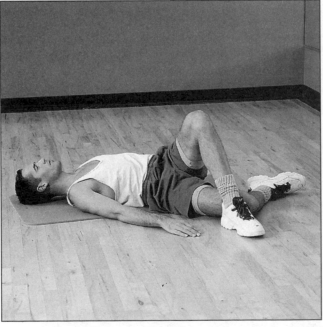

Roll your hips toward the right side of your body until the side of your right thigh and the bottom of your left foot touch the floor. Your lower back and left hip will rise off the floor, but keep your upper back and shoulders pressed firmly down. Hold for 30 seconds, then switch sides.

Seated Hamstring-
and-Gluteus Stretches
RATING: MODERATELY DIFFICULT

If after endless hours in a meeting you find that your butt has fallen asleep, but you can't get up and stretch, this exercise will help. It mainly targets the hamstring (back thigh) and gluteal (butt) muscles.

With your feet flat on the floor, sit upright in a chair with the small of your back firmly against the back of the chair. Rest your right ankle on your left leg above the knee.

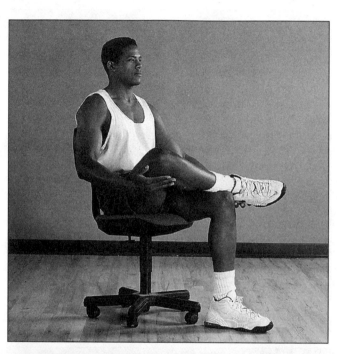

DO IT BETTER
• You can do this stretch without using a chair by sitting on the floor with your back against a wall and your feet straight in front of you.
• Another way to increase the stretch is by pulling your leg closer to your chest.
• Keeping your back straight will help reduce pressure on the lower back.

Using both hands to support the ankle and knee, lift your right knee toward your chin. Then lift the heel until your lower leg is parallel to the floor. Stretch and hold for 30 seconds. Then repeat with the other leg.

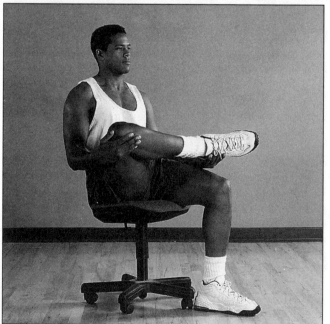

Front-to-Back Leg Extensions

RATING: EASY

This stretch is particularly recommended for runners because it increases flexibility and range of motion in the hips. This translates into a longer stride, greater ease of movement, and possibly more speed. It works the quadriceps (front thigh), hip flexor (front hip), and hamstring (back thigh) muscles.

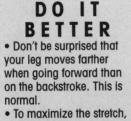

DO IT BETTER

• Don't be surprised that your leg moves farther when going forward than on the backstroke. This is normal.
• To maximize the stretch, don't use momentum to lift your leg. Do the movement slowly and with constant muscular control.
• Avoid jerking movements, which can easily result in groin pulls.

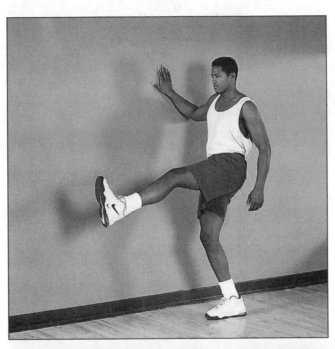

With one hand on a wall for balance, raise the leg farthest from the wall straight in front of you. Don't swing the leg, but use the thigh muscles to steadily lift it.

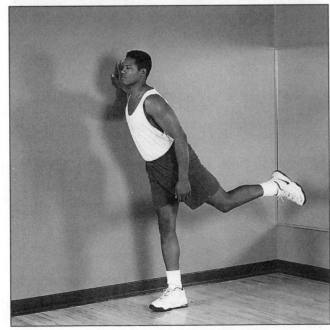

Lower the leg and let it fall back, using the hip and gluteal (butt) muscles to raise it behind you as high as is comfortable. You will need to lean forward a bit to keep your balance, but keep your back as straight as you can. Lower the leg and repeat, moving it forward and back in a slow, rhythmic pace. Repeat with the other leg.

Side-to-Side Leg Extensions

RATING: EASY

Whenever you move your upper legs—for example, while running, jumping, or weight training—the hips come into play. This exercise stretches the adductor (inner thigh) and abductor (outer thigh) muscles, which allow the legs to move from side to side.

With your hands on a wall for balance, slowly raise your right leg to the side as far as you comfortably can, while keeping the left leg slightly bent.

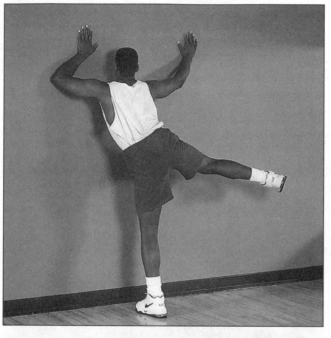

DO IT BETTER
• Don't sway your body or lean into the opposite direction of the leg lift. This may help you lift the leg higher, but it does not aid in stretching the designated muscles more.
• Hold on to a table or other object that is between waist and shoulder height if this is more convenient.
• You may find it more comfortable to turn the toes of your supporting foot slightly outward as you lift your other foot.
• Use ankle weights to increase the difficulty of the lift and strengthen as well as stretch your muscles.

Slowly bring the leg back down, swinging it past the starting point and in the opposite direction, going as far as you comfortably can. The foot should be slightly flexed, not pointed. Continue moving the leg back and forth. Then do the other leg.

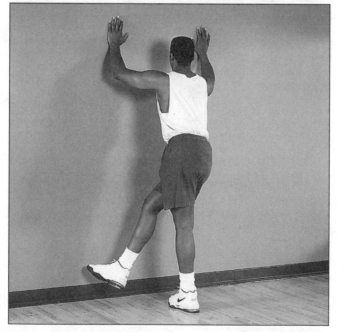

Kneeling Hip-and-Groin Stretches

RATING: MODERATELY DIFFICULT

Lower back problems are often related to hip stiffness. This stretch helps loosen muscles in front of the hips and thighs. You may want to do this exercise with the squatting groin stretch (see page 359), which helps loosen the opposing muscles behind the thighs.

DO IT BETTER

• Keeping your chest up will help increase the stretch.

• To further stretch the hip flexors, straighten your back leg by raising your knee off the ground. To also stretch the Achilles tendon, attempt to push your heel to the ground from this position.

• This stretch puts a lot of strain on the knee, so move cautiously if you have had knee problems in the past.

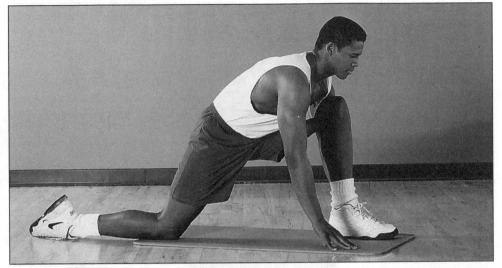

Get down on all fours. Raise one knee off the floor and move the foot between your hands until the knee is directly over the ankle and touching your chest. Stretch the front of your kneeling hip downward until you feel slight resistance. Your back leg should be nearly straight. Hold for 30 seconds. Repeat with the other leg.

Seated Groin Stretches

RATING: EASY

Sometimes called a butterfly stretch, this is a great way to limber up your inner thigh muscles and protect them against groin pulls. Skaters, skiers, gymnasts, and dancers find it especially useful since they make heavy use of these muscles to maintain good balance. This stretch will also improve your range of motion for squatting or side-to-side movements.

Sit up straight with your back against a wall. Put the soles of your feet together. Put your hands on the insides of your thighs just above the knees and gently push downward until you feel resistance. Hold the stretch for a count of 10, then relax.

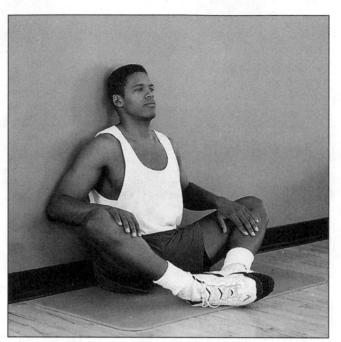

DO IT BETTER

• To increase the stretch in the inner thighs—and to stretch the lower back—use your elbows instead of your hands to gently push down on your upper thighs.
• To further increase the stretch in the inner thighs and groin, pull your heels closer to your groin.
• Avoid bouncing your knees up and down, which can lead to groin pulls.
• Keeping your back flat will help reduce the risk of back strain.

Squatting Groin Stretches

RATING: MODERATELY DIFFICULT

This relaxing squat stretches all the muscles in the groin and inner thigh. It also stretches muscles in the lower back and butt. It is often recommended for soccer and football players as well as those who ride horseback, since all of these activities tend to make the thigh muscles tight. This stretch is also good for relieving lower back stiffness.

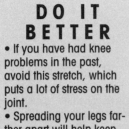

DO IT BETTER

• If you have had knee problems in the past, avoid this stretch, which puts a lot of stress on the joint.
• Spreading your legs farther apart will help keep you balanced. You can also lean your back against a wall for support.
• Squat down slowly and with control; bouncing on the knees can cause muscle damage.

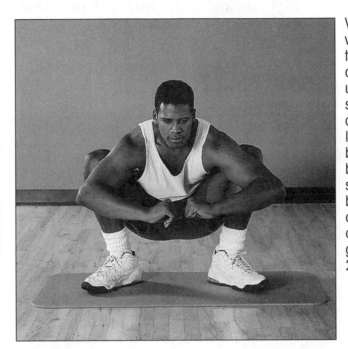

With your feet shoulder-width apart and the toes pointing slightly outward, squat down until your knees are spread apart. Let your arms fall between your legs. Lean your upper body a bit forward but keep your back straight. Lean your elbows against the inside of your knees and push outward, stretching the groin muscles. Hold for 20 seconds, then relax.

Lying Groin Stretches

RATING: EASY

If doing seated or squatting groin stretches is difficult, try using this simpler stretch as a warm-up. Since it depends on gravity rather than muscular force, it's not quite as effective as the other groin stretches. But for people with limited flexibility, it's a good place to start. And because it's done lying down, this stretch is easier on the back and knees. It works muscles in the inner thigh, including the adductor, pectineus, and gracilis muscles. You can do this stretch before getting out of bed in the morning.

Lie flat on your back with your knees bent and the soles of your feet together. Then relax: Gravity will pull your knees down, stretching the groin muscles. Hold for 30 seconds.

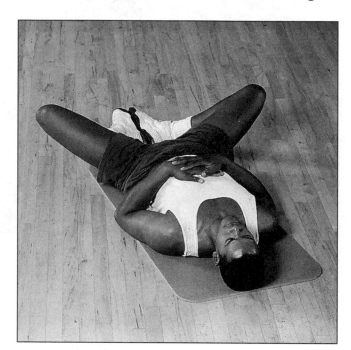

DO IT BETTER

- For extra support, place a towel or small pillow under the small of your back.
- Here's a dynamic variation to increase the stretch: While lying down, gently rock your legs back and forth at the same time, starting from the hips. Keep the movements small—about an inch in each direction.
- Don't bounce the knees, which can cause muscle pulls.

Wall Groin Stretches

RATING: MODERATELY DIFFICULT

Although groin muscles are among the most powerful muscles in the body, they tend to get stiff from lack of use, making them prone to injury. To prevent groin pulls, which often occur when lifting the legs out to the sides quickly, it's a good idea to use this stretch as a warm-up. It's particularly good if you're a catcher or volleyball player or if you spend a lot of time in the yard squatting or stepping sideways.

DO IT BETTER

- Moving your butt closer to the wall will increase the stretch in the groin muscles.
- Don't get up quickly after having your legs raised because it can cause light-headedness.
- To make the stretch more comfortable and to reduce the risk of back strain, put a pillow under the small of your back.
- To stretch more of the butt muscles, bend your knees slightly instead of keeping them straight.

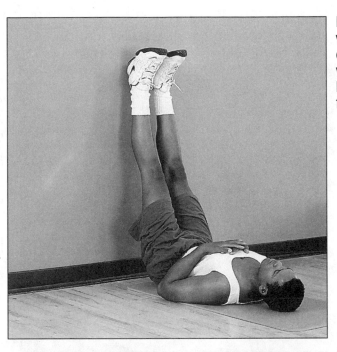

Lie flat on your back with your legs together and your heels on the wall. Your butt should be about 10 inches from the wall.

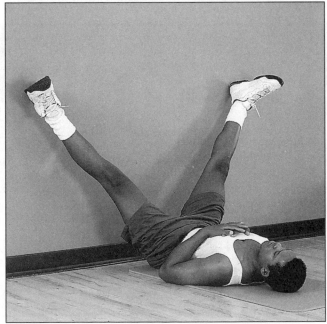

Slowly separate your legs and allow gravity to bring them down to the sides as far as they will comfortably go. Hold for 30 seconds, then relax.

UPPER-BODY STRETCHES
Four-Way Neck Twists and Tilts
RATING: EASY

Long hours hunched in front of a computer can lead to neck stiffness and fatigue. This simple stretch hits all the major muscles in the neck. It is often recommended as part of a pre-lifting warm-up. It's also a great on-the-job stress reducer.

Stand with your back straight and your legs shoulder-width apart. Your neck should be straight and your shoulders relaxed. Slowly turn your head to the right as far as it will comfortably go. Hold for 10 seconds. Then repeat going to the left.

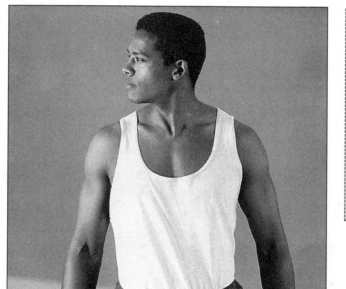

DO IT BETTER
• To increase the stretch in each direction, look with your eyes in the direction of the stretch.
• If turning your head makes you feel unsteady, do this exercise while sitting.
• Nerves and muscles in the neck are easily injured, so always do this exercise slowly and with control.

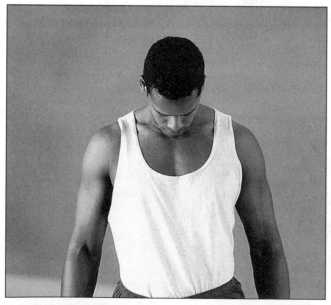

Return to the starting position. Without bending your upper body, tuck your chin into your chest until you feel a mild pull. Hold for 10 seconds.

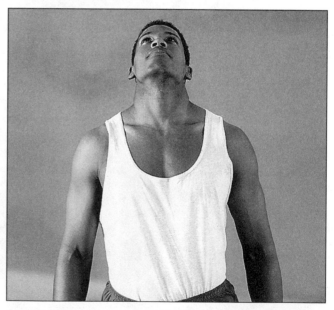

Slowly tilt your head upward until you are looking straight up. Don't let your head go so far back that it rests on your shoulders. Hold for 10 seconds; relax.

Lying Overhead Arm Stretches

RATING: MODERATELY DIFFICULT

This stretch is great for all sports that emphasize arm strength and flexibility, such as basketball, baseball, racquet sports, softball, swimming, and climbing. It increases the overhead flexibility of your shoulders and works the latissimus dorsi (mid and lower back) muscles.

DO IT BETTER

• A good measure of flexibility is being able to touch your hands to the floor while keeping your back flat.

• Moving your hands closer together will increase the effectiveness of this stretch.

• If one of your arms is more flexible than the other, hold a stick or towel with both hands, placed more than shoulder-width apart, over your head. By keeping both arms at the same distance, this will help keep the flexibility equal.

• To decrease difficulty, keep your hands farther apart at first. Then move them closer together as flexibility improves.

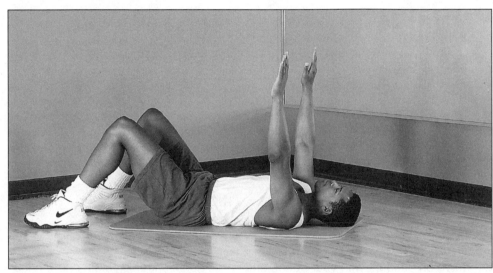

Lie on your back with your knees bent at a 45-degree angle, feet flat on the floor. The small of your back should be pressed firmly against the floor. Extend your arms straight up over your chest with your palms facing your feet.

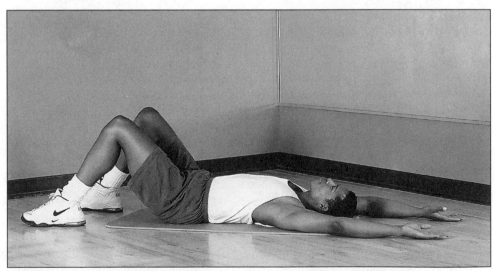

Slowly lower your arms straight back over your head. Try to press the back of your hands and arms flat on the floor. Hold for 10 seconds, then release. Slowly bring your arms back to the starting position before repeating the stretch.

Bowing Shoulder Stretches

RATING: EASY

You have seen how dogs and cats stretch when they first wake up. This stretch puts you in a similar position, minus the mouth-gaping yawn. It is a great way to stimulate a large part of your body at one time. It hits the outsides of the latissimus dorsi (mid and lower back) muscles as well as the shoulders and arms.

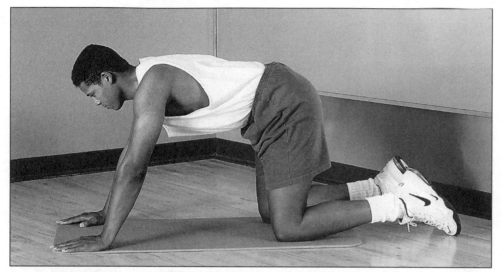

Get down on all fours with your hands and knees about shoulder-width apart. Keep your back flat, your neck straight, and your eyes on the floor.

DO IT BETTER

- Doing one arm at a time will allow you to control the stretch on each side of your torso.
- To get more stretch in the back, shoulders, and upper arms, push down on the heels of your hands.
- Another way to get more stretch is to reach forward and grab the end of a carpet or heavy mat before pulling backward. This provides additional resistance, making the stretch more effective.
- Using the weight of your torso to push your chest to the floor will increase the stretch along the sides of your back and shoulders.

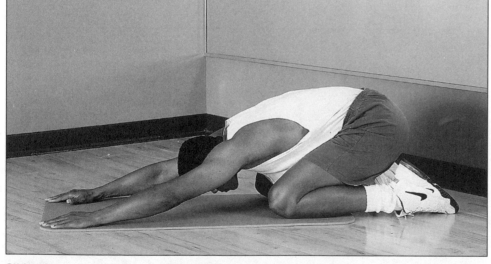

Sit back on your heels, allowing your arms to trail in front of you. Push down slightly with your palms until you feel a stretch in your arms and hips. Hold for 30 seconds. Relax, then repeat.

Triceps-and-Shoulder Stretches

RATING: EASY

The shoulder houses the most flexible joint in the body. Despite this, many people have stiff shoulders because they never stretch them. This stretch works the deltoid (shoulder), the outsides of the latissimus dorsi (mid and lower back), and triceps (back of upper arm) muscles.

DO IT BETTER

• To increase difficulty, reach down between the shoulder blades with the fingers of the arm being stretched.

• To increase the stretch and to stretch your waist, bend your torso sideways toward the arm that is pulling.

• To decrease difficulty, lean the upper arm to be stretched against a door-jamb. Use the resistance to push your elbow up to a vertical position, then hold for 15 seconds.

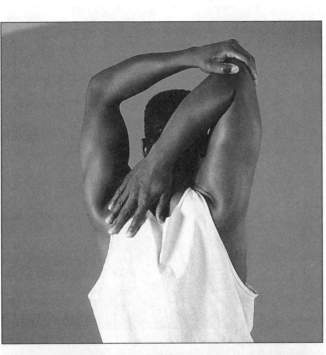

Stand straight with your feet shoulder-width apart and your knees slightly bent. With both arms overhead, hold the elbow of one arm with the hand of the other.

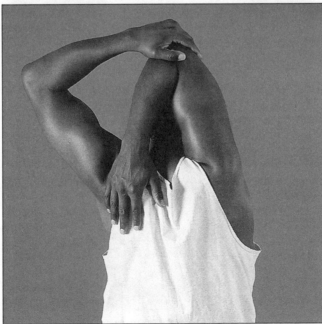

Slowly pull the elbow toward the other arm, feeling the stretch along the outside of the upper arm and shoulder. Hold for 15 seconds, then do the other arm.

External-Rotator Stretches

RATING: MODERATELY DIFFICULT

You're going to play tennis after all these years? Better work on your shoulder and external-rotator flexibility. Even if you aren't Wimbledon material, this stretch is good for any shoulder activity, including swimming and martial arts.

Stand straight with your feet shoulder-width apart. Place the back of your left hand behind your waist at belt level with your left elbow out to the side.

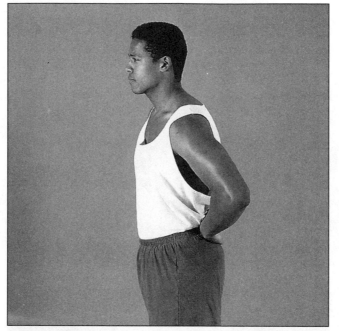

Reach across the front of your body with your right hand and grab the left elbow. Pull the left elbow gently toward the front of your body, keeping your left hand stationary. Hold for 30 seconds, then do the other arm.

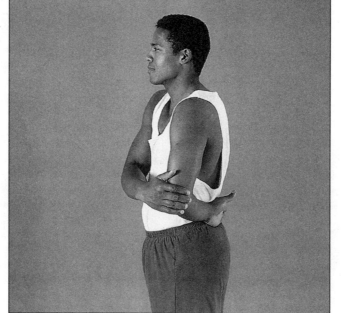

Dynamic Arm Swings and Circles

RATING: EASY

This exercise will help strengthen and improve the flexibility of all the muscles attaching to the shoulder girdle. It is recommended for those who swim or play volleyball, softball, or tennis—sports in which improved range of motion translates into more powerful performance and fewer injuries.

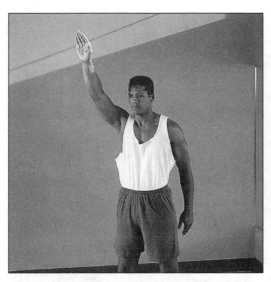

Stand straight with your feet shoulder-width apart, arms at your sides, and your palms facing behind you. Raise your right arm in front of you in a semicircular motion until it is directly overhead.

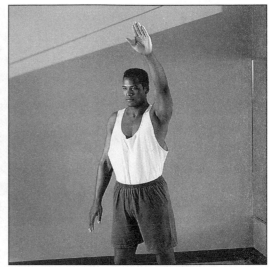

As you begin to lower your right arm, raise the left arm. Swing the arms gently, alternating them up and down in a steady, controlled manner. Do not swing them past the point of mild tension.

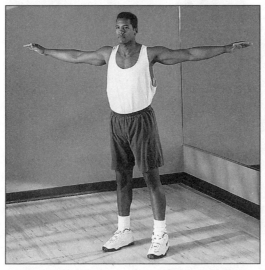

Next, lift both arms to the sides until they are parallel to the ground with the palms facing down.

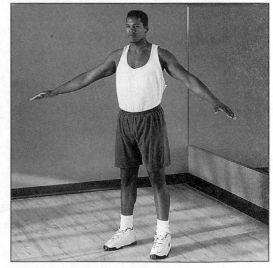

Trace small circles in the air with both arms moving in the same direction, gradually increasing the size of the circles until you're at your maximum range of motion.

Pushing Chest Stretches

RATING: EASY

Do you spend your days hunched over at a desk? If so, you need this exercise, which stretches the front of your chest, pulls your shoulders back, and helps you develop better posture. It increases arm flexibility for sports that require swinging or climbing such as golf, tennis, baseball, volleyball, or rock climbing. It mainly stretches the pectoralis (chest) and deltoid (shoulder) muscles.

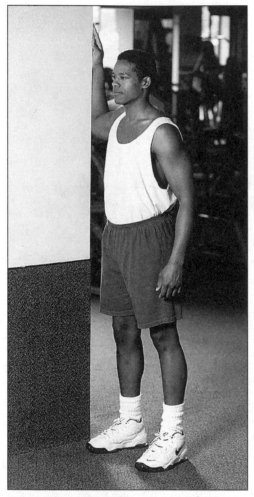

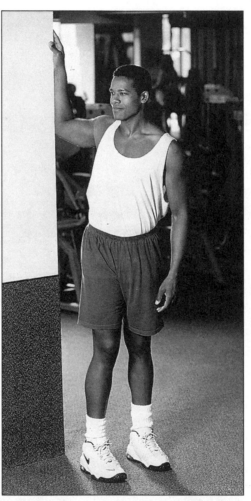

DO IT BETTER

• Leaning forward at the waist will increase the stretch of the chest and help increase external rotation. Leaning your hip in will also increase the shoulder stretch.
• This can be done using a chain-link fence, wall, or pillar in place of the doorway.
• An easy way to help loosen your shoulder joint before this stretch is by doing shoulder shrugs.
• To stretch both shoulders at the same time, stand in a doorway. Put your hands on opposite sides of the frame, with your palms facing away from you. Step forward with one leg and slowly lean forward, bending your front knee.

Stand in front of a doorway or at the end of a wall with your feet shoulder-width apart. Bend your right arm so that the upper arm is parallel with the floor and the forearm and hand are pressed against the doorway.

Slowly rotate your body counterclockwise in the direction of the opposite shoulder, stretching your shoulder and causing the arm against the door to be pulled back. Hold for 30 seconds, then repeat with the other arm.

Bending Chest Stretches
RATING: EASY

Although this stretch is similar to the down-on-all-fours version, it moves the stretch from the sides of the back and shoulders to the trapezius (upper back and neck) and deltoid (shoulder) muscles. It also works the triceps (back of upper arm) and chest. It is recommended for people who spend prolonged periods standing or sitting down.

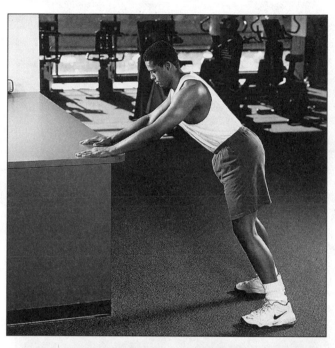

Stand a few feet away from a table, your feet shoulder-width apart. Extend your arms and lean on the table, bending forward at the waist. Don't round your back or hunch your shoulders forward.

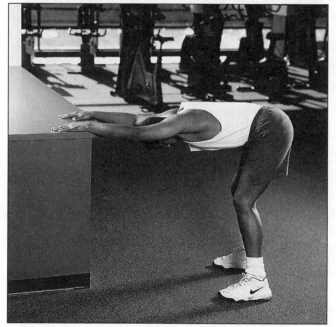

Continue bending forward until your arms and back are parallel to the ground, keeping your knees slightly bent. Push your chest and head toward the ground until you feel slight tension. Hold for 30 seconds.

Chest Pull Stretches

RATING: EASY

Swimmers will find this stretch particularly useful for loosening up the chest, shoulders, and upper back—all of which are used in swimming strokes.

Stand with your feet shoulder-width apart, arms extended in front of your chest and parallel to the floor, palms facing down.

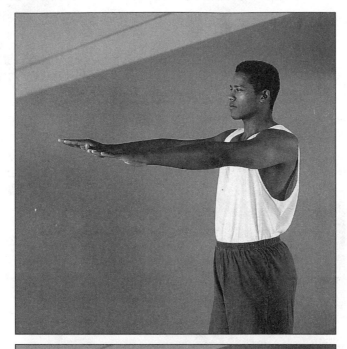

DO IT BETTER

• To increase the stretch in the upper back, when your arms are in front of you, reach as far forward as you comfortably can.
• Using hand weights will help increase your strength.
• To increase the stretch in the upper chest and shoulders, try to touch your elbows together behind you as you pull your arms back.
• To stretch the oblique abdominal muscles, twist your waist from side to side when your elbows are behind you.
• To make this stretch a bit easier, try alternating your arms—one extending forward as the other one is pulled back.

Keeping your arms horizontal, pull your elbows back on the sides until they're behind your shoulders. Try to bring your shoulder blades together. Hold for 30 seconds.
    Then bring the arms forward again to the starting position, straightening the elbows and allowing the wrists to cross.

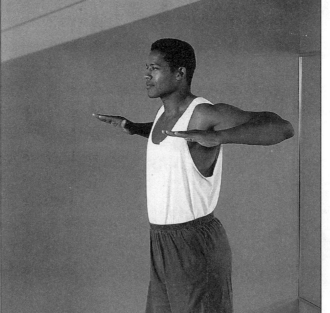

Wrist Abductor Stretches

RATING: EASY

Your wrists take a lot of strain. This stretch is a great way to keep them limber and loose—either before picking up a tennis racket or just to break up the monotony from working on a keyboard. You will feel the stretch all the way from your hand to the underside of the forearm. This stretch works the finger and wrist flexor muscles (both in the underside of the forearm) and the hand abductors (inside of forearm).

DO IT BETTER

- To get the most benefit, do this stretch with the wrist adductor stretch (see page 372), which works the opposing muscle.
- To decrease difficulty, do the same stretch, but let the left fingers bend over the right hand while pulling the left hand toward your body.
- To get more stretch in the wrist, hand, and fingers, move the right hand up so that you are pulling the fingertips (rather than the whole hand) back.

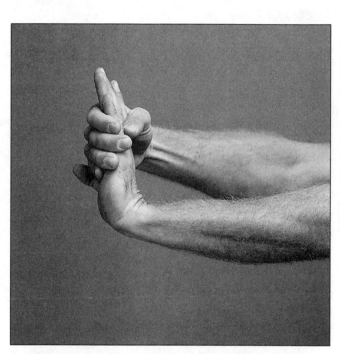

With your hand up, extend your left arm in front of you, as though you were stopping traffic.

Use your right hand to grasp your left. Gently pull back with your right hand, keeping your left arm extended. Hold for 15 to 30 seconds, then switch hands.

Wrist Adductor Stretches

RATING: EASY

There probably isn't a sport or hand motion that doesn't require the use of the finger and wrist flexor muscles (both in the underside of the forearm) as well as the hand adductors (outside of forearm). Because this exercise thoroughly stretches each of these muscles, it is often recommended for those people whose jobs involve repetitive motions, like keyboard operators and assembly line workers. This stretch is often done with wrist abductor stretches (see page 371).

Extend your left arm and let your hand drop so that your fingers are pointing down.

Use your right hand to grasp the top of your left hand. Gently pull your left hand toward your body. Hold for 15 to 30 seconds before switching sides.

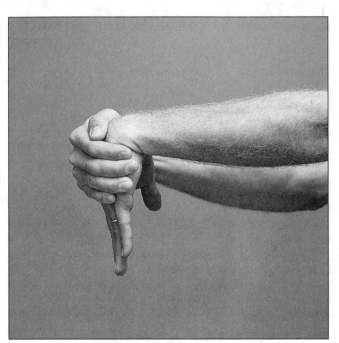

DO IT BETTER

• To get more stretch in the fingers, bend your fingers up and in toward the wrists while pulling your left hand toward your body.

• To decrease difficulty, bend your left arm across the front of your upper body and start with the fingers on your left hand pointing down. Cup your left wrist so that the fingers of your right hand are on top of your left forearm. Use the palm of your right hand to push the left hand toward your body.

Praying Wrist Stretches

RATING: MODERATELY DIFFICULT

As the name suggests, this stretch is done by putting your hands together, fingertips to palms. It stretches the finger flexor (underside of forearm) muscles as well as the brachioradialis (upper forearm) muscle. It is recommended for anyone doing a lot of hand movements such as typing or playing basketball.

DO IT BETTER

• To increase the stretch in your right fingers and wrist, press to the left and gently push the right hand back. Then do the same with the left hand.
• To get more range of motion in your wrists, do this stretch while lowering your hands a little more each time.
• To incorporate more muscles into the stretch, turn your hands out so that your fingertips are pointing away from your body. Then, as you stretch, turn the fingertips toward your body.

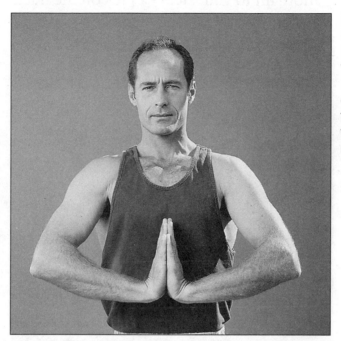

Put your hands together at about chest level. Lower your hands until you feel a stretch in the underside of the wrists and throughout the forearms. Hold for 10 to 15 seconds, then relax.

LOWER-BODY STRETCHES
Standing Calf Stretches

RATING: EASY

This exercise hits not only muscles in the calf but also muscles at the front of the lower leg. Stretching and strengthening these muscles will enable you to push off from your toes with more force, getting more lift to your step—a plus on the track or basketball court.

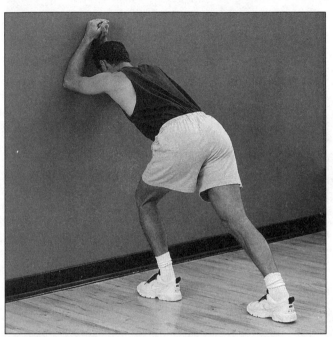

DO IT BETTER

- To get more stretch in the Achilles tendon, try this variation: From the final position, slightly bend the knee of your back leg, keeping the heel in contact with the ground.
- Keeping your toes pointing forward will maximize the stretch in your calf.

Stand a foot away from a wall and lean on it with your forearms, keeping your upper arms parallel to the floor. Extend one leg about 2 feet behind you, keeping the heel in contact with the floor. Your front knee will naturally bend; make sure it doesn't extend over your foot. Keep your back straight. Hold for 30 seconds, then repeat with the other leg.

Kneeling Calf Stretches
MODERATELY DIFFICULT

This provides a terrific stretch for your calf and Achilles tendon as well as for the hip extensor (butt and groin) and hip flexor (front hip) muscles. Maintaining balance can be a challenge, however. You may want to skip this stretch if you have had knee problems.

DO IT BETTER

- Hunching your back or leaning too far forward will throw off your balance. It's okay, however, to put one of your hands on the floor for support.
- Leaning with your side on a wall will provide further support. (If you are kneeling on your right knee, lean the left side of your body.)
- To increase the stretch in the hip muscles, pull your chest back and keep your body more erect.
- For added comfort, put a towel beneath your knee.

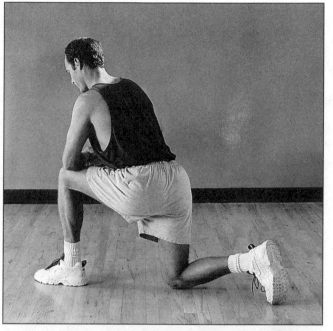

Kneel on your right knee, resting your left forearm on your left thigh. Lean forward slightly at the waist, keeping your back straight.

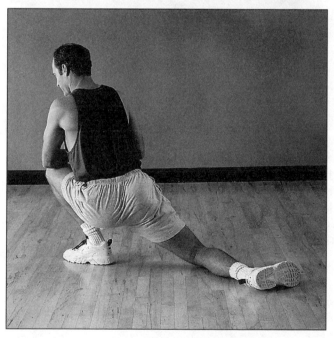

Shift your weight to the front knee, bending it as far as it will comfortably go. Keep your front heel on the ground. Shift the weight on your kneeling leg: The inside of the knee and lower leg should be flat on the floor. Hold for 30 seconds, then switch legs.

Ankle-Extension Stretches

RATING: EASY

When your calves feel tight, try this basic stretch. It works the gastrocnemius (calf) muscle, the soleus (muscle below calf), and the Achilles tendon. You can do it anywhere by holding on to a stationary object like a stair rail or street sign.

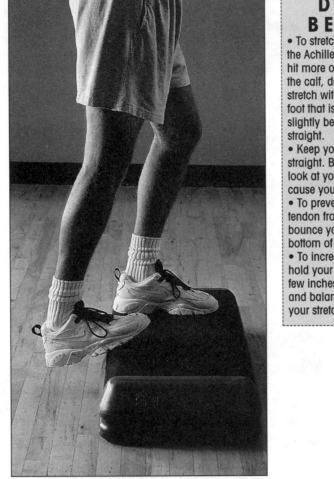

DO IT BETTER

• To stretch higher up on the Achilles tendon and to hit more of the soleus in the calf, do this same stretch with the knee of the foot that is off the curb slightly bent instead of straight.

• Keep your upper body straight. Bending over to look at your heel can cause you to lose balance.

• To prevent the Achilles tendon from tearing, don't bounce your weight at the bottom of the motion.

• To increase difficulty, hold your supporting foot a few inches off the ground and balance on the ball of your stretching foot.

Stand straight with your heels on the edge of a curb or step. Step back slightly with your right leg so that the ball of the foot is on the edge of the curb, with the heel hanging over the edge. Your left leg should be slightly bent, and your right leg straight. Slowly lower the heel of the right leg below the level of the curb as far as you can. Hold for 20 seconds, then repeat with the other leg.

Standing Thigh Stretches
RATING: MODERATELY DIFFICULT

Every time you use your legs—while walking, running, or even sitting down—you use the quadriceps (front thigh), hip flexors (front hip), and the muscles and tendons in the knee. This basic stretch will help keep these muscles strong and limber.

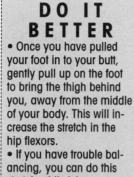

DO IT BETTER

• Once you have pulled your foot in to your butt, gently pull up on the foot to bring the thigh behind you, away from the middle of your body. This will increase the stretch in the hip flexors.

• If you have trouble balancing, you can do this stretch while lying on your stomach.

• It might be easier, for balancing purposes, to hold your left leg with your left hand and place your right hand on the wall for support.

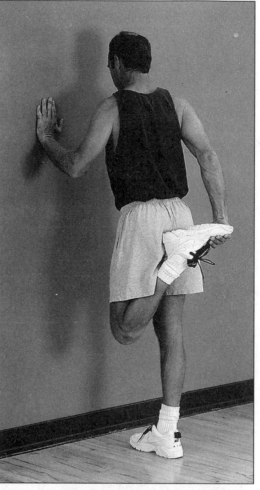

Stand facing a wall with your feet hip-width apart. Place your left hand on the wall for support. Bend your left leg behind you and grab the top of your foot with your right hand. Gently pull your heel toward your butt. Hold for 30 seconds, then relax and switch legs.

Front Hip Stretches

RATING: MODERATELY DIFFICULT

This hip stretch targets the hip flexors (front hip) as well as the quadriceps (front thigh) and ligaments at the front of the hip and thigh. What makes this stretch unique is that it hits muscles that rarely are put through their full range of motion—and which consequently are at risk for injury.

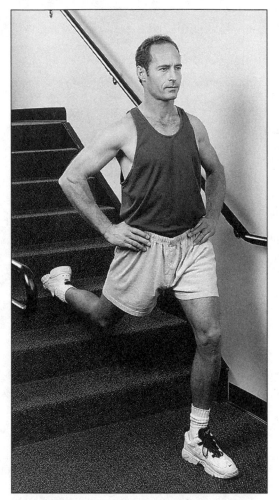

DO IT BETTER

- To stretch the inner and outer thigh muscles, turn to your right so that the inside of your right foot is on the table. (You should be facing in the same direction as your toes.)
- To stretch the hip, hamstring, and butt muscles, turn completely around to face the table, with your right heel resting on the table. Slightly bend the left leg.
- For a stretch that requires less balance, place a chair in front of you and hold on to it while doing the same movements. This time, though, bend your left leg as you push your thigh down toward the floor.
- To effectively stretch the hip flexors and thigh muscles, use standing thigh stretches (see page 377) to warm up the muscles, and then optimize the effect with front hip stretches, which provide a more severe angle of the thigh for an optimal stretch.

Extend your right leg behind you, placing the top of the foot on the third step on a flight of stairs, a table, or chair. Place your hands on your hips and support most of your weight on your left foot.

Try to pull your right thigh forward, keeping your foot secure on the step. Hold for 30 seconds. If you're doing the stretch correctly, it will feel as though you're applying pressure to the step with your right thigh rather than the right foot.

Kneeling Quad Stretches

RATING: DIFFICULT

Unlike most stretches for the quadriceps (front thigh) and hip flexors (front hip), this one is done kneeling down. While it is not an easy stretch, it is one of the most comfortable to do.

DO IT BETTER

• For greater comfort, place a towel under your left knee.
• Resting your left arm on your thigh will raise your torso, increasing the stretch in the lower back.
• To increase the stretch in the hips, try this: When you're at the end of the movement, with your left foot near your butt, lean forward by pushing your hips toward the floor.
• To decrease difficulty, get in the original position, then completely extend the right leg while bending the left, keeping the right foot firmly on the floor. Your hips should be closer to your left leg; you may be able to grab your foot.

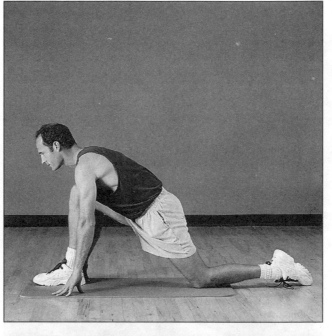

Get down on all fours. Bring your right leg in front of your body and bend it at a 90-degree angle. Extend your left leg behind you so that the knee, shin, and the top of your left foot are on the floor to help support your body.

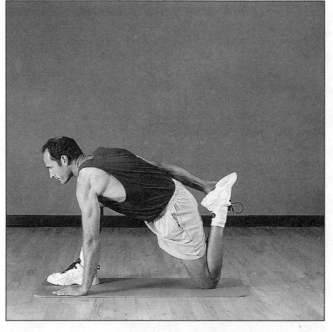

Keeping your left hand flat on the floor, use your right hand to reach behind your back to grab the top of your left foot. Pull the heel toward your butt as far as you comfortably can. Keep your back flat and your head in line with your torso. Hold for 30 seconds, then relax and switch legs.

Standing Hamstring Stretches

RATING: EASY

Tight hamstrings are a common cause of lower back pain. They can also make an existing problem worse. This exercise gives a good stretch to the hamstring (back thigh), adductor (inner thigh), and gluteal (butt) muscles.

Stand with your right leg slightly bent and toes pointing straight ahead, feet spaced more than shoulder-width apart. Extend your left leg behind you with the toes pointing at a slight angle to the left. Place your hands in the middle of your right thigh and lean into the leg, keeping your back straight.

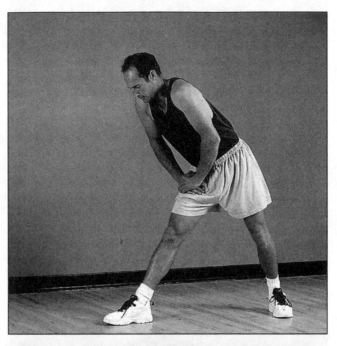

DO IT BETTER

• To increase the stretch in your hamstrings, tighten the thigh muscle in the front leg.
• To stretch the inner thigh as well as the hamstrings, turn your toes out to the side as you raise the ball of your front foot.
• To stretch the outer thigh and hamstrings, turn your toes in while keeping the ball of your front foot off the floor.

Bend your back leg as you push your hips back and down. Lower your torso until it is parallel with the floor, or as close to parallel as you can comfortably get. Extend your right leg and raise the ball of your right foot off the ground, while maintaining pressure on your front heel. Hold for 30 seconds, then switch legs.

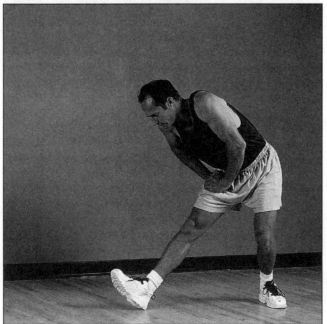

Standing Lower Back Stretches

RATING: EASY

Sitting for hours can really tire your lower back. Most affected are the erector spinae (lower back) muscles. This stretch is a great way to relax these muscles, particularly where they end in the lower back region. It also works the hamstring (back thigh) and gluteal (butt) muscles.

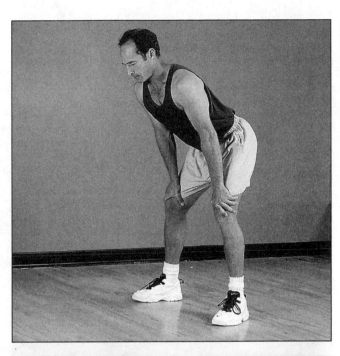

Stand with your feet hip-width apart, knees slightly bent. Bend at your waist and place your hands on your thighs, just above the knees. Keep your head in line with your torso.

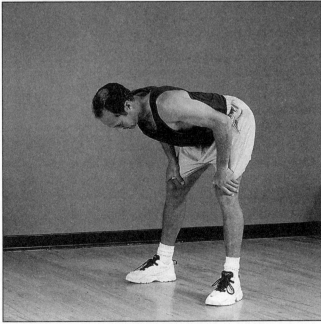

Keeping your back flat and knees unlocked, push your hips back and slowly lower your chest. Hold for 30 seconds.

Standing Hamstring-and-Butt Stretches

RATING: MODERATELY DIFFICULT

This stretch is often recommended for hurdlers, who need to fully extend the leg while still moving with explosive power. It works the hamstring (back thigh) and gluteal (butt) muscles.

Extend your left leg and place the back of your heel on a table or stair at about waist height. Your right foot should be flat on the ground and your right knee slightly bent. Keep your torso straight and your head in line with your spine.

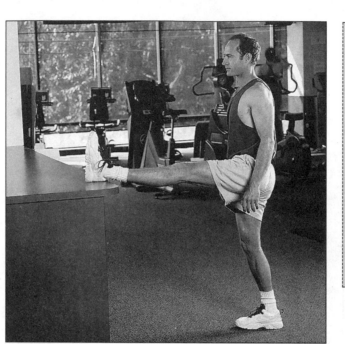

Slowly bend at the waist while keeping your back flat. Grab your shin with both hands and pull your upper body toward the leg, going as far down as you comfortably can, while maintaining a flat back. Hold for 30 seconds, then repeat with the other leg.

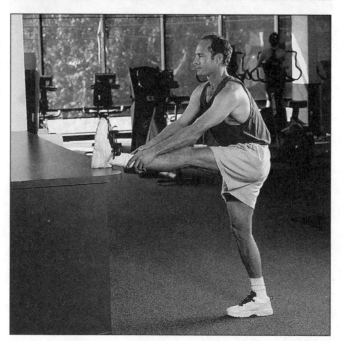

Lying Hamstring Stretches

RATING: MODERATELY DIFFICULT

The hamstring (back thigh) muscles are extremely prone to injury. This exercise works them thoroughly, keeping them strong and limber. It's a versatile stretch, meaning it can be done in a variety of ways to get different results.

DO IT BETTER

- To stretch the butt and lower back, bend your right leg and bring the left knee into your chest, extending the left leg straight up. This version is ideal for people with lower back problems.
- To stretch the hamstrings closer to your butt, begin with both legs bent. Bring your left leg as far into your chest as you comfortably can, while keeping the leg bent.
- To increase the stretch in your hamstrings, pull your thigh closer to your chest before extending the leg. Then straighten the leg.
- Contract the quadriceps of the raised leg to improve the stretch in the hamstrings.

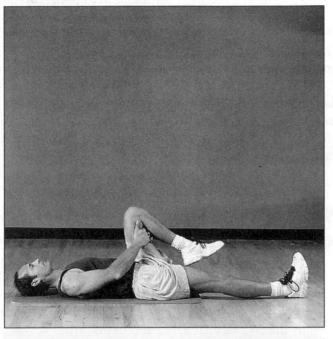

Lie flat on your back with your right leg fully extended, your hands clasped behind your left thigh, and your left knee brought to your chest.

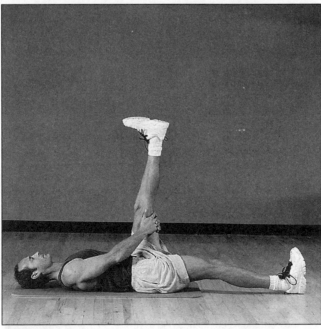

Extend your left leg straight up, knee slightly bent, keeping your hands behind the thigh. Your lower back should be pressed to the floor. Hold for 30 seconds.

SCENARIO 1: A Complete Routine

AGE: 35
WEIGHT: 160
HEALTH: Excellent
EXERCISE ROUTINE: This man is an all-around athlete. He spends at least 4 hours a day being physical: swimming, running, in-line skating, and playing volleyball.
LIFESTYLE: A freelance writer who's single, he has time to pursue his interests, which include camping, canoeing, and mountain climbing.
FITNESS GOALS: Wants to achieve maximum flexibility for pursuing his latest passion, rock climbing. He wants more arm and leg strength, along with the ability to stretch and hold for long periods of time.

He seems to have it all: youth, vigor, an interesting career, the physical wherewithal to pursue a life of outdoor adventure—plus the lack of attachment to actually be able to go do the things he wants whenever he pleases. His activities and the fact that he's in superior condition dictate a higher order of routine.

"If anyone needs dynamic stretches, this is the guy," says Frank Eksten, strength coordinator in the Department of Athletics and visiting lecturer in kinesiology at Indiana University in Bloomington. The reason is simple: He is involved with a lot of sports, which themselves are dynamic: swimming, running, volleyball.

Yet his interest in rock and mountain climbing also dictates a regimen that includes static stretches, which will help improve flexibility in sustained, difficult positions. What he needs, in a word, is variety, Eksten says. Many of the movements in the following program, while seeming similar, attack a variety of muscles from different angles, preparing them for a lot of different activities.

GROUP ONE

This first group of stretches will ensure excellent flexibility in the upper body, especially for overhead movements in sports like swimming, volleyball, and rock climbing.

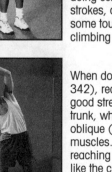

Pushing chest stretches (page 368) move the arms in an external rotation, which is critical for movements in which the wrist is positioned behind the elbow, such as when hitting a volleyball, doing certain swimming strokes, or performing some tougher types of climbing moves.

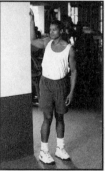

When doing **side bends** (page 342), reach overhead to give a good stretch to the side of the trunk, which is important for the oblique (side) and lower back muscles. This helps when reaching in swimming strokes like the crawl, blocking a volleyball at the net, or straining for high handholds when climbing.

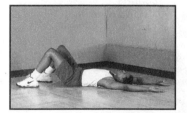

Lying overhead arm stretches (page 363) stretch the shoulder and upper back/shoulder girdle, but they are more than shoulder stretches. They also hit the upper arm to some extent and basically work all the muscles around the armpit. This is an important one for overhead flexibility and strength.

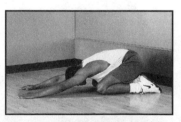

Bowing shoulder stretches (page 364) are sometimes called cat stretches. In addition to stretching the shoulders, they hit the rib cage, upper back, chest—the entire upper torso. Their specific benefits are their emphasis on the ribs and front of the body.

GROUP TWO

This second group of stretches will prepare the upper body for dynamic movement using dynamic stretches.

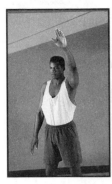

The motion in **dynamic arm swings and circles** (page 367), which emphasizes the front of the shoulder, helps prepare for volleyball, swimming, and climbing. It should be done immediately before the activity in a controlled manner so that muscle power, not momentum, carries the joint through its range of motion.

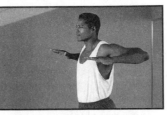

Chest pull stretches (page 370) stretch both the chest and upper back and warm up the shoulder and rotator cuff, all of which are particularly important for swimming.

GROUP THREE

This third group of stretches will develop range of motion in the lower body for rock climbing and volleyball and will reduce post-workout soreness.

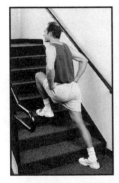

Hip flexion stretches (page 350) hit the groin in addition to the hips and gluteal (butt) muscles. They are great stretches for climbing, which often requires reaching up with one leg while keeping the other in a fixed position.

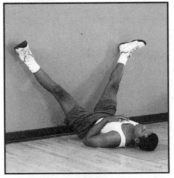

Wall groin stretches (page 361) are good for the groin and inside of the thigh. They are particularly important for getting into low squats during volleyball.

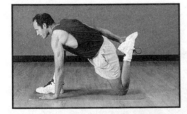

Kneeling quad stretches (page 379) are highly targeted stretches for the quadriceps (front thigh) and hip flexor (front hip) muscles, which are crucial for leg movements. The angle of the stretch isolates the quadriceps muscle without putting stress on the knee. Strong and resilient hip flexors and quadriceps are important not only for climbing and volleyball but especially for in-line skating.

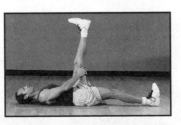

The first part of the **lying hamstring stretches** (page 383) stretches the middle of the hamstring (back thigh). The second movement stretches the hamstring closer to the butt. Flexibility all along the hamstring is important for lunging in volleyball, reaching for footholds in climbing, and controlling movements in in-line skating.

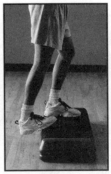

Ankle extensions (page 376) hit the calf in a flat, wide swath from the Achilles tendon to the muscles that are under the knee. They are important for posture, stability, and balance.

SCENARIO **2**:Relief from Pain

AGE: 46

WEIGHT: 190

HEALTH: He has been experiencing lower back pain and stiffness almost every day, especially with vigorous activity. Has also started getting wrist pain from working on a computer.

EXERCISE ROUTINE: Takes a 20- to 30-minute walk almost every day. Has tried lifting weights at the company gym but hasn't stuck with it.

LIFESTYLE: A sales representative for a medical instruments company, he works long hours behind a desk. Blows off steam in his home workshop making furniture. With two teenage sons, however, he sees his only true "free" time as being lunch hour.

FITNESS GOALS: Gain flexibility in his back and wrists, both to relieve pain and to make it easier to handle lumber. Time is of the essence: He would like a routine that takes 15 minutes or less and can be done in the office during lunch.

He sits at a desk all day, doesn't do much vigorous exercise, then spends a lot of time bending over saws and picking up tools and materials in his shop. No wonder this guy is in pain.

It's great that he walks, but that doesn't seem to be enough, and he knows it. According to Frank Eksten, strength coordinator in the Department of Athletics and visiting lecturer in kinesiology at Indiana University in Bloomington, a well-rounded workout routine of both strength and aerobic conditioning would be ideal. But he's already shown a lack of commitment to exercise, mainly because of time constraints.

Flexibility must accomplish a lot for this man, and because of that, he needs more help than he can get in a short lunch-hour break that's already half taken with a daily walk, Eksten says. But there are ways to consolidate time: First, he can do some stretches immediately after the walk, which will eliminate the need for an additional warm-up; he can steal 10 minutes from the 30-minute walk, if necessary. Second, he can perform a wide range of stretches right at his desk while contemplating spreadsheets.

GROUP ONE

Done immediately after walking, these stretches will help relieve lower back problems and enhance flexibility in the shoulder girdle and neck.

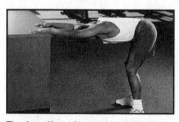

The **bending chest stretch** (page 369) is a standing version of the cat stretch—it's just as good as the down-on-all-fours version at stretching the back, chest, and shoulders but avoids a person's being caught in a strange, supplicating stance when the boss is around. A good stretch for someone who spends lots of time at a computer.

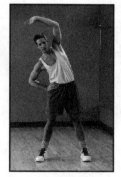

Side bends (page 342) stretch the sides of the trunk, helping ensure good mobility in the spinal column, which will help alleviate lower back pain and stiffness from prolonged sitting.

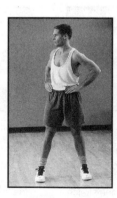

Side twists (page 343) will help relieve lower back stiffness from sitting in a chair. They will also limber up the oblique (side) muscles, which are important for supporting the spine.

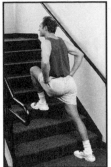

Hip flexion stretches (page 350) are good all-around stretches for the hip, gluteal (butt), and groin muscles. They help with lower back pain and with muscles needed for bending and picking things up. A good choice for after a walk, when stairs will probably be along the route to the office.

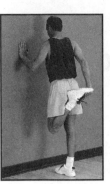

Standing thigh stretches (page 377) are just as effective as lying stretches for the same muscle but are a bit less conspicuous in an office setting. They isolate the quadriceps (front thigh), which are important in eliminating and preventing lower back pain.

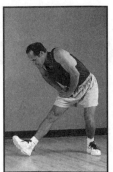

Standing hamstring stretches (page 380) are great for loosening up the hamstrings (back thigh), which are often tight in people who have lower back pain.

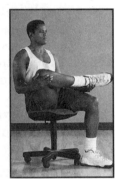

Standing lower back stretches (page 381) hit the area where the hamstrings (back thigh) come together with the gluteal (butt) and lower back muscles, improving range of motion in bending movements.

GROUP TWO

To address problems with wrist pain and enhance overall flexibility, these stretches can be done while working at a desk.

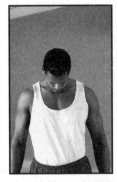

Four-way neck twists and tilts (page 362) loosen the neck and alleviate possible nerve impingement which can produce pain.

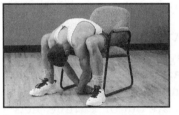

Lower back leans (page 344) provide a great stretch for the lower back and can easily be done at the office since they are performed while seated.

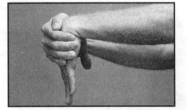

Seated hamstring-and-gluteus stretches (page 354) give an extra stretch to the lower back and, while the sitting is still going on, alleviate the effects of sitting in a chair.

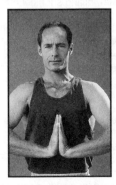

Praying wrist stretches (page 373) help stretch muscles in the wrist that can become stiff and sore from computer use.

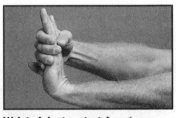

Wrist adductor stretches (page 372) extend the wrist muscles, helping relieve impingement from repetitive motion.

Wrist abductor stretches (page 371) also flex wrist muscles to help relieve pain from nerve impingement, only they hit the muscles from another angle.

SCENARIO **3**: Making the Commitment

AGE: 26

WEIGHT: 170

HEALTH: Suffers soreness from even light sessions as a casual weight lifter.

EXERCISE ROUTINE: Goes to the gym two or three times a week. He leaves after 30 to 45 minutes and often doesn't work out the entire time. Gets no aerobic exercise, which he suspects is the reason why he becomes easily winded.

LIFESTYLE: A pilot for a major airline, he works about 32 hours a week and spends a lot of time in hotels.

FITNESS GOALS: Plans eventually to devote more time to lifting, perhaps even entering local bodybuilding competitions. Wants to reduce soreness, improve wind, and maximize flexibility to prevent muscle injury.

"The first thing I ask of this guy is 'What do you really want?' " says Frank Eksten, strength coordinator in the Department of Athletics and visiting lecturer in kinesiology at Indiana University in Bloomington. His goals and behavior are out of sync in a number of ways: He wants to improve his wind but does no aerobics. He dreams of competitive bodybuilding but sloughs off his workouts. He only works 30 hours a week but seems unable to find time to exercise.

If he is serious about someday competing as a bodybuilder, the first order of business is to start an aerobics routine, Eksten says. That's right, aerobics. It will boost his exercise energy level and bring his body fat levels down for maximum chiseling of muscles when he lifts.

As for stretching, the fact that he is bodybuilding, albeit halfheartedly, is key: He needs a complete routine to ensure adequate overall flexibility. If he's doing the kind of incomplete lifts that bodybuilders often employ to isolate specific muscles, he is best off stretching after his workout rather than before to ensure that worked muscles get taken through a complete range of motion.

Since he plays no sports beyond lifting and has no problems related specifically to flexibility, the goal is to provide a good overall program that he can easily do in a hotel room. "Because his needs are broad and he seems to have a fair amount of time, he should use a variety of stretches," says Eksten.

GROUP ONE

These stretches will help develop flexibility in the upper body.

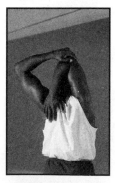 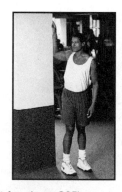

Pushing chest stretches (page 368) are helpful for men doing lots of bench presses or inclined presses, especially if they're doing fewer exercises for the shoulders and upper back—a tendency among beginners and noncommittal lifters. The reason is that heavy chest exercises tend to build muscles in a way that hinders external rotation, the kind of mobility that this move promotes.

Triceps-and-shoulder stretches (page 365) are good for preventing soreness in the shoulders, which they are especially prone to, from the motion of lowering weights to the starting position during exercises such as lat pull-downs, dumbbell rows, and seated pulley rows.

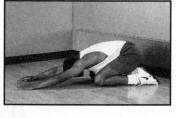

Bowing shoulder stretches (page 364) are good overall upper-body stretches to start with, hitting shoulders, rib cage, upper back, and chest. They are particularly valuable for offsetting soreness from bench presses and dumbbell flies.

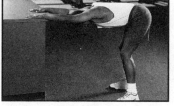

Bending chest stretches (page 369) not only work the chest but also incorporate the shoulders and upper back. They are particularly good for avoiding soreness in the upper back from lat pull-downs and dumbbell rows.

GROUP TWO

These are designed to help work a variety of muscles in the midbody.

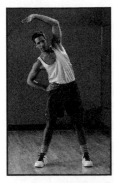 **Side bends** (page 342) promote good overall mobility in the spinal column (important for all types of lifting), in addition to stretching the shoulders and upper back, which helps prevent tightness under the arms from exercises such as chin-ups, dumbbell rows, lat pull-downs, and bent-over rows.

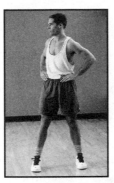 **Side twists** (page 343) help stretch the oblique (side) muscles, which provide critical support for the spine. They will prevent lower back pain, which occurs in people who are largely inactive but lift weights occasionally.

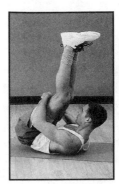 When doing **lying leg pulls** (page 345), pulling the knees into the chest works mainly the lower back, hips, and hamstrings (back thigh); extending the legs incorporates the gluteals (butt)—all muscles important for leg exercises such as squats, lunges, step-ups, and leg presses.

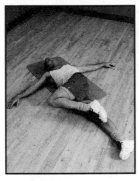 **Lateral lower back stretches** (page 347) are aggressive stretches for the torso, hips, and lower back. They are good for muscles involved with squats, lunges, and dead lifts.

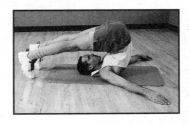 Like lying leg pulls, **legs-overhead stretches** (page 346) work the lower back, hips, and hamstrings (back thigh). This exercise is a bit more versatile, however. If the legs are spread in their final position, it's also a good groin stretch. This stretch is the most difficult in this group of stretches and should be attempted after warming up with the other stretches.

GROUP THREE

These stretches will help develop flexibility in the lower body.

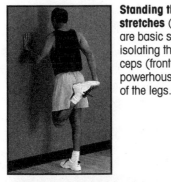 **Standing thigh stretches** (page 377) are basic stretches for isolating the quadriceps (front thigh), the powerhouse muscles of the legs.

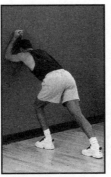 **Standing calf stretches** (page 374) are good stretches for a hotel room, where there is no step or curb from which to drop the heel. It puts pressure on the lower calf, near the Achilles tendon.

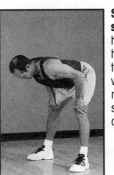 **Standing lower back stretches** (page 381) hit the area where the hamstrings (back thigh) come together with the gluteal (butt) muscles, preventing soreness from leg curls and lunges.

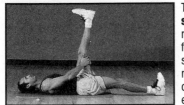 The first movement of the **lying hamstring stretch** (page 383) works the middle of the hamstring (back thigh) from the motion of trying to straighten the leg. The second movement stretches the hamstring closer to the butt. It's an important exercise since it hits so many areas.

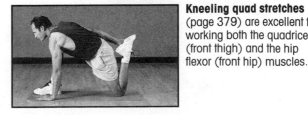 **Kneeling quad stretches** (page 379) are excellent for working both the quadriceps (front thigh) and the hip flexor (front hip) muscles.

SCENARIO **4**: Making Do with Less Time

AGE: 38

WEIGHT: 170

HEALTH: He frequently has muscle strain from lifting, carrying, and playing the part of a jungle gym for his three young kids. Gets a severely stiff neck almost monthly, which takes about two days to unwind.

EXERCISE ROUTINE: Doesn't work out, but is generally active—figures he logs about 2 miles a day walking around the house and yard.

LIFESTYLE: He works on a circuit board assembly line. Dedicated family man (has one toddler, two school-age children), he comes home right after work and devotes all free time to the kids. The only quiet time he gets is early morning.

FITNESS GOALS: Would like increased muscle tone, particularly in the back and torso, to support his active and affectionate children. Wants to prevent his neck problems.

"Despite what he thinks, this guy is basically sedentary," says Frank Eksten, strength coordinator in the Department of Athletics and visiting lecturer in kinesiology at Indiana University in Bloomington. "He does no aerobics, no strength training, and no real heavy labor." What's more, with an assembly line job, he probably spends much of his day using muscles in extremely constrained, repetitive motions.

More exercise would help alleviate some of his neck and back problems, but he lacks time. What he needs is a stretching program that both promotes overall flexibility and addresses his specific problems and can be accomplished in 10 to 15 minutes before work.

GROUP ONE

These stretches will improve flexibility in the neck and shoulder girdle, helping to reduce neck pain and stiffness.

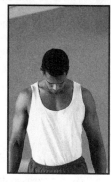

Four-way neck twists and tilts (page 362) are simple stretches that help loosen the neck and reduce the risk of nerve impingement, which can cause pain.

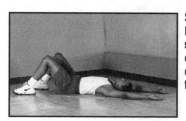

Stretching the shoulder and upper back using **lying overhead arm stretches** (page 363) may help alleviate neck pain from shoulder and upper back muscles that attach at the neck.

GROUP TWO

The following workouts will overcome the lack of broad movement typical of assembly line work and gird for sudden stresses from enthusiastic children.

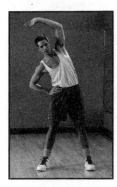

The reaching overhead motion of **side bends** (page 342) gives a good stretch in the side of the trunk, improving mobility and strength in the spine, helping prevent lower back pain caused by repetitive movements.

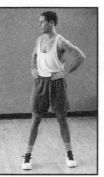

Side twists (page 343) provide an important stretch for helping to prevent and relieve muscle strain in the lower back.

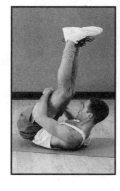

With **lying leg pulls** (page 345), a slight change of arm position alters the intensity of the stretch and the muscles affected: Pulling on the hamstrings works mainly the lower back, hips, and hamstrings (back thigh); pulling on the shins also works the gluteals (butt)—all muscles important for picking up kids and bracing them when they jump.

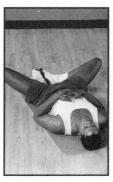

Lying groin stretches (page 360) are relaxation exercises, good for well-rounded support of the upper body. Best of all, they can be done before getting out of bed in the morning.

GROUP THREE

These stretches will relieve lower back pain and make the lower back more resilient when playing with kids.

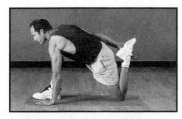

Kneeling quad stretches (page 379) are highly targeted stretches for the quadriceps (front thigh)—crucial for leg movement, picking things up, and overall flexibility.

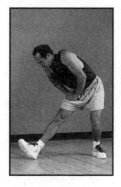

Standing hamstring stretches (page 380) hit the hamstrings (back thigh), which are stressed when someone leaps on you from the front.

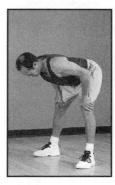

Standing lower back stretches (page 381) work the area where the hamstrings (back thigh) come together with the gluteal (butt) muscles. They also work the lower back and will improve range of motion in bending movements—important for protecting the lower back and hips.

INDEX

Underscored page references indicate boxed text. **Boldface** references indicate tables.

C

Cable cross-overs, for upper-body workout, 285
Cable crunches, for midbody workout, 212
Cable curls, for upper-body workout, 260
Calf raises, donkey, for lower-body workout, 329
Calf stretches
    kneeling, for lower-body stretching, 375
    standing, for lower-body stretching, 374, 389
Calisthenics, 130–32
Calorie burning, 4
    from exercise, 10, 115
    exercises for
        boxing, 127, 129
        cross-country skiing, 133, 135
        running, 29
        walking, 153
    leg strength and, 311
    for reducing belly fat, 195
    in Stone Age vs. modern times, 5, 7
    27 effortless methods of, 85–88
    for weight loss, 115–16
Calorie intake
    in Stone Age vs. modern times, 55
    weight gain and, 9–10
Calories
    in alcohol, 65, 68
    calculating number of, needed, 54–55
    controlling intake of, 54–55
    stored as fat, 10
    tracking, 24
Canola oil, monounsaturated fat in, 58
Carrots, for snacking, 64
Checkups, annual, for finding weight-related problems,
    17
Cheese
    in fast food, 64
    fat in, 58
    lean, 52
Chest pull stretches, for upper-body stretching, 370,
    385
Chest stretches
    bending, for upper-body stretching, 369, 386,
        388
    pushing, for upper-body stretching, 368, 384, 388
Chewing gum, for avoiding eating, 60
Chicken, skinning, 51, 58
Children, obesity in, 13
Chin-ups, for midbody workout, 185, 189, 225, 249
Chocolate, baking, substitute for, 53
Cholesterol
    effect of alcohol on, 66
    reducing, with weight loss, 17
Chopping wood, calorie burning from, 87–88
Circuits
    lower-body, 334
    midbody, 249
    upper-body, 306
Circuit training, 160
    guidelines for, 126

Clothing
    achieving lean look with, 95–98
    types to avoid, 96
Cocoa powder, as chocolate substitute, 53
Comfort, overeating for, 70
Concentration curls, for upper-body workout, 179,
    264
Confrontation, for avoiding eating, 60
Cookbooks, recommended, 53
Cooking
    fat-cutting strategies for, 50–53
    staples for, 48–49
Cookware, no-stick, for cooking with less fat, 49, 50
Cooldown
    after exercise, 30
    after running, 143
Cravings, driven by psychological needs, 12
Cross-country skiing, as exercise, 133–35
Cross-country ski machines, 134
Cross-country skis, selecting, 134
Crossed-leg rolls, for midbody stretching, 353
Cross-overs, cable, for upper-body workout, 285
Cross-training, 90
    advantages and disadvantages of, 124
    aerobic exercise in, 123–25
    avoiding injuries from, 124
    starting, 124
    weight loss from, 123–26
    weight training in, 125–26
Crunches
    abdominal strength from, 192–93
    cable, for midbody workout, 212
    guidelines for, 195–96
    oblique, for midbody workout, 201
    raised-leg, for midbody workout, 181, 187, 200
    rowing, for midbody workout, 175, 206
    side, for midbody workout, 201
    straight-leg, for midbody workout, 170, 198
    twisting, for midbody workout, 208
    variations of, 197
Curling overhead dumbbell presses, for upper-body workout, 295
Curls
    alternating biceps, for upper-body workout, 181, 187, 261,
        306
    barbell, for upper-body workout, 175, 257
    cable, for upper-body workout, 260
    concentration, for upper-body workout, 179, 264
    forearm, for upper-body workout, 189, 273
    French, for upper-body workout, 265
    hammer, for upper-body workout, 172, 262
    inclined dumbbell, for upper-body workout, 263
    leg, for lower-body workout, 179, 320, 334
    preacher, for upper-body workout, 258
    reverse grip biceps, for upper-body workout, 259
    standing triceps, for upper-body workout, 266,
        306
Curl-ups, for midbody workout, 177, 184, 187, 199
Cycling. *See* Bicycling; Mountain biking
Cycling, in weight lifting, 160
Cycling gear, for mountain biking, 140

Jump rope, for boxing, 128
Junk food
    late-night eating of, 69
    sacrificing, 105

K

Kickbacks
    dumbbell, for upper-body workout, 181, 271
    standing, for midbody workout, 238
Kicking, in swimming, 151–52
Kitchen
    staples in, 48–49
    tools for, 49–50
Knee injury, leg strength for preventing, 311
Kneeling calf stretches, for lower-body stretching, 375
Kneeling hip-and-groin stretches, for midbody stretching, 357
Kneeling leg kicks, for midbody workout, 240
Kneeling leg raises, for midbody workout, 243
Kneeling quad stretches, for lower-body stretching, 379, 385, 389, 391
Knee raises, hanging, for midbody workout, 177, 185, 205
Knee-to-chest lower back stretches, for midbody stretching, 351
Knives, as kitchen tool, 50

L

Labels, food
    reading, 72
    understanding, 57
Lapses in dieting, how to deal with, 32
Late-night snacking, 69
Lateral lower back stretches, for midbody stretching, 347, 389
Lateral lunges, for midbody workout, 170, 172, 182, 236
Lateral raises
    bent-over cable, for upper-body workout, 299
    lying, for upper-body workout, 179, 187, 301
    standing, for upper-body workout, 179, 181, 298, 306
Lateral squats, for lower-body workout, 316, 334
Lateral step-ups
    bench, for lower-body workout, 184, 323
    for midbody workout, 172, 237
Lat pull-downs, for midbody workout, 184, 219, 249
Lawn mowing, calorie burning from, 87
LDL cholesterol, effect of alcohol on, 66
Leaf raking, calorie burning from, 87
Leanness
    attitude of, 99–100
    dressing for, 95–98
    lifestyle and, quiz about, 78–79
Leg and upper-body raises, for midbody workout, 174, 230
Leg curls, for lower-body workout, 179, 320, 334
Leg extensions
    front-to-back, for midbody stretching, 355
    for lower-body workout, 181, 319, 334
    reverse, for midbody workout, 185, 241
    side-to-side, for midbody stretching, 356

Leg kicks
    kneeling, for midbody workout, 240
    lying, for midbody workout, 248
Leg lifts, for measuring abdominal strength, 193
Leg lunges, alternating, for midbody workout, 172, 235
Leg-overs, for midbody workout, 217
Leg presses, vertical, for lower-body workout, 318
Leg pulls, lying, for midbody stretching, 345, 389, 391
Leg raises
    kneeling, for midbody workout, 243
    lying, for midbody workout, 247
    lying inside, for lower-body workout, 325
    for measuring abdominal strength, 193
    for midbody workout, 181, 207
Legs-overhead stretches, for midbody stretching, 346, 389
Leg strength
    importance of, 310–11
    quiz for rating, 308–9
Leg swings, standing back, for midbody workout, 242
Leg workouts. See Lower-body workouts
Lentils, as low-fat food, 52
Lifestyle
    changes in, for permanent weight loss, 25
    diary of, for weight loss, 106
    lean, quiz about, 78–79
Lifting, importance of leg strength in, 311
Light box, for seasonal affective disorder, 101
Low-density lipoprotein cholesterol, effect of alcohol on, 66
Lower back, protecting, in midbody workouts, 197
Lower back leans, for midbody stretching, 344, 387
Lower back pain
    from abdominal weakness, 193
    lying leg pulls for relieving, 345
    stretching routine for, 386–87
    upper-body strength for preventing, 255
Lower back squats, for midbody stretching, 348
Lower back stretches
    knee-to-chest, for midbody stretching, 351
    lateral, for midbody stretching, 347, 389
    standing, for lower-body stretching, 381, 387, 391
Lower-body circuit, 334
Lower-body strength
    importance of, 310–11
    quiz for rating, 308–9
Lower-body stretches
    ankle-extension stretches, 376, 385
    front hip stretches, 378
    kneeling calf stretches, 375
    kneeling quad stretches, 379, 385, 389, 391
    lying hamstring stretches, 383, 385, 389
    standing calf stretches, 374, 389
    standing hamstring-and-butt stretches, 382
    standing hamstring stretches, 380, 387, 391
    standing lower back stretches, 381, 387, 391
    standing thigh stretches, 377, 387, 389
Lower-body workouts
    bench lateral step-ups, 323
    donkey calf raises, 329
    feet flexions, 332, 334
    freehand squats, 317

P

Pain
- back, workout for preventing, 186–87
- joint, workout for overcoming, 183
- lower back
    - from abdominal weakness, 193
    - lying leg pulls for relieving, 345
    - stretching routine for, 386–87
    - upper-body strength for preventing, 255

Paperwork, organizing, 93–94
Parallel dips, for upper-body workout, 170, 179, 184, 189, 272, 306
Pasta, low-fat, 58
Pepperoni, fat in, 64
Phantom chairs, for lower-body workout, 324, 334
Pineal gland, eating regulated by, 6
Pizza, homemade, 53
Planning
- exercise time, 103
- healthful meals, 103

Plateauing, in weight lifting, 160
- avoiding, 167–68

Plateaus, exercise, 121, 132
PNF stretching, 340
Pollution, avoiding, when running, 144
Pork, fat in, 51
Poultry, skinning, 51
Power lifting, 160
Praying wrist stretches, for upper-body stretching, 373, 387
Preacher curls, for upper-body workout, 187, 258
Prejudice, against fat people, 19–20, 21
Presses
- behind-the-neck, for upper-body workout, 293
- bench (see Bench presses)
- curling overhead dumbbell, for upper-body workout, 295
- dumbbell military, for upper-body workout, 172, 179, 181, 294
- inclined dumbbell, for upper-body workout, 179, 182, 280
- overhead, for upper-body workout, 292, 306
- toe, for lower-body workout, 326, 334
- vertical leg, for lower-body workout, 318

Protein, animal, overeating, 43, 44
Prunes, pureed, as fat substitute, in baking, 53
Psychological needs, food cravings to satisfy, 12
Psychological problems, from obesity, 16, 20
Pull-downs
- lat, for midbody workout, 184, 219, 249
- neck, for upper-body workout, 288
- triceps, for upper-body workout, 270

Pulling, in swimming, 151
Pullovers, bent-arm, for upper-body workout, 182, 284
Push-downs, triceps, for upper-body workout, 269
Pushing chest stretches, for upper-body stretching, 368, 384, 388
Push-ups
- bench, for upper-body workout, 287
- as measure of upper-body strength, 252–53

neck, for upper-body workout, 289, 306
for upper-body workout, 170, 174, 189, 286
Pyramiding, 160

Q

Quad stretches, kneeling, for lower-body stretching, 379, 385, 389, 391
Quizzes
- about eating habits, 40–41
- about lifestyle, 78–79
- for rating
    - abdominal strength, 192–93
    - aerobic fitness, 110–11
    - belly fat, 2–3
    - belly strength, 192–93
    - endurance, 110–11
    - flexibility, 336
    - lower-body strength, 308–9
    - upper-body strength, 252–53
    - workouts, 156–57

R

Racewalking, as exercise, 154
Raised-leg crunches, for midbody workout, 187, 200
Raking leaves, calorie burning from, 87
Reading, calorie burning from, 88
Recovery time, after aerobic exercise, 111
Red wine, health benefits of, 67
Repetitions, in weight lifting, 159–60
Repetitive-stress injuries, upper-body strength for preventing, 254–55
Resistance training, 160
Resting heart rate
- calculating, 120
- as measure of aerobic fitness, 110

Resting metabolic rate
- decrease in, from dieting, 29
- lean body mass and, 30

Reverse grip biceps curls, for upper-body workout, 259
Reverse leg extensions, for midbody workout, 185, 187, 241
Rice, as low-fat food, 52
Roller skis, 134
Roman chair sit-ups, for midbody workout, 177, 187, 204, 249
Romanian dead lifts, for midbody workout, 232
Rotator cuff external rotations, for upper-body workout, 302
Rowing, as exercise, 145
Rowing crunches, for midbody workout, 175, 206
Rowing machines, selecting, 146
Running
- calorie-burning from, 29
- as exercise, 142–44
- for measuring aerobic fitness, 111

Running shoes, buying, 143

S